The Structure of Individual Psychotherapy

THE STRUCTURE OF INDIVIDUAL PSYCHOTHERAPY

BERNARD D. BEITMAN
University of Missouri–Columbia

Foreword by Irvin D. Yalom

THE GUILFORD PRESS
New York   London

© 1987 The Guilford Press
A Division of Guilford Publications, Inc.

Printed in the United States of America

Last digit is print number 9 8 7 6 5 4 3 2

Library of Congress Cataloging in Publication Data

Beitman, Bernard D.
  The structure of individual psychotherapy.

  Bibliography: p.
  Includes index.
  1. Psychotherapy.   I. Title. [DNLM: 1. Psychotherapy.
WM420 B423s]
RC480.B357   1987   616.89′14   86–3160
ISBN 0–89862–461–4

To the memory of
Karl Beitman, my father
Harry Levine, my father-in-law

Acknowledgments

A book 16 years in the making is a summation of a life. The influence of many people and institutions is etched on these pages.

My mother knits beautiful sweaters and my father worked long hours as a manager of a five and ten cent store. Their examples have served me well. I have attempted to knit the yarns of the psychotherapy schools into an attractive and useful piece (as my mother's sweaters are handsome and warm). The effort required perseverance like that which my father showed in his daily repetitive grind in his store.

My brother Allen sharpened me for competition. Although I received more press as an athlete than he, when we played one-on-one he invariably emerged the winner. I knew there was always someone better than I was.

The Moreland Elementary School of Shaker Heights, Ohio, provided challenges to my inquisitive and competitive mind. Mount Pleasant High School in Wilmington, Delaware, provided a context in which I could grow as an athlete as well as a student. Mr. Schomborg helped bolster my confidence as a writer and Mr. Michaelwicz, as an athlete and leader. In Wilmington, I was bar mitzvahed to carry into future generations the culture of my Jewish heritage. I was connected to generations preceding me and feel the continuity in which I am a link. I also learned from these times in the synagogue to question religious dogma and discovered a yearning for unity. I came to respect the similarities among religions and nurtured the hope that religious ideologies could give way to a unifying concept. Later, I found that I could apply this hope to the schools of psychotherapy.

Swarthmore College and I fit well together. I loved the love of ideas embraced in that sylvan atmosphere. The college was small enough that a football player of my stature could emerge a star. I felt important and believed that I could contribute something. Leaving Swarthmore for Yale Medical School was one of the biggest losses of my life. I hated being without that supportive, encouraging atmosphere, having to try once again in a larger and more impersonal arena to make something of myself. I wanted to be good at something again. This book is the product of that desire.

At Yale I met Gerry Klerman, who has, over the years, served as a mentor and supporter. He supervised my medical school thesis, which has served as a springboard for some of the ideas expressed in this book. At Stanford, during my psychiatric residency, Irv Yalom served as a role model for the writer–psychotherapist. How often his image bolstered my perseverance at the typewriter! The Stanford program was also well suited for me because there was little structure and few service demands. I had the time to pursue the ideas incorporated in this book and write the basic outline upon which it stands during my first year of training. I also spent days on Haight Street learning about and experiencing that short-lived peace explosion engineered by mystic-seeking flower children. They showed me that the world of institutions is often far removed from the concerns of the street and the planet.

At the University of Washington, Carl Eisdorfer, then chairman of the department, made it possible for me to continue work on these ideas by helping to protect my time. The moody, introspective atmosphere of the Pacific Northwest aided in their development.

The University of Missouri Department of Psychiatry was an excellent place to finish the book. Jim Weiss, David Davis, and Armando Favazza have warmly supported this endeavor. Bob McCallum offered some excellent thoughts that helped me to clarify the text. Joe Lamberti graciously helped with the final proofreading.

Seymour Weingarten, Editor-in-Chief of The Guilford Press, secured Leslie Greenberg to critique an earlier version. The book is much improved as a result of his constructive criticism.

Of the many psychotherapy writers I have not personally known, I am most indebted to George Kelly and Sigmund Freud. Kelly showed me the potential variability of thought. Freud gave me practical observations of the psychotherapeutic process and the unconscious. Freud also served for me, as he has for many others, as a model of commitment and courage.

At various times, numerous friends have expressed a confidence in me that has helped me to believe in myself. These include: Dan Lederer, Hap Peele, Dan Hunt, Randy Weingarten, Don Stanford, Steve Walsh, Esme Hammond, Bill and Carol Nicklos, Connie Johnson, Ed Goldenberg, Glenn Leichman, Elizabeth Morris, Gail O'Connell, Susan Jackson, Mai Ting, Andy Weil, Winnie Rosen, Thaddeus Golas, Frances Haselsteiner, Carol Ricker, Jane Isay, Judy Greissman, and the many psychiatric residents at the University of Washington who supported my efforts, contributed cases, and taught me more about psychotherapy.

Over 16 years, many people have allowed me to try to help them. A few I have hurt; their lessons stay with me. Some have helped me to understand myself. To many of these people who for some part of their lives were called my patients, I am grateful for their involvement with me.

Most dear to me are my wife, Paula, and my sons, Arie and Karlen. Through them I have learned to love.

Foreword

The psychotherapies continue to increase in numbers and diversity. A few therapies, like direct analysis, will therapy, marathon groups, and primal scream may disappear, but, like troops from the teeth of the dragon in the golden fleece legend, a multitude of others spring up in their place.

There are so many therapies that several publishers have issued guides for the perplexed consumer. Much confusion reigns about the criteria for selection of a therapy. No longer can we rely on "effectiveness," the obvious criterion, since contemporary outcome research, which Dr. Beitman ably reviews, has failed to demonstrate the difference in outcome between any of the therapies scrutinized.

Much confusion too, for the student. Nietzsche said that if you want to learn about a man's philosophy, ask first, "What are his values?" Is this true, too, for the psychotherapist? Do values determine the developing therapist's decision about specialization? Which of the therapies shall the student embrace? The "deeper" forms which require long bondage, but offer prestige and the certainty that radiates from orthodoxy? The humanistic or philosophic therapies for students who search for wisdom? The briefer, behavioral therapies that offer cost effective and chi square efficiency (if one is willing to endure the catcalls of "superficiality")? The transpersonal approaches that appeal to those on a spiritual quest? The baffling, trickster cures for those who wish to paradox and dazzle? Cognitive approaches for the rationalist? Somatic approaches for the materialist?

Let us consider for a moment psychotherapy outcome research. Psychotherapy has been proven to be more effective than no therapy. In a number of studies psychotherapy has proven to be equally or more effective than drug therapy for anxiety and depression. Psychotherapy and drug combinations are more effective than drug therapy alone. But when we examine the studies that pit one psychotherapy against another or when we compare by meta-analysis all the outcome studies of various

forms of psychotherapy, the conclusions are clear: Of all the psychotherapies studied, none demonstrates a clear superiority over the other!

Keep in mind that this research refers primarily to symptom relief,
that is, to feeling and functioning better. It does *not* mean that patients
obtain the same personal education in each of the therapies. Every therapist knows that is not the case. Yet the overall contribution of these effects to the final quantitative accounting of therapy—that harsh adjudica-
tion made by outcome researchers or insurance or DRG boards—appears
to be the same. There are many different types of learning produced by
many, many therapies, but in the contemporary climate of professional accountability they all lead to a single, final common pathway of
outcome.

Dr. Beitman's position is that, given the diverse and overripe state
of our pluralistic field, the last thing we now need is any new therapies.
Instead, what the moment demands is an integration of contemporary
psychotherapies. Rather than simply explicating the differences among
the various schools in order to enable the student to differentiate one from
the other or to produce an encyclopedic or historical survey (a tired task
attempted many times), Dr. Beitman has assumed the task of unveiling
the similarities among the therapies. If, after all, all therapies produce
similar outcomes, perhaps it is because, at a fundamental level, they
operate in the same way! Of course they do not appear to do the same
thing, but let us not be misled by external appearances. Dr. Beitman asks
us to perform the difficult intellectual task of recognizing the basic foundation upon which all therapies appear to be built while also recognizing and respecting each school's unique contributions.

What do the diverse psychotherapies hold in common? Dr. Beitman
observes that all therapies consist of four discrete stages: engagement; pattern search; change; and termination. These four stages constitute the
skeleton of this integrative attempt. Beitman discusses each stage from
an extraordinarily unbiased and cosmopolitan vantage point. To take one
example, consider the stage of pattern search. Every therapy attempts
to define patterns of thought, feeling, and/or behavior—patterns that the
client is able to alter and that, if altered, would result in favorable outcome. The author analyzes a large number of therapies and describes a
variety of modes to elicit clinical data and organize that data into comprehensible patterns. The range of psychotherapies studied is exceptionally
wide; have they ever been housed in a single dwelling before? They include cognitive therapy (Beck); interpersonal therapy; rational–emotive
therapy (Ellis); psychoanalysis; Morita therapy; Naikan therapy; existential therapy; Gestalt therapy; Jungian therapy; behavioral therapy (Ban-

dura, Lazarus); Rogerian therapy; therapies described by Kopp, Langs, Cashdan, Driscoll, Hart; and many, many others. The patterns used to organize clinical data include visual data filters such as stimulus–organism–response models (e.g., the cognitive therapy ABC sequence of Activating event, *B*elief, *C*onsequence), the Lazarus "BASIC I.D." acronym, "spirals" of Watzlawick and other communication theorists, psychodynamic triangles, parent–adult–child ego states, and "parts of the self" models. Other patterns emphasize culture, biocultural stages of development, problem analysis, patterns of emotional expression, expectations, major interpersonal styles, intrapsychic conflict, self–other boundary weakness, and deep unconscious.

Dr. Beitman fleshes out this outline with a discussion of pattern search methodology and resistance to pattern recognition. Every step is studded with analyses drawn from a host of therapies. He often swings away entirely from Manhattan and Boston — the bastions of traditional psychotherapy — and makes excursions into the barbarian psychotherapeutic colonies of the Far West. But each time he returns, his arms are laden with intellectually illuminating commentary on the commonalities between therapies. What is particularly refreshing is that the author has no ax to grind, no ideological school to defend, no jargon to impose. He is an intellectually honest and dedicated integrationist. Virtually every major concept is graphically illustrated by some clinical vignette — examples that are delightfully uncensored. Not since Harold Searles has an author presented his own countertransference and therapeutic foibles in such a disarming — some might say foolhardy — fashion.

I dislike writing forewords and usually deftly duck when I spot an invitation coming. But I greatly respect Bernie Beitman's work and, as he reminds me, he is a former student. Given these conditions, I could find no gracious way to refuse. And as I immersed myself in his writing, gradually my attitude changed. No longer do I feel imposed upon; instead, I am proud to be associated with this work. This is no ordinary book on psychotherapy: It is a life-labor filled with the maturity and wisdom that come only from many years of deep personal and professional reflection.

Irvin D. Yalom
Stanford, California

Preface

On the weekend of June 7–8, 1985, in Annapolis, Maryland, the Society for the Exploration of Psychotherapy Integration (SEPI) held its first annual meeting. Many of the participants had been working alone or in small groups on the question of bringing together the conflicting schools of psychotherapy. They may have felt a rising tide of interest in their objectives, but the evidence had been meager. During that Annapolis weekend, many of those gathered there sensed the beginning of a movement. Perhaps the time of ideological polemics was closing. Here, in this place, was evidence that a group of dedicated psychotherapists was earnestly searching for a framework to bring together the divergent schools.

Many were drawn to the integration movement because of the sobering immediacy of psychotherapeutic failure. Not only have research trials failed to prove the superiority of one form of therapy over another, but individual practitioners have been forced by the weight of their own clinical experience to recognize that no single approach is always better. Patients vary; therapists vary; problems vary; resources vary. Can the best be selected from the variety of approaches in order to increase overall effectiveness?

Some debate arose regarding the objectives of SEPI. Were we working toward a systematic eclecticism or an integration? One participant declared that systematic eclecticism was an oxymoron — the juxtaposition of two impossibly related characteristics. Others thought that integration was too broad — too ill defined. Practical concepts were needed.

This book is a contribution to integration and systematic eclecticism.

In working toward integration, I have attempted to describe the common factors that define the nature of psychotherapy. Each psychotherapeutic relationship may be divided into stages; each stage may be defined by its objectives: engagement, pattern search, change, and termination. In addition to having objectives, each stage has characteristic content, techniques, and distortions or blocks. The stages and their subdivisions serve to organize the chapters of the book. I have subordinated the theories of psychopathology to the psychotherapeutic process, recognizing our limitations in understanding human personality and psychopathology. Instead I offer outlines of key content areas in which maladaptive patterns are most likely to be found and couple them with two useful organizing concepts: Stimulus (S) → Organism (O) → Response (R) and reciprocal causation.

In working toward systematic eclecticism, I have outlined the contexts that codetermine choices, placing the greatest emphasis upon psychotherapy stages. I have described many of the specific technical choices available at the many choice points of therapy, but I am unable to say what technique should be selected at what time. Too many other variables influence the specific choice, not the least of which is the therapist's own personality.

Ultimately systematic eclecticism and integration should converge into a practical description of the psychotherapeutic enterprise. Psychotherapists no longer need new schools of psychotherapy. Instead we require an adequate, useful definition of what we are doing. It is to this end that this book is dedicated.

Contents

The Structure of Individual Psychotherapy

1. *Introduction*

A graduate student in psychology was struggling through his oral examinations. The head of his committee recognized that his strengths lay in clinical work and shifted the questioning to clinical decision making.

PROFESSOR: If you had a choice between two therapeutic techniques, positive reinforcement or shock, how would you decide which to use?
STUDENT: I'd look at the data.
PROFESSOR: What if the data don't exist for this situation?
STUDENT: I'd read well-respected therapists on the subject to get their opinion.
PROFESSOR: What if these authorities were contradictory and unclear?
STUDENT: I'd check to see if I had a shock generator or candy pellets available.
PROFESSOR: Let's say you have both in your desk.
STUDENT: Then I could use either one.
PROFESSOR: How could you decide?
STUDENT: I'm not sure what you are getting at, Sir.
PROFESSOR: What would keep you from using the aversive condition?
STUDENT: If I didn't think it would help.
PROFESSOR: Is there any other reason you wouldn't?
STUDENT: I don't know. I really don't know.
PROFESSOR: C'mon! Shock hurts!

Therapeutic choices are forced by multiple factors beyond scientific data and advice from authority. Clinicians must often make decisions in the absence of sufficient predictive information. Knowingly and unknowingly we fall back on values, experience, and expediency to select the range of alternatives.

Dogmatic declarations about the correct way to perform psychotherapy have provided therapists with guidelines by which to judge their actions. Freud's insistence upon the pure gold of transference interpre-

tation and Wolpe's insistence upon relaxation for systematic desensitization, once generally accepted, have given way to other concepts. Transference may be interpreted for many years without change and psychoanalytic
change may take place without attention to transference (Horwitz, 1974).
Relaxation is unnecessary for in-imagination exposure to feared situations
(Yates, 1975). Techniques have not yet been shown to have a consistently
powerful effect on the outcome of psychotherapy (Orlinsky & Howard,
1978). Some technique is necessary to establish therapeutic alliances, to
gather information, and to promote change. That no single clinical approach is clearly superior has created a paradigm strain among many
psychotherapy theorists and practitioners.

The search has begun for a better conceptualization, an integration,
a systematic eclecticism. Many authors are rushing to fill the breach with
their notions about how to solve this increasingly evident problem (Beutler, 1983; Driscoll, 1984; Garfield, 1980; Hart, 1983; Prochaska & Di-
Clemente, 1984). The problem, however, appears to be beyond the competence of one person to solve. To redefine psychotherapy in terms more
compatible with clinical and research experience requires the efforts of
large groups of therapists working together to determine its nature. No
one person is capable of defining the "true" form of psychotherapeutic
practice because it is being defined daily through the activities of hundreds of thousands of therapists. Models of psychotherapy must therefore
begin with general descriptions of what psychotherapists do every day
rather than with the theories and experience of one persuasive writer and
speaker.

In constructing this book, I have tried to stay close to what happens
and what can happen. "What happens" is that patient* and therapist
meet, decide to work together, attempt to find psychological patterns to
change, to change them, and to stop seeing each other. "What can happen" refers to the numerous alternatives available to therapists at these
recurrent choice points. Consequently, theory is replaced by description
of fundamental elements of the psychotherapeutic process. The "glue"
holding this description together is the human relationship proceeding
through time. Theory in psychotherapy has become closely aligned with
ideology, and ideology obscures many practical considerations.

---

*A note on word choice: Among the problems in writing a psychotherapy book are
whether to use "client" or "patient" and whether to use "he/she." I have opted to use client
in some places and patient in others. Rather than use the masculine pronoun (or the feminine
pronoun) I have opted to use *he or she* and *him or her*.

THEORIES OF PSYCHOPATHOLOGY
AS IDEOLOGICAL DISTORTIONS

The schools of psychotherapy have provided great impetus to the growth and proliferation of psychotherapy in the United States. Their theories of psychopathology have provided individual therapists with prescriptions about the correct way to practice psychotherapy and strong beliefs to justify these practices. In addition, the schools have provided professional organizations through which members can seek out like-minded colleagues to gain support for their shared theories. The rigid doctrines that compose the school walls provide protection from hostile forces but also limit the range of perceptions of those cloistered inside.

The greatest controversies among psychotherapy schools concern theories of human psychological functioning and dysfunctioning. Each has taken a slice through the complicated tangle that is the human psyche and declared its version superior. Theorists have divided the unconscious into many competing sections, drawn boundaries in preconscious activity, and placed varying maps upon behavior in the interpersonal environment. Humans are all these psychological territories and psychotherapy directly or indirectly touches each area. If these ideological illusions are stripped away, the actual daily interaction between therapists of different schools and their patients show considerable overlap. In this book, I offer a general model of psychopathology that does specify certain techniques and is subordinate to the requirements of the psychotherapeutic process.

The names and purported purposes of techniques from different schools also veil similarities. The techniques are embedded in theoretical propositions and therefore appear to support the theories. I, in company with Pentony (1981), argue that the theories are often elaborated after the technique has proved useful. Freud found catharsis useful and built his theories of strangulated affect from this observation. Rogers found empathic reflections useful and around it constructed his notions of individuation. The successful technique provides a vehicle for the elaboration of the author's own psychological theory but does not necessarily explain its usefulness in the psychotherapeutic process. Both catharsis and empathic reflections serve as useful engagement techniques by which the patient comes to appreciate the skills and interests of the therapist. These techniques also served to engage other therapists' interests in their practice of psychotherapy.

This pragmatic approach to technique helps to define the similarities among the psychotherapies. Each school has different justifications for its techniques, but each therapist must accomplish similar subgoals of the therapeutic process with each patient. The pragmatics of interventions (the purpose, objectives, intended outcomes) pull the diverse approaches together. Each patient must be engaged, encouraged to define maladaptive patterns, helped to change, and disengaged. Up to now therapist–writers have warned followers to avoid certain goal-seeking techniques because they might be harmful. For example, Langs (1973) strongly limited the use of questions and prohibited the involvement of a significant other on very clearly described theoretical grounds. In the future, such caveats need to be substantiated on pragmatic rather than theoretical grounds. Until that happens, therapists may be encouraged to experiment with multiple methods for accomplishing the goals of each therapy stage.

THE SEARCH FOR COMMON FACTORS

Among those who have searched for unity in complexity are Jerome Frank (1976) and Judd Marmor (1976). Their pioneering efforts sought to illuminate what therapists *actually* do instead of what they *say* they do. Their influence has been restricted because much of their work was published before the current peak of interest in defining common principles. In addition, they did not pair their presentations of common factors with discussions of differences in ways that could be readily incorporated into clinical practice. Frank placed great emphasis upon the "demoralization" hypothesis. Demoralization results from the persistent failure to cope with internally or externally induced stresses that patients and those close to them expect them to handle (1976). A major function of all psychotherapists is to combat demoralization by instilling hope and providing the opportunity for self-mastery. Marmor and Frank agreed upon a number of common factors:

1. *A Good Relationship.* An intense, emotionally charged, confiding relationship built on trust is recognized as an essential element of most psychotherapy.

2. *Emotional Release.* In a wide variety of ways, therapists encourage their patients to express and experience pent-up feared feelings. Emotional release may strengthen the therapeutic relationship and may increase the potential for change.

3. *Cognitive and Experiential Learning.* Therapists teach their clients new information directly through verbal instruction and indirectly through experiment and other opportunities for self-discovery. Therapists may provide situations in which maladaptive beliefs about the self and others may be examined.

Through the strength of the patient's attachment to the therapist, a variety of influencing methods become available. These include positive and negative reinforcement (smiling, compliments, interest in certain topics) and identification with the therapist as a model for a better way to consider oneself.

4. Practice. Built into most therapies is the practice opportunity. Called "working-through" in psychodynamic therapies and related to maintenance and generalization in behavior therapies, the practice phase enhances the patient's sense of mastery over the new learning.

While Frank and Marmor placed themselves outside psychotherapy schools to look at the whole of psychotherapy, others have used the basic notions of their chosen orientation to discern common factors. Raimy (1975), for example, presented evidence that all psychotherapies attempt to challenge and change misconceptions about the self. The means by which these misconceptions are challenged may be selected from four basic methods: (1) self-examination — the therapist encourages the client to evaluate beliefs; (2) explanation — the therapist provides verbal evidence intended to change the misconception at issue; (3) self-demonstration — the therapist maneuvers the client into situations to demonstrate the misconception either in the therapeutic relationship or through real-life experiments; (4) modeling — the client observes one or more models performing activities thought to be impossible to perform.

Dewald (1976) asserted that "all psychotherapy, regardless of specific form or technique, is viewed as an interpersonal or intrapersonal process, and should be understandable from a psychoanalytic perspective" (p. 283). He described the various ways in which therapists of different schools manage the therapeutic relationship, anxiety, the drives and their derivatives, defense mechanisms, regression, identification, catharsis, and reinforcement.

THE "HYPHENATED" ECLECTICS

Concurrent with the search for common factors, other writers have sought to meld the "best" elements from two apparently contrasting schools of therapy. The most widely accepted of the hyphenated eclectics is cognitive–behavioral therapy. While a few diehard radical behaviorists may still have difficulty with speculations about the unmeasurable events that take place within the black box called the skull, many therapists are comfortable with the union. Some writers have attempted to bring together the very divergent schools of psychoanalysis and behavior therapy. While

numerous books and articles have endorsed this marriage (Birk & Brinkley-Birk, 1974; Fensterheim & Glazer, 1983; Marmor & Woods, 1980;
Wachtel, 1977) there is little evidence that this form of hyphenated eclecticism has enjoyed widespread practice.

Any time two schools of therapy are concurrently popular, some
therapists are likely to hyphenate them. Existential psychoanalysis, for
example, at one time was popular enough to receive its own section in
the *Comprehensive Textbook of Psychiatry* (Weigert, 1967) but since then
has lost its place. During the heyday of transactional analysis (TA) and
Gestalt therapy, many practiced a hyphenated form. Gestalt therapy
provided access to emotions and the TA provided a conceptual grasp of
interpersonal relationships. There are therapists practicing any number
of hyphenated variables: Gestalt–Reichian (Brown, 1974), humanistic
RET (Ellis, 1973a); Behavioral–Gestalt (Harper, Bauer, & Kannankist,
1976), and cognitive–psychoanalytic (Bieber, 1980).

THE SYSTEMATIC ECLECTICS

More psychotherapists define themselves as eclectics than as adherents to
a specific school (Beitman, Chiles, & Carlin, 1984; Garfield & Kurz,
1974; Norcross & Prochaska, 1982). One of the personal advantages of
this self label is the ambiguity associated with the term, which gives the
practitioner license to practice his or her own idiosyncratic approach. In
recognizing the need for a more systematic eclecticism, a number of
writers have attempted to organize the diffuse practices of their colleagues
according to a variety of schemes. Are they offering methods to integrate
the psychotherapies or are they describing systematic eclecticism?

An integration of the psychotherapies is a splendid ideal through
which the warring factions may come together to heal the gaping breaches
between and among them. Integration implies the continued existence
of each of the many schools of psychotherapy, now bound together by
a common spirit of understanding and working with the group toward
commonly agreed upon objectives. However, should it be possible for
therapists of different schools to find a common meeting ground, then
school boundaries will likely be threatened. There is little scientific basis for these ideological differences; only shared and mutually supported
opinion. Should it happen, integration would be a temporary phenomenon giving way to a yet newer paradigm.

Systematic eclecticism, according to Wachtel (1985), is an oxymoron — a hybrid of two incompatible elements. How can one be systematic
about haphazard choosing? In my view, both integration and systematic

eclecticism are transitional concepts that will give way to objective descriptions of the psychotherapeutic process with its key choice points and alternatives. Younger therapists are likely to find the conflicting ideologies distasteful and lean toward objective approaches. As with most paradigm shifts in scientific revolutions, the older ideas will die with the older therapists, as younger ones replace them with new perspectives (Kuhn, 1962).

Some of the systems offered by psychotherapists for organizing an eclectic approach will be described in the rest of this section. Each is the product of the mind of one or more people, and each makes a useful contribution to our total understanding of psychotherapy.

Arnold Lazarus

An early major contributor to behavioral therapy and theory, Lazarus developed a content eclecticism that stretched the bounds of behaviorism but did not break them. He could not accept many basic psychoanalytic ideas (Lazarus, 1971, 1976; Lazarus & Fay, 1982). Lazarus, recognizing that *behavior* in the environment is but one essential source of psychotherapeutic data, added *affect*, *sensation*, *imagination*, *cognitions*, *interpersonal*, and *drugs* (physiological variables) to form the acronym BASIC I.D. (Lazarus, 1976). He continued the behavioral form of questioning — what, where, when, who, and how — and insisted that long-lasting change required attention to all modalities, a claim echoed by numerous other founders of schools who believed that they, too, had found the necessary and sufficient means for psychotherapeutic change. His position has likely helped numerous behavioral therapists to increase the range of content of their therapeutic investigations.

Sol Garfield

After 35 years as a psychotherapy researcher, teacher, and clinician, Garfield (1980) felt the need to crystallize his own views on the subject. Garfield noted the proliferation of psychotherapy schools and speculated about its meaning: Are some approaches better, are some better for some patients, or does this diversity express our relative ignorance? (p. 1). He set out to order the significant variables and phenomena of psychotherapy.

Garfield's book records the wisdom of a psychotherapist who has been immersed in the details of psychotherapy research, behavioral practice, psychoanalytic practice, and teaching. But it has no organizing theme except for the underlying notion that their must be one. The reader can see the author struggling with decision making during psychotherapy, trying to make sense of the data, trying to generalize for the reader's benefit. Garfield's effort seems to represent the mind of many experienced psychotherapists who have broken away from specific schools and have consequently felt free to search in diverse places. He has some notion of what he does, of ideas he believes important, of basic elements of psychotherapy. But he has no system to impart, no general framework to guide his presentation.

Larry Beutler

In stark contrast to Garfield's unsystematic eclecticism is Beutler's (1983) highly systematic approach. More than any other eclectic to date, he has attempted to answer the question: what technique with what type of patient? The critical patient variables for Beutler are: (1) monosympto-matic or complex symptom, (2) reactance level (highly reactant people rebel against external direction), (3) external defensive style (project blame outward, somatize) or internal defensive style (exaggerates self-blame or avoids thinking about it). These variables then codetermine the therapist's approach. Beutler has carefully defined the techniques from the major schools in terms compatible with the general styles he believes to be best matched with each of these three patient characteristics. For example, clients with low levels of reactance should be directed, while those with high levels of reactance must be extended much greater self-direction. Monosymptomatic patients should be treated with narrow-band (e.g., behavioral) treatments, while complex symptoms need a broad-band approach (e.g., insight). Externally defensive patients require behaviorally oriented, externally focused treatment, while internally defensive people should have an internally focused (e.g., insight) treatment.

The obvious breadth of Beutler's system, and the wealth of the evidence he has marshaled to support it, make his ideas very compelling. Nevertheless, the presentation contains obvious gaps. Shouldn't diagnosis enter the algorhythm? What about the patient's own view of how treatment should proceed? Shouldn't some people who are internally focused learn to get out of that defensive style and act? Said Beutler (1983) about his work: "The problem with publishing ideas is that one frequently feels compelled to defend them rather than allowing them to evolve. In the best of all possible worlds, the written word could be viewed as a developmental process rather than as a collection of sacred truths" (p. *xi*).

James Prochaska and Carlo DiClemente

As a result of their work with smokers, with particular attention to those people who changed without help from therapists, Prochaska and DiClemente (1984) outlined the stages of change in their transtheoretical approach. People suffer without thinking about change (precontemplation); they think about change (contemplation); they act; and they maintain the change. Some relapse. These patterns are particularly highlighted in the addictive behaviors, in which the pattern to be changed is quite obvious. The authors tie together eight processes of change with each of the four stages of change. Contemplation requires "consciousness raising." The transition between contemplation and action requires self-reevaluation. Action requires self-liberation, a helping relationship (not necessarily a therapist), and management of reinforcement. Maintenance requires counterconditioning and stimulus control.

They added to this meshing of technique with stages, five levels of content generally to be discussed in the following order: (1) symptom/situational, (2) maladaptive cognitions, (3) current interpersonal conflicts, (4) family/systems conflicts, (5) intrapersonal conflicts. (If sufficient change does not occur at one level, then they advise therapists to proceed to the next level.)

The stages of change described by Prochaska and DiClemente may reflect a hidden consensus among many psychotherapy writers (see Chapter 7). Their processes of change as tied to the stages of change are thought provoking and deserve further analysis, but their levels of change run against the same stone wall that similar propositions tend to hit. No therapist can say what content should be discussed or in what order it should be discussed for all therapist–patient pairs. Some patients jump right into intrapsychic discussion because for them this level of analysis fits their theory of what is wrong. Like most schemes for organizing the data of the search for critical patterns, the transtheoretical hierarchy of content levels will be useful for some therapists and some patients.

Richard Driscoll

Beutler's system and the transtheoretical approach of Prochaska and DiClemente grew out of formal research in psychotherapy. Driscoll's (1984) pragmatic eclecticism is based upon the convergence of several philosophical systems and direct clinical observation. The term "pragmatic" is the fulcrum around which his ideas spin. The term refers to one of the three major aspects of language, the other two of which are syntax (rules for ordering sentences) and semantics (the meanings of words). Pragmatics refers to the purpose or function of words, namely their intent to influence the listener. Driscoll, then, emphasized the increasingly recognized fact that therapists are attempting to influence their clients (see Chapter 9). Pragmatic also implies practical, utilitarian, atheoretical. As described by Driscoll, this approach also carries two other major features: (1) the use of common language instead of idiosyncratic terminology to structure observation and understanding of the data of therapy, and (2) emphasis on the "in order to" aspects of client as well as therapist behavior (p. 8).

He uses the notion of purposive action to develop a scheme for filtering and organizing the search for patterns. Each actor is motivated by some "want" (motivation, desire, craving, reason). Associated with the want is a "know" (a cognition, perception, understanding, belief) and a "know how" (competency, skill, ability). The "want," "know," and "know how" come together into a "performance" (movement, action) that has an "achievement" (effect, impact, change, influence) (pp. 28–29). This scheme has much in common with other often-used organizing methods, from the Stimulus→Organism→Response (S→O→R) approaches to the activating Event→Belief→Consequences of the cognitive therapists (Beck, 1976; Ellis, 1973b) to the systems analysis of family therapists.

Driscoll does not attempt to define what to do with which patient at what time in therapy but leaves those decisions to the individual situation. His emphasis is upon the personal experiences of the practitioner rather than on the elucidation of superordinate principles for each to follow.

Joseph Hart

After an introduction and historical review, Hart's *Modern Eclectic Psychotherapy* (1983) challenges the limitations therapists place on their role possibilities. In Hart's opinion, the usual doctor–patient, teacher–student, and scientist–subject roles could be extended to many others. His list includes: coach–athlete, attorney–client, manager–employee, minister–church member, master artist–artist, business representative–customer. After arguing that role plurality is an excellent model for clinical eclecticism, his arguments become more narrowly focused. His ideas come to represent an attempt to form a new school of therapy masquerading as eclecticism. More than the other eclectics described in this section, Hart "knows" that his form of therapy is the correct one. His central word is "functional," the definition of which resembles Driscoll's use of "pragmatic." The functional level of discourse asks what is happening around the person and in the person's experience and how is the person responding. After summarizing the ideas of his precursors (William James, Pierre Janet, Trigant Burrow, Jessie Taft, and Frederick Thorne) he declares that "functional eclecticism must be considered the core eclectic position around which all others diverge as peripheral viewpoints" (p. 28). What emerges is a highly refined approach to therapy based upon his notions of what content is to be discussed. His stages of change, on the other hand, are quite compatible with the sequence outlined in Chapter 7 of this book.

PSYCHOTHERAPY RESEARCH

Psychotherapy researchers have long pondered their lack of influence on psychotherapy practice (Garfield, 1980; Goldfried & Padawar, 1982). The schism appears to be narrowing. Clinicians are likely to increasingly rely upon researchers to justify expenditures by third-party payers for psychotherapeutic services. Psychotherapy may be becoming more definable; the work of psychotherapy researchers is leading to more specifiable research questions having definite bearing upon psychotherapeutic practice. The breakdown of psychotherapy schools is likely to allow practitioners to utilize the evaluation techniques employed by researchers in their own practice.

In my view, psychotherapy research has functioned like another school of psychotherapy. Its adherents shared similar belief systems, were dedicated to the operations defining its practice, and were cloistered away from other practitioners. Like each of the many schools of psychotherapy, some useful ideas have emerged from psychotherapy research. But the future of psychotherapy understanding is likely to belong increasingly to the careful delineation of the psychotherapy enterprise. With the dissolution of ideology, the emphasis on what works, and increases in understanding of the nature of human psychological functioning, the knowledge will be better defined. Careful and controlled observation will come to replace speculation.

Despite the volumes of data generated by psychotherapy researchers, firm conclusions have been difficult to reach. The question "Does psychotherapy work?" has become as meaningless as the question "Does surgery work?" Does it work for whom, done by whom, by what means, is the more compelling query. Generally speaking, psychotherapy seems useful. This conclusion is drawn from major overviews of psychotherapy research.

Comparative Sets

Luborsky, Singer, and Luborsky (1975) examined all "reasonably controlled" comparisons of psychotherapies by scoring wins, losses, and ties. The main sets of comparisons included group versus individual, time limited versus unlimited, client-centered versus other traditional psychotherapies, and behavior therapy versus psychodynamic psychotherapy. The authors suggested that the equivalent results could be explained by the fact that each psychotherapy provides patients with some plausible system of explanation for their difficulties and with principles that may guide future behaviors.

Meta-analysis

Smith, Glass, and Miller (1980) undertook a yet more massive project by systematically examining most of the controlled research in psychotherapy according to accepted methodological criteria. They treated each outcome study in a manner similar to the way single-subject data would be analyzed in a single controlled experiment. They included 475 studies comprising 1,766 different effects and including the magnitude of each effect and characteristics of the treatments, clients, therapists, settings, research design features, and outcome measures. The major findings were that psychotherapy was beneficial, that different psychotherapies do not yield benefits of different types or degree, and that differences in how psychotherapy is conducted (group vs. individual, length of treatment, experience of therapist) make very little difference in outcome. Of interest is the percentage of types of therapies examined: 21% systematic desensitization, 11% behavior modification, 9% vocational–personal and undifferentiated counseling, and 11% a variety of placebo treatments. Also, the clients tended to be young (mean age 23), had been solicited by the experimenter (46%), or came in response to an advertisement (16%). Therapists had modest experience (mean of 3.2 years). These data give an idea of the tremendous difficulty of performing research on standard clinical psychotherapy and also indicate that such research is necessary, especially on the long-term treatment of more difficult patients (Cohen, 1981).

APA Commission

The American Psychiatric Association's Commission on Psychotherapies (1982), concluded that psychotherapy was effective for a variety of symptomatic and behavioral problems. These include chronic moderate anxiety states, simple phobias, depressive symptoms, sexual dysfunction, adjustment disorders, family conflicts, and communication difficulties. Psychotherapy may also be useful for postillness psychosocial rehabilitation. The commission report also mentioned that the most extensive review of the literature concluded that approximately 5 % of patients in psychotherapy get worse because of the psychotherapy (pp. 222–225).

Other Research Contributions

The question concerning the relationship between specific psychotherapeutic approaches and specific diagnostic categories has received increasing attention. The lure of a diagnosis-related treatment has been influenced by the many instances in medicine in which a specific diagnosis implies a specific treatment with a high probability of successful outcome.

The treatment of the simple phobias (snakes, heights), is the clearest example of treatment specificity. A wide variety of treatments have proven successful in the treatment of simple phobias. The first and most celebrated was Wolpe's (1976) systematic desensitization. In this approach, anxiety-evoking situations are presented to the imagination of the deeply relaxed patient in rank order of their capacity to disturb. Each image is repeated until it totally fails to evoke anxiety. Other approaches include having another person carry out the feared behavior, either in real life or in imagination; rapid exposure to the feared situation, either in imagination or in real life; and gradual exposure in real life. Each approach has been shown to be of some utility. The key ingredient is exposure (Marks, 1978). The more complex phobia, agoraphobia, is also treatable through a variety of exposure methods. For longer lasting improvements, however, gradual exposure *in vivo* with the help of the spouse appears most useful (Barlow & Beck, 1984).

In reviewing the various forms of psychotherapy for depression, Weissman (1984) was unable to conclude superiority of one approach over any other. However, in a number of controlled trials, cognitive therapy (Beck, Rush, Shaw, & Emery, 1979) has been shown to be the equal of antidepressant medication (Blackburn, Bishop, Glen, Whalley, & Christie, 1981; Murphy, Simons, Wetzel, & Lustman, 1984; Rush, Beck, Kovacs, & Hollon, 1977). While interpersonal therapy (Klerman, Weissman, Rounsaville, & Chevron, 1984) has also been shown to be useful in depression, the results of current and future studies will define its relative efficacy. In one study, social skills training, time limited psychodynamic psychotherapy, and amitriptyline were each effective and none was superior (Hersen, Bellak, Himmelhoch, & Thase, 1984). Is there a specific factor (like exposure in the treatment of phobias) that underlies cognitive, interpersonal, social skills training, psychodynamic theory, and drug therapy in the treatment of depression?

THE LIMITS OF PSYCHOTHERAPEUTIC KNOWLEDGE

Since Freud's thunderous pronouncements about the nature of psychotherapy, many other writers have proclaimed their true and correct ways to conduct the psychotherapeutic relationship. Each writer appears convinced of his or her beliefs. Each maintains that therapists are negligent if they fail to follow the prescribed approach. How can such contradictory pieces of advice be fully correct?

Perhaps the psychotherapies are truly different. Each has its own change mechanisms, its own data-gathering strengths, and its own powers of influence. To use a pharmacological analogy, each one may resemble a different class of medications, each of which can effectively treat subclasses of the same disorder. Depression, for example, may respond to lithium, polycyclic antidepressants and to monoamine oxidase (MAO) inhibitors, as well as to placebos. Each has a different mechanism of action that may yield the desirable positive outcome.

This perspective does not appear to be the majority view. The predominance of eclectics among psychologists (Prochaska & DiClemente, 1984) and psychiatrists (Beitman *et al.*, 1984) suggests that many therapists assume the existence of a common base onto which the variety of contributions from other schools may be placed. This common base has yet to be elucidated.

The overview of research studies described earlier has substantiated the general efficacy of the endeavor. Other work has demonstrated the lack of efficacy of individual psychotherapy without medication in the treatment of schizophrenia (Goldstein, 1984). Psychological help may prove to be cost-beneficial in the treatment of certain medical problems (Mumford, Schlesinger, Glass, Patrick, & Cuerdon, 1984). But these outcome studies do not define the nature of psychotherapy. Increasing attention has been paid to the nature of the therapeutic alliance (Docherty, 1985) thereby suggesting a growing consensus about the importance of this element of the psychotherapeutic process.

The cacophony of claims to psychotherapeutic supremacy and the small amount of clinically substantive data from psychotherapy research highlight the extent of our ignorance. Yet it is hardly a total ignorance. Professional psychotherapy is a complex process that is a unique subdivision of that problematic class of human activity known as interpersonal relationships. To study ourselves being ourselves requires emotional and cognitive distance. To be objective about our subjective selves requires that we transcend ourselves.

Has enough information been gathered to define psychotherapy?

2. The Stages of Individual Psychotherapy

The proliferation of descriptions of psychotherapy offers the possibility of defining psychotherapy by consensus. Each version of psychotherapy seems to have characteristics that it shares with all other approaches, some other characteristics that it shares with a few other approaches, and characteristics that are significantly unique. This chapter is concerned with commonalities because it is these characteristics that define the basic nature of psychotherapy. If a number of different observers, each with a distinct perspective, describe the same or similar phenomena, then they are, by consensus, defining psychotherapy.

After outlining fundamental principles (the therapist's ability to choose, the therapeutic relationship time as a unifying concept, and stages as contexts for choices), I describe the stages of psychotherapy as a basic organizing principle for defining psychotherapy. This concept serves as the framework for this book and as a way to bring conceptual order to individual psychotherapy. It may also help to stimulate new research directions and to further our understanding of supervision.

CONSENSUS AS A METHOD FOR DEFINING PSYCHOTHERAPY

In attempting to understand psychotherapy, I began with the bias that each writer has something to offer the psychotherapeutic procedure and that something basic underlay all approaches. The more I read, the more I noticed that writers often used different terms to describe what seemed to be the same phenomena. The differences in terms were important to the schools that the writers represented because they were embedded in certain theoretical concepts essential to each school. If the theories could be stripped from the observation, then a basic underlying reality might be grasped. The more writers from different schools seemed to describe a specific element, the more likely it was that this element was a basic part of the psychotherapeutic process.

To use a visual analogy: Reading the books of psychotherapists of different schools produced in my mind a series of plastic slides on each of which was drawn a diagram of the author's concept of the psychotherapeutic process. The process was drawn linearly on a time scale, with a beginning, middle, and end. I placed these slides together and shone a light through them looking for places of overlap in their linear models. These points of overlap became the defining elements of the psychotherapeutic process.

There are many problems with this approach. Are the psychotherapies similar enough that they can be compared? Can a few sessions of brief therapy be compared to 5 years of psychoanalysis? Is time the best organizing principle? What about the books and articles I didn't read? Did I miss something crucial? How can I keep my own biases out of the picture? Even if a consensus can be stated, how accurate is it to psychotherapeutic reality? Perhaps most of the therapists are misperceiving the process themselves.

To reply to these criticisms: I think the psychotherapies are similar enough. Time is an excellent organizing principle for an attempt at clinical description. It is fundamental to the definition of psychotherapy. I wonder about the books I didn't read. I do not keep my own biases out of the presentation because they supply some of the personal quality that each therapist brings to his or her approach. However, I am unable to delineate where the consensus information blurs into my own idiosyncratic beliefs.

I looked at technique in much the same way as I looked at process. The Venn diagram in Figure 1 illustrates the form of this approach. The three overlapping circles could represent the three major schools of psychotherapy: psychodynamic, cognitive–behavioral, and existential–humanistic. The blackened area represents the convergence of the three schools; the lined areas represent the convergence of two but not the third; and the white areas signify the sectors of uniqueness for each one.

The circles might also represent three supposedly different observations having something in common. For example, therapists commonly encounter blocks to therapeutic intent or flow. Behavioral therapists might call them "noncompliance to behavioral assignment"; psychoanalysts might call them "resistances"; and Gestalt therapists might call them "awareness blocks." The terms share the description of a metaphorical wall and differ in the arenas within which the wall is constructed. The block in behavioral therapy is in the requested or expected behavior. In

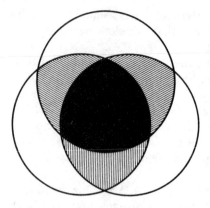

Figure 1. Intersection of concepts and techniques among major schools of psychotherapy.

psychoanalysis it is in the production of unconscious material or hidden emotion. In Gestalt therapy, it is the cutting off of immediate experience and its consequences. Areas of overlap between behavioral and psychoanalytic therapies include the psychoanalytic patient's refusal to free associate or to bring in dreams when requested. Areas of overlap between behavioral and Gestalt therapies include refusal to role-play. Areas of overlap between psychoanalytic and Gestalt therapies may include blocks to emotional awareness.

Another phenomenon fitting the Venn diagram is the concept of self-observation. Most therapies require that clients observe themselves and report their findings. Behavioral therapists might ask for self-monitoring of target behaviors (e.g., number of cigarettes smoked). Cognitive therapists ask that automatic thoughts be recorded. Psychoanalysts want patients to observe their in-the-office thought flow and to report it along with dreams and fantasies. Gestalt therapists want reports of ongoing experience in the affective, experiential realms. Areas of overlap between behavioral self-observation and psychoanalytic observing ego include the analytic patient's observation of his or her own inappropriate behavior toward the therapist. Convergence between behavioral self-observation and Gestalt awareness includes the Gestalt patient's observation of a repeated sign of blocked emotion (e.g., a clenched fist). Convergence between Gestalt therapy and psychoanalysis is illustrated by the Gestalt patient's report of a spontaneous image from childhood triggered by an affective exercise.

A final illustration concerns technical responses to therapeutic blocks. Psychotherapists differ from most other social contacts by the manner in which they handle strongly charged ideas. Where friends and relatives tend to say, "Stop that!" "Don't worry so much!" therapists tend to accept them and take them a step further. When confronted with a strange behavior, Gestalt therapists might ask that it be exaggerated. When confronted with an irrational belief, cognitive therapists might say, "So what?" When confronted with a defense in therapy, psychoanalysts will tend to analyze it. Each approach accepts the therapeutic target and carries it further into the patient's experience without demanding that it suddenly be changed according to the therapist's wishes.

THE INTENT OF THIS BOOK

Psychotherapy no longer needs a prophet from the mountains to bring down from exalted heights a message of the true and correct way of doing psychotherapy. Under the ideal of some integrated theory of psychotherapy, some writers have attempted and will attempt to do so. No new schools of psychotherapy are necessary. The integration that is necessary is less in terms of a new theory than in terms of the relationships between and among psychotherapists. Can psychotherapists agree that they are all in the same general enterprise? Differences must be respected but can commonalities be accepted? The framework described in this book is intended to provide a construct by which psychotherapists can come to see their similarities. If psychotherapists can begin to agree upon their common enterprise, then they may come together to more accurately define it. Accurate definition will lead to better teaching, better research, and probably better outcome.

For practicing psychotherapists, the intent is twofold. By defining the common factors of the psychotherapeutic process, practitioners may come to understand more fully that part of their efforts that is unique to their own personalities. By becoming more confident about their own approaches through understanding common factors, they may feel less threatened by other contributions and therefore more able to consider them. Experienced therapists probably will not be able to give up the theoretical and practical basis of their current practices even if such a transformation were desirable. Perhaps though, this book and the movement of which it is a part will help to develop a more flexible element in their current therapeutic constructs. This flexible element will permit each therapist model to accommodate to and assimilate new and different psychotherapeutic ideas. It will provide a metaprogram for reprogramming (Lilly, 1972) the therapist's existing concepts. In this way, current practitioners will come to be defined, for example, as psychodynamically based, behaviorally based, cognitively based, or Gestalt based systematic eclectics (or integrationists).

A less likely but highly desirable outcome would be the provision of practicing psychotherapists with a set of concepts that enable them to talk with each other about patients. Except for those therapists who belong to organized schools, most therapists have little opportunity to discuss their cases with colleagues. Professional isolation appears to be common among psychotherapists. It will take more than a single book to increase dialogue—a strong national organization may be more effective. If psychotherapists are able to agree that they have much in common, then a step has been taken in this direction.

For beginners, the intent is to provide a clear structure by which to organize their readings and experiences of psychotherapy. Some may be angry at the limited amount of "cookbook" description, since beginners often want to be told by authorities what is the best technique or best concept. It is in the nature of being a student to want direction. It is also in the nature of being a teacher to describe the limits of knowledge of his or her discipline. While some will state dogmatic rules about proper therapist behavior, I am limited by current knowledge to defining recurrent choice points and the associated alternatives. Those students who want to be told what to do will be unhappy with this book. Those who desire understanding of the limits of our knowledge through description of choice points and their alternatives will find this book to be a good place to start.

Ultimately, the intent of this book is to help in the process of therapist liberation from dogma. In the same way that therapists help their patients to develop autonomy within a social structure, therapists should also be encouraged to develop their own skills and intuitions against the background of basic psychotherapeutic principles. Individuals in society must develop within certain constraints and so must psychotherapists. Within these rules is room for the expression of much individuality.

INTRODUCTORY PRINCIPLES FOR
THE PSYCHOTHERAPY STAGES

Before outlining the stages of psychotherapy, I describe four underlying or introductory principles that guide and inform the stage concept. (1) Most fundamental is the therapist's ability to make choices based upon influences that transcend any theory of psychotherapy or requirement of a specific patient. (2) Closely associated is the fact that no matter what theory one holds, individual psychotherapy is primarily a relationship between two people that is subject to the distortions common to any dyadic relationship, especially those in which the pair is working together toward a mutually agreed upon goal. (3) The relationship, like all relationships, is strongly influenced by time. (4) The time line through which the dyad exists may be broken up into stages; stages provide contexts for decisions made about the relationship and its potential directions.

The Therapist's Ability to Choose

Psychotherapy is generally not practiced as a technical procedure applied in a uniform way by uniform agents. Unlike robots designed for specific jobs, psychotherapists have varying past histories that influence their choices in the present. Specifically trained robots are highly predictable. Automobile mechanics and surgeons are also more predictable because they are confronted with relatively predictable problems. Psychotherapists are confronted with free-willed beings called patients whose actions are less predictable than that of cars or anesthetized bodies and who tend to seek certain responses from others. By confronting two highly variable beings with each other, the alternatives multiply.

Scientifically minded therapists (e.g., Freud, Wolpe) have tended to ignore the free wills of their patients, at least in the presentation of their theories and methods. In the scientific ideal, the therapist applies procedures from theory and research that would result in the desired outcome. Patients are simply passive recipients of these ministrations. In clinical practice, however, one cannot ignore the freedom to choose available to each patient. In viewing the psychotherapeutic process, one also cannot ignore the influence of the therapist's personality on the choices he or she makes. The variety of personality-based therapy styles becomes most obvious when one watches videotapes of therapists in action but also may be inferred as a result of observing therapists describe their therapeutic activities. Within the same school, some therapists may be aggressive or passive, intellectual or emotional, intuitive or rational and still fit within the broad lines of the school's practice. Therapists-in-training may be attracted to particular leaders because their therapeutic personalities have much in common. I contend that essential ingredients of optimal therapy include a balanced blending of therapist personality with effective technique. One intent of this book is to encourage therapists to recognize when they are choosing and to learn to explain their choices as functions of their personalities and therapeutic intent. This procedure will help to sharpen clinical observation and intuition (Strauss & Hisham, 1981).

The Therapeutic Relationship

Stripped of its contrivances, individual psychotherapy is a relationship between two people over time. Human beings bring to all relationships expectations and behavior patterns based upon previous experiences. These expectations and behavior patterns may not mesh with each other, especially if a cooperative arrangement is required. The result can be friction. Psychoanalytic practice from the time of Freud to the present is the study of these frictions. Its practitioners use the term "resistance" to describe the patient's tendency to subvert the process of therapy, "transference" to refer to the patient's misperceptions of and inappropriate behaviors toward the therapist, and "countertransference" to refer to the therapists own distortions of his or her perception of the patient. Perhaps there are better terms, less ideological in nature, to describe these common elements of human relationships. "Parataxic distortions," "characteristic interpersonal styles," and "coping strategies" are among the alternative terms. I will use the term "distortion" to cover all three terms, thereby implying that the participants are not seeing each other as they truly are. What "they truly are" is philosophically problematical but practically refers to perceiving each other in ways that lead to the most constructive change in the most efficient manner. Correction of these distortions may play a useful part in psychotherapeutic change.

In addition to distortions, patients and therapists bring to the encounter previously established patterns of cooperative behavior. The desire to work toward cooperation and the ability to carry out mutually agreed upon objectives are essential ingredients to any psychotherapy success. The client's experience of having done so with the therapist may provide the basis for future similar experiences with others.

Finally, patients and therapists come to like each other. Liking can become excessive and occasionally leads to unethical interactions, but for the most part is to be an expected by-product of the therapeutic interaction. Two people work together, get to know each other well, and come to appreciate and respect each other. These responses are not distortions but rather are another set of expectable reactions to this human interchange.

Time as a Unifying Concept

In this three-dimensional terrestrial existence, time is a constant to which humans must accommodate. Each life is a river born in tiny springs, rushing, meandering, constantly moving toward the sea of dissolution.

For some moments, the streams of two lives blend; occasionally the relationship is defined as psychotherapy. The confluence creates a series of events through time that may be called a process. The process may arbitrarily be divided into stages. Stages can be defined by their objectives, the alternatives by which these objectives may be reached, and the likely impediments to achieving the objectives.

Stages as Contexts for Choices

Context implies a limitation on alternatives. Context provides a boundary for the activities taking place within it. A baseball game is played on a three-sided field enclosing a diamond shape. Certain rules govern the behavior of players within these geometrical configurations. At various choice points of the game, there are a limited number of alternatives defined by the field, the rules, and the specific situation. The field, the rules, and the situation are contexts within which alternatives emerge. The contexts limit the range of available choices. If, for example, the bases were loaded in the bottom of the ninth inning with a tie score, the pitcher could choose to intentionally walk the batter, could walk off the field declaring that he was satisfied with the tie, or could try to strike out the batter. Within the rules, he could intentionally walk the batter, but his team would then lose. He could ask for the tie, but the rules do not permit that alternative; only the umpire can call the game at this point. Striking out the batter would be the best for his team at that point. Context has limited his alternatives.

The beginning of a movie or play sets the context for the drama by defining the setting, the players, and their interactions. The setting of the drama limits the choices geographically and by era. If the setting is a small white settlement in the 1600s near what was to become Boston, Massachusetts, handguns will not be available as instruments of influence, and religion is likely to dominate the lives of the settlers. Personalities are defined by their characteristic reactions in a variety of social settings. Therefore, character sketches provide limitations for interactions within the contexts of time and place. As the drama unwinds, the outcome becomes more predictable, particularly since it takes place within the finite context of a time limit for its presentation. The movie must have an ending as well as a beginning and middle.

The various stages of the psychotherapeutic process provide contexts for the therapeutic interaction. The need to establish a therapeutic alliance provides a limitation to the therapist's choices because there are a limited number of ways in which to engage patients in therapy. The need to gather information provides another context for there are a limited number of ways to define psychological patterns. The process of change provides yet a different context because the methods by which change may be initiated are also limited. Other variables that limit choices include the therapist's own predispositions and capabilities, the client's expectations and understanding of psychological change, and the kind of problem the patient brings.

The Stages of Individual Psychotherapy

The process of psychotherapy may be arbitrarily divided into four stages: engagement, pattern search, change, and termination. The process of change may be divided into three substages: giving up the old pattern, initiating the new pattern, and practicing/maintaining the new pattern. The value of using stages in psychotherapy may be compared to the value of dividing the year into four seasons. Stages provide smaller units by which predictions of likely occurrences may be made. Their names and the specific points in time at which boundaries are drawn are somewhat arbitrary.

The use of stages to present concepts of psychotherapy is time-honored. Psychoanalysts have described the stages of development of the transference (Greenson, 1967) and have often employed a general three-stage concept for the psychotherapeutic process (e.g., Langs, 1973, 1974). Sullivan (1954) subdivided the early stages into "formal inception" and "reconnaissance" and labeled the middle stages the "detailed inquiry." In his early formulations of client centered therapy, Rogers (1942), listed the following stages that he felt made up the psychotherapeutic process: (1) the creation of the counseling relationship, (2) releasing expression, (3) the achievement of insight, and (4) termination. Wolpe's (1973) description of systematic desensitization also followed a clear sequence that he labeled orientation, correction of misconceptions, relaxation training, establishing the hierarchy, and pairing relaxation with the steps of the hierarchy. Behavior therapists may not formally acknowledge an engagement stage but observations of their therapeutic conduct reveal that they demonstrate skill similar to that of psychodynamic therapists in managing the therapeutic relationship (Sloane, Staples, Cristol, Yorkston, & Whipple, 1975).

Stages represent a common organizing principle because psychotherapy can be considered a form of problem solving. The pair must come to know each other, to trust each other. The problem bearer must convey information useful for the helper's attempt to define a solution. The solution must then be carried out (e.g., Mahoney & Arnkoff, 1978).

One of the consistent similarities found among four of the six systematic eclectics reviewed earlier is in their description of the therapeutic process. Prochaska and DiClemente (1984) build their presentation around stages. Beutler's (1983) greatest emphasis is upon matching therapist and patient with technique, but his description of the process of therapy is quite compatible with that of Prochaska and DiClemente. His terms are different and convey a somewhat different emphasis: identify (patterns), comply (request patient to collaborate), magnify (awareness of the maladaptive pattern), validify (test out new insights through behavioral and interpersonal change), solidify (gain social supports and reinforcements for changes), and good-bye. Garfield (1980) devotes much of his book to events common during the process of therapy without making specialized definitions of stages. Nevertheless, these elements appear in his examples. Driscoll's (1984) procedural guidelines, which compose the bulk of his contribution, are organized along the stages of psychotherapy. He describes methods to build the therapeutic alliance, to assess and clarify the problem areas, to help define alternatives, and to motivate change. Hart's (1983) presentation is not explicitly organized by the stages of the process, but this organizing principle seems to have aided in the structure of his book. In an early chapter, he defines the multiple roles available to each therapist and therefore to each patient–therapist pair. This element is an essential part of the engagement stage. Much of his theoretical review concerns methods and content for defining patterns. Then he describes stages of change as the need step, the choice step, the action step, and the image step. The need step involves helping the client isolate, recognize, and verbalize a need or want. Choosing is then required to affirm the need or want through new action. This sequence can result in a new personality image to replace the old one. Although other terms may be more useful, Hart describes a series of steps common to psychotherapeutic change across schools (see Chapters 7 and 8).

THE STRUCTURE OF EACH STAGE

Each stage may be seen to be composed of six elements: goals, techniques, content, resistance, transference, and countertransference. These elements serve as the organizing scheme for this book.

Goals

Goals define the boundaries of the stages. Once a goal is accomplished, the stage associated with it has been traversed. However, patient–therapist pairs must often retrace their steps to firm up their engagement or to clarify and develop patterns. The goals of engagement include the patient's development of trust and confidence in the therapist as well as a willingness to be influenced. The pattern-search goal is generally the development of a pattern or set of patterns that, if changed, will bring about a satisfactory psychological shift. One pattern may not be sufficient; multiple patterns may be examined and discarded before some elements that can lead to an adequate resolution are defined. The goals of change are tied to its subgoals: the relinquishing of the old pattern, the initiating of the new, followed by practice and maintenance. The goals of termination include separating early enough to maintain goals already achieved while not extending the relationship unnecessarily.

Techniques

A wide variety of techniques may be used to accomplish the goals of each stage. Some techniques are most useful in the engagement stage (e.g., empathic reflections) and others are better suited for change (e.g., behavioral rehearsal), although many techniques may be useful in all stages. The critical question is what techniques may be most useful for accomplishing the goals of each stage in therapy for what clients. For patients who see themselves as students of the therapist, homework assignments may prove excellent engagement techniques. For patients who are unable to describe their daily life with efficiency and accuracy, homework assignments may be superior pattern-search techniques.

Content

The content of therapy is the least predictable aspect of psychotherapeutic process. The wide variety of personality and psychopathology theories attests to the uncertainty therapists have in knowing what to talk about. There appear to be some general themes. Engagement is concerned with trust and competence. Pattern search is most often associated with problems in daily living surrounding interpersonal relationships. Termination is concerned with trying out new actions alone and having to say good-bye.

Resistance

During the early years of psychotherapy when the overreaching fact was psychotherapeutic ignorance, Freud and his followers required of themselves that they listen with minimal intervention. But allowing the patient to determine much of the process while confronted with a silent listener resulted in the patients beginning to distort the person of the therapist and the process of the therapy. The therapist became more than just a physician listener; therapy became a threatening enterprise. Patients began to subvert the therapeutic intent. They failed to free associate, chose to talk about inconsequential matters. The form and content of these blocks to therapeutic flow were first thought to be great nuisances. Gradually Freud and his followers found that these resistances offered useful ways of understanding the person and his or her problems. The manner in which patients avoided problems in therapy resembled the ways in which they avoided problems outside the office.

Transference

People enter into new relationships with perceptions and attitudes derived from previous relationships. The more intimate the new relationship, the more likely old, idiosyncratic attitudes will emerge. During the engagement stage, clients tend to react to the surface appearance of the therapist (age, sex, dress, manner, accent). As intimate self-revelation takes place, more stereotyped attitudes are likely to be disclosed. They may be derived from past interpersonal experiences; they may also be samples of the patient's intrapsychic dynamics. For example, a person who criticizes herself for any feeling of self-compassion may react critically to demonstrations of concern by the therapist. Apparent distortions of the person of the therapist may not have their primary source in the previous experience of the client. Therapists themselves may trigger realistic responses by their own distortions of the person of the patient. For example, a sexually stimulated therapist may unwittingly induce a feeling of being helplessly in love in a susceptible client who otherwise would have remained grateful with feelings of affection.

Countertransference

Therapists also perceive their clients in terms of their own previous relationships. In addition, patients may induce responses in susceptible therapists that are similar to reactions other people have to these patients. Once the therapist's own idiosyncratic personal responses are distinguished from the effects the patient is creating, some very useful information can emerge. First, the therapist has the opportunity to further explore the personal sources of neurotic distortions. Second, the therapist can explore the reasons for his or her own personal vulnerability to such people. Third, the therapist can gain a richer appreciation of the reasons other people have trouble relating to these patients.

Table 1 contains an outline of the stages and their basic elements.

THE PROBLEM OF
THEORIES OF PSYCHOPATHOLOGY

I am not advancing a new theory of psychopathology nor offering an integration of the cacophony of existing ones. The extreme variety of claims of correctness attests to the limitations of our knowledge of ourselves. Instead, I am choosing to emphasize two "process configurations" that seem to have general support from many different types of therapists: (1) the notion that a stimulus triggers an intrapsychic response connected to a consequence is an integral part of the practices of many psychotherapists (Driscoll, 1984; Hart, 1983); (2) the notion of reciprocal causation, especially deviation-amplifying feedback, while relatively new in science as well as in psychotherapy, has great potential utility.

$S \rightarrow O \rightarrow R$

Therapists usually start with symptoms, with complaints, with pain. Symptoms may take the form of arguments, unwanted feelings, maladaptive behavior, or undesired fantasies or thoughts. Therapists usually work backward to environmental–interpersonal triggers and often search for the thoughts and feelings that connect the unwanted consequence with the unrecognized trigger.

This basic notion emerges in different forms in different therapies. Yet most therapists gather information by noting the consistent, repeated patterns of patient behavior triggered by a variety of other people and situations. In so doing, therapists also note aspects of the patient's intrapsychic experience that conform with their favorite ideas of cerebral processes (e.g., automatic thoughts, defenses, emotions, fantasies). Driscoll (1984) suggested the formula: Behavior $= f$ (Situations and Individual Characteristics); that is, behavior is a function of situations and individual characteristics. Hart (1983) described the "functional" level of clinical discourse in a similar way: "The functional level of discourse always asks *what* is happening (around the person and in the person's experience) and *how* is the person responding" (p. 21). Both Driscoll and Hart claimed that this thought process underlay the practice of most clinicians.

Vicious and Virtuous Cycles, Deviation Amplifying Feedback (DAF)

Among the newer ways to understand how things change is the notion of deviation amplifying feedback (DAF). For much of human history, cause and effect has dominated our concepts of influence. A single finger moves a single pencil. A single surgeon removes a blood clot. A single therapist cures a patient. In the older style of thinking, cause flowed unidirectionally to effect.

In this century, the notion of homeostasis was introduced. A deviation from a desired standard is dampened by a mechanism geared to counterbalance the deviation. This process is also called deviation *dampening* feedback. Two parts of the system operate on each other to reduce the change introduced into the system. The same mechanism may be operating in stalemated psychotherapeutic relationships, as well as in firmly entrenched intrapsychic and interpersonal problems. Deviation *amplifying* feedback refers to a deviation that sends the system out of its current equilibrium toward another equilibrium. The deviation is amplified through mutually effecting responses (reciprocal causation). For example, a new consultant to a system wants to make a quick and effective impact (to make a favorable impression) in order to have the system members think well of him. This positive attribution increases his self-confidence, increasing the likelihood that he will perform well on his next task. A new element is introduced into a system, the effect snowballs and forces the system toward a new equilibrium. Consider this example: A person is governed by the rule: "I must be superior, perfect and excellent in all my endeavors or else I'm worthless." Into his life is introduced an additional burden (wife threatening miscarriage) so that he cannot function up to his standards for himself. He notices that his functioning is diminished; he feels guilty. His guilt decreases his ability to concentrate, which leads to further self-perceived erosion in performance that further increases his guilt. This vicious cycle, begun by a relatively small deviation in his self-perceived performance, then leads to increasing guilt, concentration loss, and finally the need to take a leave of absence from work. He becomes acutely depressed because he sees himself as a failure at work.

The notion of deviation amplifying feedback is relatively new to science and to psychotherapy, perhaps first reaching active use in 1960 (Pentony, 1981). The idea appears to be fundamental to both intrapsychic and interpersonal–environmental concepts of psychological dysfunction. A single event or series of events sets out a sequence of responses that lead to a new uncomfortable equilibrium that for the therapist is defined as the focus of treatment. The therapist then formulates the difficulty in terms that are acceptable to the patient and that provide a way to intro-

Table 1.
The Stages of Individual Psychotherapy

	ENGAGEMENT	PATTERN SEARCH	CHANGE	TERMINATION
GOALS	Trust Credibility Ground rules Self-observer alliance Motivation	To define patterns of thought, feeling, and/or behavior that, if changed, would lead to a desirable outcome	1. Relinquish old pattern(s) 2. Initiate new pattern(s) 3. Practice new pattern(s) 4. Maintain and generalize	To separate without unnecessarily prolonging contact but with sufficient time to maintain change. To practice separation
TECHNIQUES	Empathy Role definition Managing the contract Specialized knowledge Effective suggestions	Questionnaires Listening Questions Homework Role-playing Incongruities	Placebo response Exhortation Interpretation Reframing Modeling	Mutually agreed Patient initiates Therapist initiates
CONTENT	Presenting problems Underlying fears Distrust Therapist decisions about type of treatment	S→O→R Deviation amplifying feedback Emotion Expectations Interpersonal style Intrapsychic conflict	Specifying patterns Responsibility awareness Responsibility assumption Therapist's lessons on coping and values	Separation themes Fears of relapse Mourning

[handwritten note: teaching stress mgt Child dev examples]

30

RESISTANCE	To trust competence ground rules self-observer motivation	To ground rules self-observer pattern-search methods —pattern-search content	To change itself Patient limitations Therapist limitation Patient–therapist impasse	Recurrence of symptoms New symptoms Impulsive behavior (marriage, pregnancy)
TRANSFERENCE	To therapist's surface presentation (age, sex, dress, accent, race, physical attractiveness, style of therapy)	As samples of key interpersonal and key intrapsychic patterns. As products of previous therapy, expectable events of current therapy, or therapist countertransference	Fear of losing therapist Sample of behavior to be changed and responsibility for creating it	Interpersonal attempts to hold on to or push therapist away
COUNTER-TRANSFERENCE	To patient's surface presentation (age, sex, dress, accent, race, attractiveness, diagnosis)	Therapist-induced Patient-induced (informs therapist how patient affects others)	Fear of losing patient Use understanding of how patient affects therapist in intervention (e.g. self revelation)	Interpersonal attempts to hold on to or push patient away

31

duce a deviation, the amplification of which may lead to a more desirable equilibrium.

In the preceding perfectionistic example, some maladaptive patterns may have originated in the person's childhood attempt to adapt to an early environment (e.g., "You are our only son, you must be strong and perfect"). Any demonstration of excellence may have been rewarded, leading to further attempts at excellence, any failures simply ignored. In such a case, the person would have experienced his existence with his parents only when he was perfect or excellent. When he confronted a failure at work or love later in life, he became a non-person.

Psychoanalysts might demonstrate how he attempts to use the therapist to confirm his excellence. Behaviorists might prescribe homework to demonstrate his value without perfection. System therapists might bring in his wife or employer to help shift his self-concept and behavior. Cognitive therapists would attempt to introduce a deviation through his thinking about himself. Existential therapists might refer to his desire to overcome death through perfection (an impossible effort) or attempt to meet him in the here-and-now through an I–Thou existential encounter to demonstrate his person-value. Each of these efforts may be construed as attempts to set in motion a positive feedback loop leading to a more enjoyable homeostatic equilibrium. Vicious and virtuous cycles may theoretically be initiated by any intervention, whether it be directed at unconscious defenses, transference distortions, behavioral change, or change in self statements. The amplification of a well-placed deviation or a series of deviations will lead to a more desirable equilibrium.

DAF is an outline of an idea for grasping psychological difficulty and psychological change within the psychotherapeutic context. It is a "process configuration" devoid of content. It may have implications for understanding human nature, childhood development, and theories of psychopathology, but these implications are not essential to a process description of psychotherapy. DAF is subordinate to the process description. Among many psychotherapy theorists, there is a demand that psychotherapy practice be derived from a theory of personality and/or a theory of psychopathology. The inadequacy of our current understanding of human nature and the limits of theories of psychopathology now challenge the wisdom of this requirement.

Not only does reciprocal causation have implications for understanding how people can get into and out of psychological difficulty, but it also has applications to the psychotherapeutic relationship. The purpose of the engagement stage is to set in motion a series of events in each client's mind that lead from apprehension and uncertainty to confidence and hopefulness. The unwinding of doubt and fear leads to the second stage, in which unfolding of internal and external events is required. This unfolding, too, requires sequential interventions leading to a laying out of critical patterns and a firming of the therapeutic bond that renders it relatively impervious to breakage. This temporary homeostatic equilibrium provides a platform from which change may be initiated. Ideally change will perpetuate itself until a new stable equilibrium is reached from which continued growth may be initiated. As patients build their own platforms, the need for the therapeutic one dissolves.

Unwanted reciprocal causation and unwanted homeostasis that occurs during the psychotherapy relationship may also be called "therapeutic stalemate." Again using the DAF idea, therapists may examine how they contributed to the mutually caused state and how they are maintaining it.

OTHER LIMITATIONS OF THIS STAGE CONCEPT

The concept of psychotherapy presented here is limited in some major ways:

1. The reader is not instructed in what to do when: As mentioned earlier in the section on the limits of psychotherapeutic knowledge, there appears to be insufficient information about how or when to do what in psychotherapy. Therapists, readers, and writers who do not believe in a single theory would like this information. Unfortunately, the question has yet to be adequately formulated. At what level of intervention (strategy, tactic) is this question being asked? Should the reader be instructed about what to do at a specific point with a specific type of patient? But how is the specific point to be described? How much context needs to be delineated? What is sufficient data to define a specific type of patient? Is age, sex, marital status, diagnosis sufficient? Should not symptom complexity, characteristic defense mechanisms, medical history, previous psychotherapeutic relationships, and patient expectations also be included?

The easiest advice centers around the therapist's own reactions to patients. This information appears relatively manageable. If the therapist feels threatened, excessively angry, deeply in love, or very confused, consultation with a colleague is an easy recommendation to make. A considerable amount of introspection about the sources of these dysphoric reactions might also be useful exercise. How much is this reaction my own problem and how much of my reaction would be shared by other therapists?

2. The concept might be accused of being "grab bag" eclecticism: Since I am not telling therapists what to do when, is this not grab bag eclecticism, according to which anything may as well be tried? While it is true I have not told therapists what to do, I am trying to define the choice points and their objectives, along with the range of alternatives available to achieve those objectives. The delineation of choice points is a new contribution requiring refinement, and there are likely to be more alternatives available than I have been able to find and describe. Furthermore, each therapist may be predisposed toward certain responses at certain choice points. One set of predispositions may be more effective for one therapist than for another with different predispositions. It is results that count. The concept of this book is caught between having abandoned the insufficient ideologies of psychotherapy while not yet having achieved a reliable and valid way of determining outcome effectiveness. While flexibility at choice points is likely to increase effectiveness, this flexibility still must take place within a general structure governing the conduct of psychotherapy.

3. *Written descriptions of stages are only rough approximations:* Written descriptions of the psychotherapeutic process are but rough approximations of clinical reality. The linear nature of the print medium constricts descriptions of the ebb and flow of movement, fear, trust, unfolding, change, and battles against change. Print and time bear superficial resemblance to each other; the pages of the book follow one after the other as do minutes in the hour; seconds follow each other as do words on a page. Written descriptions have difficulty capturing the boundaries between stages, particularly those between the pattern-search and change stages. On paper they may appear to be discrete, but back and forth movement between them is closer to clinical reality. The boundaries between the stages are relatively permeable. The clearest demarcation is the beginning of engagement. The second clearest boundary is termination, although therapeutic relationships are frequently resumed.

4. *Couples, group, and family therapy are not emphasized:* Mixed therapy modalities have a definite place in the general practice of psychotherapy. To limit oneself to individual psychotherapy is to eliminate some potentially useful approaches. Nevertheless, I have spent most of my reading and practice time with individual psychotherapy and am therefore restricted in the presentation of ideas from group, marital, and family therapy.

STAGES AS A FRAME FOR
UNDERSTANDING THERAPY PROCESS

Certain events common in psychotherapy may be more clearly comprehended through the use of the stages concept. By placing the events under examination within the framework of the stages process, therapists may develop some better idea about how to proceed. Following are some examples.

Stages as an Outline for the Single Session

Hill (1985) noted that during the middle sessions of psychotherapeutic relationships, therapists and clients appear to move through the same general sequence. During the first third they attempt to clarify their focus for that hour and during the second third they work on insight, catharsis, and/or change. Beutler (1983) suggested that the process of the individual session seems to recapitulate the treatment process as a whole. Generally speaking, each session begins with an introductory or low-intensity period that gradually progresses to greater intensity and then tapers off near the end. This pattern follows that of therapy in general, from an initial relationship-building period through the resolution of acute struggles to the tapering off toward the end of treatment. More specifically, the early minutes are spent in reengagement; this leads to a definition of patterns to be changed, and is followed by an attempt at change and then termination. During the engagement stage of therapy, more of the session is likely to be spent in trust and confidence issues; during the pattern search, more of the session is likely to be spent exploring the variety of patterns to be changed. During the change substages, more time is likely to be spent on the process of change and its difficulties. During termination, separation issues are likely to predominate. When the therapist is aware of these patterns, each session may become more predictable and possibly more easily controlled.

If it is true that the individual session recapitulates the psychotherapeutic process, then it should be possible to select one session during engagement or pattern search from which to predict the course of therapy.

Making Sense Out of Patient's Behavior

The stages form a context for the therapeutic interaction that predicts or explains patient as well as therapist behavior. If, for example, a patient engages in small talk, remains silent, or attempts to elicit personal information from the therapist, the stage of therapy will provide increased understanding of the meaning of these actions. During the pattern search, they are clear resistances to the work of that stage. Later in therapy these actions imply a readiness to stop.

Predicting Stalemates

Patients who have left their previous therapist without satisfactory resolution of their problems may tend to recapitulate their difficulties with the new therapist. Knowledge of the patient's and the therapist's contributions to the stalemate and the stage in which it happened may allow the new therapist to predict when the problem will recur. For example, a middle-aged man had seen numerous therapists in his life, ending each relationship when he felt betrayed by the current therapist. The sense of betrayal was tied to his increasing trust and dependence upon the therapist. Therefore, it could be predicted that a firm engagement would likely lead to a stalemate.

Accepting Previous Therapeutic Gains

On the other hand, patients with previous therapy experience may have learned their roles sufficiently well that instead of reaching stalemate after stalemate each therapeutic relationship moves them further along their own therapeutic stages. Each therapist is simply an adjunct to that process. Occasionally therapists are referred patients who have been in therapy for years with many different therapists who have been apparently unable to help them. The final therapist is somehow associated with a dramatic change. Not only do such events bolster the self-pride of the therapist but they may serve to affirm cherished techniques. A more humbling explanation would suggest that the previous therapists had helped to develop engagement and the pattern search to the point at which the patient was prepared to change by the time the final therapist was reached.

Patient — Therapist Behavior after Breaks in Therapy

Breaks in the regular frequency of therapeutic contact often create a need for reengagement. Therapists may expect to pick up just where the pair left off, but holidays, vacations, and agreed trial separations may create the need for some patients to go slowly in their recontact. Therapists too may go slowly because the time lapse has somewhat decreased their familiarity with the patient.

STAGES AS A WAY TO CHARACTERIZE
THE DIFFERENT FORMS OF THERAPY

Schools of therapy may be defined by the range of alternatives selected for the common choice points that occur during the stages of the process. All therapists must perform some engagement behaviors, develop certain patterns, and initiate change. The differences are marked by the probability that one set of alternatives will be chosen over another. Independent judges blind to the therapist's intended approach have been able to distinguish certain forms of treatment. Twelve raters, for example, were able to distinguish between cognitive therapy and interpersonal therapy (DeRubeis, Hollom, Evans, & Bermis, 1982). Independent judges were also able to distinguish among cognitive–behavioral, supportive–expressive psychoanalytically oriented psychotherapy, and drug counseling (Luborsky, Woody, McLellan, & O'Brien, 1982).

Each of the forms of therapy rated by the judges in these studies had been described by a manual that defined the range of techniques and the range of content suitable for that specific form of therapy. Certain content clearly defines the form of therapy. If the therapist encourages discussion of the past, the probability is high that the therapy being performed is psychodynamic. If the therapist asks about specific thoughts in specific situations, the probability is that the form of therapy is cognitive. If the therapist insists upon clear definition of current social roles and minimizes the past, then the form of therapy is likely to be interpersonal.

Certain techniques are also highly associated with specific forms. The recording of automatic thoughts in homework assignments is a high probability marker of cognitive therapy; the interpretation of transference reactions of psychoanalytically oriented therapy; and the encouragement of new social roles of interpersonal therapy.

These forms of therapy are also distinguished by the range of alternatives prescribed for accomplishing the goals of each of their stages. Each form directly or indirectly encourages during the engagement stage the conveyance of some form of empathic understanding. For cognitive–behavioral therapy it might be expressed as "You seemed anxious as you came in today, I wonder what thoughts were going on in your mind while you were in the waiting room." This empathic question not only shows that that therapist is interested in the patient's current ongoing state but also defines the content area of greatest interest to the therapist. A psychoanalytically oriented therapist making the same observation in the first stage might offer a simple interpretation after sufficient data gathering: "I notice that you were quite anxious when you came in. I see the similarity between that reaction and your fears of your parents' criticism whenever you began to speak." Again the therapist outlines the content areas of greatest interest, thereby introducing the patient to his or her therapy form.

The problem of defining the range of alternatives for therapists in practice is more complex. Many, if not most, do not follow manuals in their treatment, but instead tailor their behavior to the needs of their patients as perceived through their own personalities and experiences.

One approach to this problem is to rate a series of interviews by one therapist with a number of different patients in order to discern the range of alternatives at major choice points. These ratings could determine the probability that any one of them would be selected.

A FUTURE DIRECTION OF PSYCHOTHERAPY RESEARCH: STAGES AS MINI-OUTCOMES

Stages represent a concept of potential convergence between process and outcome research. Each stage has a goal that represent mini-outcomes. A variety of measures for the therapeutic alliance have been well established (Hales & Frances, 1985) and may therefore serve as outcome measures for the engagement stage. What techniques, in the hands of what kind of therapist, with what patients, with what kinds of problems lead most quickly to effective therapeutic alliances? Can the influence of therapist training and belief be isolated from technique? Is diagnosis the critical variable or is the patient's tendency to react positively or negatively to authority the most critical variable? The answers to these questions are likely not to be framed in yes and no terms but instead in terms of percentages of influence. For example, a 36-year-old feminist psychologist trained in cognitive–behavioral methods and philosophically against most psychiatric medications may have the highest probability of engaging a 21-year-old passive agoraphobic woman by directing her into imagery exercises that elicit powerful affective discharge. On the other hand, she might best engage a rigid, authoritarian, 45-year-old agoraphobic man by suggesting a medication consultation for his panic attacks. Whether or not the consultation takes place is another question.

Similar research for the pattern search is more problematic since there have yet to be developed generally accepted measures of specificity for patterns requiring change. Researchers would have to develop measures for identifying when in the therapeutic process patient and therapist had developed a clearly defined set of patterns that, if changed, would lead to the desired outcome. Furthermore, these patterns would need to be within the range of the patient's comprehension and offer alternatives within the patient's potential. Some general patterns appear to be more suitable to certain classes of patients than others. Some seem more easily managed by certain therapists than others. What is the best matching? What techniques seem to accelerate or retard the cooperative elucidation of patterns?

The substages of change each present the possibility of mini-outcome objectives for which measures could be developed. How can researchers measure ways in which clients give up their old maladaptive patterns? How can researchers reliably define when a new pattern is being initiated and then practiced? What techniques aid in the giving up of old patterns and in initiating the new patterns and practicing them? While I have outlined possible answers to these questions in the chapters on change, questions of therapist and patient variables must also be considered.

As is discussed in Chapter 9 on change content, therapists communicate lessons in living and values to their clients. Some are as simple and direct as "face your fears," "the past is not the present," and "emotional awareness is useful." Can psychotherapy researchers specify which lessons are most suitable for which patients? Can the series of coping strategies and values conveyed by psychotherapists be better delineated?

Termination is perhaps the most predictable stage of therapy. Some research is already available to describe the relationship between process of termination and outcome (Horowitz, Marmar, Weiss, Dewitt, & Rosenbaum, 1984). Which patients should discuss their reactions to the separation and which ones should not, in order to improve outcomes? When is maintenance of change better served by stretching out meeting frequencies and when is it better served by a final ending at the same frequency? Do follow-up appointments increase the likelihood of continued change?

ANOTHER RESEARCH DIRECTION: THE STUDY OF PRACTITIONERS

Psychotherapy research has remained in the province of academics. The phrase "it's just academic" exists in our vocabulary to emphasize the often-irrelevant nature of scholarly research to daily practice. The once-astounding finding that cognitive therapy was equal to antidepressants in the treatment of depression (Blackburn et al., 1981; Murphy, Simons, Wetzel, & Lustman, 1984; Rush et al., 1977) may have encouraged psychotherapists to believe more strongly in themselves and to convince third-party payers of its efficacy, but has it changed the practices of psychotherapists?

Psychotherapy research should include practitioners who, after all, are scientists too. Like most human beings, psychotherapists are attempting to comprehend the nature of their realities, to experiment with new ideas in order to better grasp the nature of their experience (Kelly, 1955). They are trying to predict and control the small universe of their consulting rooms. These efforts should be formalized with the help of academic researchers and major professional organizations. Many questions would need to be answered before a massive effort could be undertaken. What instruments should be used? When and how should they be administered? Which should be provided as feedback to therapists and to which should the therapist remain blind? Can the superior therapists be identified? Can each therapist's strengths and weaknesses be delineated?

Practitioners strongly influence the direction of psychotherapeutic practice anyway. Their votes through book purchases, organizational membership, and attendance at symposia designate the current influential psychotherapist. Can the practitioners be more formally studied for their preferences and predispositions? Can we learn from the superior ones who do not advertise their skills? Bergin and Strupp (1972) concluded that large-scale collaborative studies were not feasible because:

- there would be a great deal of difficulty in isolating the effects of one or a limited number of variables;
- such studies would be likely to have a minimal effect on psychotherapeutic practice;
- the complex administrative machinery would be costly and likely to be ineffective.

They therefore encouraged development along other lines including systematic research on basic mechanisms, naturalistic observations of psychological change and intensive study of single cases (pp. 426–427).

A study of practitioner efficacy could start as a small-scale project begun in different locations. These pilot-project researchers could then blend their experiences into a yet larger study. But are therapists willing to test their own skills against those of their colleagues?

SUPERVISION

The stages of the supervisory relationship parallel the stages of the individual psychotherapeutic relationship. The pair must come to trust each other sufficiently that the trainee will allow the supervisor to have some impact on him or her. They will need to define an area of discourse that may provide learning experiences that can change the trainee's thinking about the conduct of psychotherapy. There are many potential roadblocks to the accomplishment of these goals. Some trainees resent supervision because they are antagonistic toward their training program or toward psychotherapy itself. Some therapists are simply frightened of the psychotherapy role, as suggested by the following example:

A third-year resident in psychiatry switched to a new training program because his old one did not offer training in psychotherapy.

During our first few sessions, he read from his extensive progress notes taken almost verbatim during the psychotherapy sessions. His patient complained, but he wished to be thorough in collecting the "data" of the hour. I gently suggested to him that perhaps his patient had a point — he did appear to be ignoring her. He insisted upon continuing to take notes. As he entered the next supervisory hour, I began taking notes of what he was saying without looking up at him. I responded to his questions but never made eye contact. He asked, "What are you doing?" I replied, "Taking notes on our interaction as it is happening." "Why?" he asked. I said, "I want to make sure I get all the details." He was satisfied with that for awhile. After a few minutes more of my note taking, he burst out with, "Hey, you're not paying any attention to me." When I suggested to him that his patient might be experiencing the same feelings, he paused. He then began to discuss his fears of being depended upon and admitted that perhaps his note taking was a way to avoid that experience.

Temporarily placing the supervisee in the role of patient is but one of many role possibilities for the supervisory relationship; others include the standard patient–therapist possibilities: authoritarian–subservient, scientist–collaborator, professional consultation, or teacher–student. What is the trainee's preferred way of relating to a supervisor? What is the supervisor's preferred way of relating to a supervisee? Can they reach a compromise satisfactory to both of them?

A similar question can be raised for each of the crucial elements of the psychotherapeutic process. What content areas are preferred by the supervisor and supervisee? What change and data-gathering techniques are most cherished? What are the supervisee's strengths? What does he or she listen for and understand well? Can the supervisor listen to the supervisee's descriptions of the interaction and/or watch the interaction on videotape to discover preferred engagement techniques, preferred pattern-search methods, and preferred change approaches? Many of these elements are beyond each supervisee's conscious knowledge but appear as reflex reactions to the needs and demands of the situation. Supervisors should consider highlighting these hidden strengths in order to define the supervisee's preferred alternatives at the common choice points of the therapeutic interaction. In this way, the pair begins to define an outline of the supervisee's form of therapy.

Prochaska and DiClemente (1984) have suggested a similar approach to supervision. In their transtheoretical model of supervision, the supervisor tends toward a consultant–client relationship but may shift into student–teacher, patient–therapist, master–apprentice. The content of their supervision centers around eliciting the supervisee's preferred stages of change (contemplation, action, or maintenance), favored levels of change (symptom, cognitions, interpersonal conflicts, family conflicts, and intrapsychic conflicts), and preferred processes of change (e.g., consciousness raising, self-reevaluation, and contingency control).

Both the transtheoretical approach to supervision and the one I am suggesting require the supervisor to match his or her style and content to the supervisee's knowledge and experience base. This flexibility requires a broad-based knowledge of many different approaches and the willingness to consider their relevance.

The more traditional view of psychotherapy supervision is to teach one approach in order to provide the supervisee with a solid grounding in the techniques of one school. As the ideological claims among current schools fade, this approach may have less appeal. There will be supervisors who insist that their methods be followed according to the letter of their manuals. Psychotherapy research studies may continue to require strict adherence to specific models. Much can be learned from restrictions on one's behavior as well as from the flexible development of alternatives.

Perhaps even more than psychotherapy itself, supervision is ultimately teaching. Teaching involves communicating ideas that can be useful to the student's future practice. Like the psychotherapist, the supervisor will impart cherished values and lessons to trainees. No matter how flexible and open-minded the eclectic therapist may wish to appear, no matter how value free the therapist may wish his treatment to be, values and lessons seem to be communicated (Beutler, 1983; Strong, 1978). Successful psychotherapy may be marked by a convergence of values between therapist and patient (Beutler, 1983) and so might successful supervision.

The ideas in this book are open to the same observation. I attempt to be open-minded and flexible, but my previous experiences have led me to favor certain ideas. Some of them I recognize. For example, my training as a psychiatrist has predisposed me to psychoanalytic words and concepts, thus the use of "resistance," "transference," and "countertransference." My training as a physician has biased me against elaborate theories and taught me to appreciate ideas that can be quickly put into useful operation, especially medications. Many of my values are also sprinkled throughout this book. I view personal factors as an inevitable part of psychotherapy to which all psychotherapists and supervisors must attend.

3. *Engagement*

A voice on the phone or a face in the waiting room signals the beginning of the subtle scrutiny that culminates in the decision to engage in psychotherapeutic work together. The time required may take a few minutes or many months; the decision may be made in gradual, sometimes agonizing, increments or may be made firmly and quickly. The commitment may be challenged by therapist errors, patient perversity, vacations, and life's unpredictable occurrences. Engagement may then need to be reexamined and renewed, perhaps at yet a deeper level. The goal of engagement is to emerge from the anonymity of the first few seconds into a pair of individuals willing to define and alter the maladaptive psychological patterns of the person designated patient. As engagement develops, the patient becomes increasingly more open to the therapist's influence.

After describing the goals or markers of engagement, (trust, credibility, acceptance of ground rules, self-observer alliance, motivation), I describe various engagement methods, including conveying empathy, defining roles, managing the contract, demonstrating specialized knowledge, and making effective suggestions. Superficially, engagement is concerned with problems, symptoms, and treatment alternatives, but the most relevant content involves indirect questions about the therapist's trustworthiness and competence. This section is followed by a discussion of the many decisions therapists must make: about medications; about the type of therapy to be used — couples, family, or none at all. The chapter ends with descriptions of common engagement distortions — resistance to engagement, early distorted perceptions of the therapist, and early inappropriate or exaggerated reactions by the therapist toward the patient.

ENGAGEMENT MARKERS

The attainment of a number of objectives seems to mark the achievement of engagement. Potential patients must come to trust their therapists,

usually must find their therapists competent and attractive,* must follow
the ground rules of therapy, must be willing to form a self-observer
alliance, and must have sufficient motivation for change. Not all patients
can be engaged. A certain minimum amount of previous human contact
may be necessary. The most important determinants of a patient's readiness to engage lie in his or her previous experiences of important interpersonal relationships (Hartley, 1985).

Trust

Trust of another seems to require three interrelated beliefs. First, the patient must recognize that the therapist will not hurt him or her. For those
people who have been repeatedly damaged by dependency upon and
openness to others, the ability to achieve this belief may take a great deal
of time. The establishment of trust can become one of the most important goals of treatment. Second, and related to the first, the patient must
recognize that the therapist is consistent and therefore predictable. Again,
those patients who have experienced the fright engendered by relationships with destructively unpredictable people may have trouble believing that stretches of kind consistency indicate continuation of this behavior. As the patient comes to believe that the therapist is consistently able
to avoid malicious harm, the groundwork is laid for belief in the therapist's willingness to help. These three elements of trust are usually not
traversed once each, but rather repeatedly in sequence as therapy moves
through its stages. Apparently, trust in one's self develops out of trusting
another and then gradually grows out of the often accompanying dependency (Strupp, 1976).

Competence and Attractiveness

Upon the foundation of trust, patients build belief in the therapist's ability
to help to solve problems (Strong, 1978, p. 106). Some clients are satisfied
by a certificate on the wall, by location in a certain building, or by the
casual comment of a friend. Others require much evidence to believe that

---

*I say "usually" because exceptions to the rules are commonplace in psychotherapy.
Perhaps there has been no greater group of rule breakers than Milton Erickson and his like-
minded therapists. Therapist incompetence, for example, may prove beneficial to change
by spurring the patient to change on his or her own (e.g., Watzlawick, Weakland, & Fisch,
1974).

this therapist is not only generally helpful in psychological matters but is also capable of helping him or her. Perceived competence (credibility) is critical to psychotherapy because it determines patient willingness to accept the therapist's influence. The notion that therapists influence clients is especially controversial among those psychodynamic therapists who view interpretations to be value free (Buckley, Karasu, Charles, & Stern, 1979). Much evidence suggests that psychodynamic therapists indirectly convey to their patients lessons and values for better living (Beutler, 1983; Buckley *et al.*, 1979; Strupp, 1976). Each patient's willingness to accept indirect as well as direct influence is determined in great part by the patient's perception of the therapist as competent and credible. Otherwise, influence would be extremely difficult to achieve.

Attractiveness as defined in social psychology arises primarily from clients' needs to find in therapists consistency and support for their values. Attraction builds as clients perceive therapists to have values similar to their own and thus as persons against whom to test the consistency of their own values (Strong, 1978). Peer counseling, for example, relies on shared values as the primary engagement method, since perceived expertness is generally lacking. Attraction also arises out of patients' need to like their therapists, to which the therapists' physical appearance, sexuality, and personal power may contribute. Patients' reported feelings of "liking" and attraction are more useful predictors of outcome than the therapists' reported feelings for the patients (Gomes-Schwartz, Hadley, & Strupp, 1978; Gurman, 1977; Marziali, Marmar, & Krupnick, 1981; Shapiro, Struening, Shapiro, & Barton, 1976). Among therapist factors, the two most predictive may be empathy and technical performance (Luborsky & Auerbach, 1985). Independent assessments of relationship climate (e.g., watching videotaped sessions) have inconsistently correlated with outcome. Independent observers may be using markers different from those of clients (Horowitz *et al.*, 1984).

Acceptance of Ground Rules

In order for therapists to conduct their business, patients must conform to the basic rules governing the therapeutic interaction. While professional psychotherapy is vulnerable to criticism as an "assembly line production" (Bart, 1974) with approximately 1 hour spent on each piece produced, cultural and economic forces have shaped the psychotherapist's working time into discrete blocks to which patients must adjust. Trust and willingness to be influenced increase each patient's predisposition to come and leave on time and pay the fee. While requests to change the fee, increase or decrease frequency, change the meeting time, or alter the length of a session may sometimes be reasonable, these maneuvers early in treatment are more likely to imply difficulty with engagement. As suggested by Langs (1973), the manner in which patients attempt to manipulate the ground rules of therapy may demonstrate their maladaptive maneuverings within other interpersonal commitments. Careful, empathic handling of patient attempts to subvert the therapeutic contract can provide an opportunity to build trust and increase credibility.

Self-Observer Alliance

The ability to observe one's inner experiences is differentially developed among patients entering therapy. Whether reporting ongoing streams of consciousness, classes of cognitions, the ebb and flow of emotion, specific groups of behaviors or reactions to the therapist, patients must have developed the ability to self-observe and be willing to report their observations to the therapist. For some patients the ability to self-observe is too well developed. Such patients may report an abundance of extraneous information because they are unable to determine what about themselves is relevant to the therapeutic task. They may also use their confusion as a way to hide from the therapist. Some may not wish to report highly charged self-observations because of fear of the therapist's using the information against them. Finally, some patients have very little notion of how to self-observe or how to report these observations to another. Often they must be instructed in how to move away from description of external events toward an integration of their own responses to these events.

When patients are capable of self-observation and understand how to report their experiences but avoid doing so, they may be said to be resisting engagement. Patient willingness to provide the therapist access to critical internal events is a major aspect of the engagement process. When the patient permits the therapist to align with his or her self-observer, the therapist then gains a window on thought–feeling patterns through which influence may be exerted. As indicated by this description, the patient must trust that the therapist will cause no harm and is competent to bring about beneficial change. For those patients who have difficulty with trust, the development of the self-observer alliance may be a long and tedious process. Patients may feel comfortable in the presence of their therapists but be unable to commit themselves to work together on their own difficulties (Dickes, 1975; Luborsky, 1976).

The self-observer alliance is constructed by therapists seizing opportunities through which the patient may be likely to acknowledge internal experience. The discussion of medication side effects, for example, provides a physiological model for self-observation and report. Discussion of the patient's response to a therapist's error may also build the self-observer alliance. In attempting to bring the self-observer into play, therapists should consider asking patients' permission to invoke it. For example, if the patient is reacting to something the therapist did or said, rather than cajole the patient to address the internal response, therapists might say, "I wonder if you would be willing to discuss your reactions to what I've just said." If the patient shows reluctance, then the critical matter is not the content of the patient's experience but rather the patient's resistance to permitting access to the self-observer.

Motivation and Readiness to Change

Motivation is a complex concept composed of many variables. Generally it refers to the amount of energy and commitment patients bring to the therapeutic encounter, but these factors seem inadequate for a full description. In what stage of the change process does the client present? Have problem patterns been defined or is the client hurting but does not have any idea what needs to change? Or does the client know what has to be changed but does not know how to go about it? (McConnaughy, Prochaska, & Velicer, 1983) Does the client find the therapeutic relationship compatible with his or her needs and expectations (Gurman, 1977)?

These factors may be most relevant to the concept of motivation, although others have been adduced to it. Sifneos (1972) has included psychological-mindedness as an important motivational construct. This characteristic is probably a relative constant through time for each patient. Motivation is an often flickering flame that must be fed by both participants to develop the energy for transformation. Rosenbaum and Horowitz (1983) argue from their data that the following variables appear most relevant to outcome: The patient actively participates in therapy by elaborating realistic goals, by communicating information, and by indicating a willingness to change. The patient also shows interest in the treatment process and experiences it as relevant to his or her concerns. Rosenbaum and Horowitz felt that these variables characterized "Active Engagement." In the following section, I will discuss some of the many methods by which therapists can enhance such "active engagement."

ENGAGEMENT METHODS

Therapists have developed numerous strategies for gaining trust and willingness to be influenced. These strategies include: conveying empathy,
providing role definition, managing the contract, demonstrating specialized knowledge, making effective suggestions, and managing the termination variable.

Conveying Empathy

The use of empathy in psychotherapy has two distinct steps that are often
blurred in the minds of those considering it. The first step, gaining empathic understanding, and the second, expressing the empathic understanding, each may be approached in various ways. The methods by
which a specific therapist gathers empathic information and expresses this
understanding will vary with the therapist's personal and professional
predisposition and the needs of the individual patient.

GAINING EMPATHIC UNDERSTANDING

Empathy is the attempt by one person to know the experiences of another,
to enter into the skin of that other, to discover what it is like to be him
or her. Because inner human experience is so complex, therapists must
choose restricted levels through which to enter the other's world. Here-
and-now emotion is the most common empathic target. Conscious cognitions, unconscious processes, and visual images are the other mental levels
into which therapists may choose to project themselves. And by what
means may therapists enter into these levels of another's experience? The
major alternatives include: by thought, by feeling, and by the combination of thought and feeling.

Therapists may use their thoughts to enter any level of the other's
experience. By avoiding use of their own feelings, therapists maintain an
objective perspective but lose some of the ongoing experience. When using objective thought to gain empathic understanding, therapists may attempt to categorize patient emotion. They may also consider patients to
be members of specific classes, inclusion in which seems to predict certain experiences. For example, age predicts biocultural milestones (Erikson, 1963; Haley, 1973), diagnosis predicts certain thought patterns (Beck,
1976; Raimy, 1975), and social role predicts common conflicts (recent
immigrant, divorcing man or woman). Theoretical assumptions about
human psychological dysfunction lead therapists to filter the data of the

patient's presentation in ways that support these theoretical assumptions and lead to a kind of empathic understanding. Ellis's Rational Emotive Therapy (1962), for example, posits 12 basic irrational thoughts that pervade neurotic functioning. Therapists using these assumptions seek out their confirmation and "discover" them in their clients. For some patients, these discoveries resonate with their inner experiences.

Therapists may also choose to permit their clients to effect them emotionally by allowing client words and nonverbal signals to enter into their ongoing experience and by noting how they are affected by these sounds and rhythms. The ability to comprehend the patient through attention to inner responses is based upon "what seems to be a universal capacity for unconscious perception and sensitivity" (Langs, 1976, vol. 2, p. 562). For Freud, therapist introspection was a kind of telephone between two worlds (Freud, 1963) by which the inner workings of the other could be grasped.

Therapists may suspend thought about themselves reacting to patients and instead attempt to climb the narrow viaduct of patients' words and nonverbal signals into the ongoing experience of the other. This "swinging boldly into the life of the other" or "imagining the real" (Buber quoted in Havens, 1974, p. 7) seeks to reduce the objective distance between the two experiences. In its complete form, it goes beyond partial or temporary identification; this reduction of interpersonal distance (phenomenological reduction) is marked by a growing community of mood in which the therapist experiences what the patient is experiencing (Havens, 1974).

"ACTIVE LISTENING"

The Rogerian technique of empathic reflection or "active listening" is probably the best known and most widely used method of expressing therapist willingness to comprehend the ongoing experience of the client. In its simplest form, active listening requires therapists to paraphrase what the patient has just said, using the emotional tone in which it was said. As Rogers (1951) taught this technique, he gradually discovered that trainees tended to parrot back client utterances without truly entering into their frames of reference. He switched to teaching therapists to enter the client's world and to describe the world from that internal reference point.

The time interval and the depth of emotion encompassed by empathic reflections are highly variable. Therapists may summarize a few sentences or, as suggested by the following example from Mann (1973), may encompass a few sessions of listening.

CASE 3.1. A 31-year-old married man was taking several university courses in an extended effort to get a college degree. His reason for seeking help was his consuming fear of failing and accompanying difficulty in studying. In his background was an alcoholic father, who one day was found hanged, a mother chronically disabled with arthritis, a one-month-old son who had been found dead in his crib five years before, a boss with whom he was very close who died very quickly of leukemia one year before, and an always-present fear that his job will suddenly end by his being fired. The central issue for the twelve treatment sessions was expressed to him as, "Because there have been a number of sudden and very painful events in your life, things always seem uncertain, and you are excessively nervous because you do not expect anything to go along well. Things are always uncertain for you." (p. 20)

When therapists construe their patients as members of categories, empathic understanding may be also conveyed by questions that reflect knowledge of the experience of others in similar circumstances. A person about to enter the role of patient may be asked, "How do you feel about being here today?" with the understanding that many people are uncomfortable with the role. A patient being forced to consider the possibility of a fourth divorce may be asked, "I wonder if you are particularly uncomfortable about this marital situation because you might then be forced to fail for a fourth time?" A 50-year-old woman may be asked about her reactions to her last child's leaving home.

When therapists monitor their own fantasies and emotions in response to patients, this information may be used as empathic reflections, questions, and also as trial interpretations.

CASE 3.2. Upon feeling sexually stimulated by a woman patient early in therapy, a male therapist suggested that her problems with men were related to her initial seductiveness, which led men to want her sexually while preventing them from seeing her as a whole person. He added that she also feared expressing herself fully, thinking that she would be rejected if she were not sexy. The patient was initially startled by this intervention but appeared to respect the therapist's grasp of her patterns.

Some psychodynamic therapists use the "trial interpretation" at the beginning of therapy to "test" the patient's psychological-mindedness for their approaches (Sifneos, 1972). As suggested by this vignette, patients may also be impressed with the therapist's understanding of them as conveyed by a trial interpretation, and thereby be helped to engage in therapy (Malan, 1979).

Therapists may also "join" patients by close attention to nonverbal processes. Visual data provide an especially important perspective about those patients who are unable to speak directly but are conveying a great deal of their inner experience in nonverbal ways. Through attention to these signals, the therapist may attempt to pace the patient, to enter into the ongoing nonverbal signals, as a way of bringing them together. No more literal example of pacing could be drawn than the following case from Milton Erickson as described by Haley.

CASE 3.3. Erickson had a patient who upon entering the office could not refrain from pacing. As he walked anxiously back and forth, Erickson asked him, "Are you willing to cooperate with me by continuing to pace the floor as you are now doing?" The patient fully agreed because he had to continue walking in order to stay in the office. The patient then agreed to let Erickson participate in the pacing by directing him here and there. Gradually the patient came to rely on his directions and Erickson began to pause during his directions and the patient began to pause. Gradually he had come to a "complete pause" and could continue to "go into the trance in a chair." (Haley, 1963, p. 52)

The nonverbal signals of silent patients may also be used in this way. For example:

CASE 3.4. As I interviewed a silent, depressed woman during an intake meeting on an inpatient unit, I noticed that she responded to my questions with slight but definite movements of her head and face. Gradually I discerned the possible meanings of these communications and stated them back to her. In response to further questions, she reacted more clearly with her mouth and eyes, and again I translated her meanings back to her. Finally, she cried and began to speak.

Other terms have been used for this approach including "going with the resistance" (Polster & Polster, 1973) and the Utilization Technique (using what the patient shows) (Haley, 1963).

In addition to the techniques described in this section, sincere, genuine, and concerned responses that touch the other's ongoing experience also draw patient and therapist together.

Empathic understanding is useful in all stages of psychotherapy because it permits the therapist to predict the patient's likely reactions to a therapist intervention by knowing the patient's current state of mind. Therefore, empathic understanding can assist with the proper timing of therapist techniques. However, as useful as empathic reflections may be during the engagement stage, patients may signal discomfort with them. As illustrated in the following case, therapists may be required to support before they probe for deeper negative emotions through the sometimes painful empathic statements.

CASE 3.5. A 40-year-old woman whose parents were seriously ill was living in their home. Her mother had metastatic cancer and her father had rapidly progressing diabetes. She had never truly separated from them — they provided her self-definition through their views of her — and was now wrestling with the effect of their impending deaths on her identity. She knew she had to become herself without them. Though she appreciated the freedom they had given her, she implied resentment for their lack of structure. After hearing numerous repetitions of this theme, I said, "You seem to be angry at them for not providing you with more guidance." She recoiled and declared how much she loved them and appreciated what they had done for her. Later I repeated the same empathic reflection and she responded similarly. I gradually realized that I needed to reflect back her positive feelings toward them first. After I empathically reflected back her love for them, she was more easily able to describe her resentment.

Providing Role Definition

Among the clear messages from psychotherapy research is the evidence that patients stay longer in therapy if, at the outset, the roles of both participants are clearly defined (Frank, Hoehm-Saric, Imber, Liberman, & Stone, 1978; Garfield, 1978; Parloff, Waskow, & Wolfe, 1978; Sloane, Cristal, Pepernik, & Whipple, 1970; see also Richert, 1983 for additional references). Practicing psychotherapists tend not to conduct formal role-induction procedures as was done in the research trials, although the therapist's style may be evident to some patients through reputation. Nevertheless, role definition is clearly a valuable engagement strategy and should be integrated into other methods.

Therapists have a wide range of mutually compatible role sets from which to choose. Perhaps more important than the types of roles selected is the impression conveyed while introducing them. Patients want to see a person who is an expert (even if they wish to defeat the therapist) and generally want to feel supported while entering and remaining in the role. Since support is an important element of engagement and is often not directly addressed, I will summarize some of its critical elements.

The conveyance of empathy demonstrates support by indicating that the therapist feels the patient is important enough to enter into his or her world. In addition, by entering the patient's world, the therapist enables the patient to feel less alone and to feel understood. Therapists also support by expressing both verbally and nonverbally personal acceptance, respect, valuing, or liking of their patients. Support may be conveyed by acknowledgment of the patient's strengths and virtues even while searching for negative elements (Yalom, 1983). The careful, judicious management of the therapeutic contract appears to be a different form of support. The "good enough holding" (Langs, 1973; Winnicott, 1965) conveyed through managing the therapeutic structure is more technical than other forms of support. Yet structure of all types is usually experienced as support because patients become confident of their limits and therefore know where they stand. Shifting limits are experienced by patients (and children) as confusing while clear "no's" define the underpinnings of the relationship and are therefore literally supportive. As therapy progresses, support is also conveyed through the therapist's willingness to respond to emergencies, persistence during rough going, a desire to remain on the patient's side, and a strong belief in the patient's ability to change (Strupp, 1975).

A therapist may select from a wide variety of roles and may implement them by direct description and/or by highlighting a specific interchange as a model for the type of interaction he or she is striving to create. Patients will also attempt to impress their own role definitions on the relationship because of their own beliefs about what therapist behaviors will be useful.

Chessick (1982b) listed five general types of therapeutic relationships moving along a continuum from very little interpersonal distance to relatively great interpersonal distance. In the *existential alliance*, the therapist aims not at judging or evaluating but toward a community of shared experience. In the *narcissistic alliance*, the therapist is included within the patient's psyche as a mirroring, idealized, or depreciated "self-object" (a mental representation of other as part of the self). The *classical transference* of psychoanalysis refers to a distorted interpersonal relationship in which the therapist represents significant people from the patient's past. The *rational alliance* is a collaboration between two separate people who together address the psychological difficulties of one of them. The rational (self-observer or working) alliance is part of many psychotherapy forms. Cognitive therapy alliances are sometimes described as *collaborative empiricism*. This latter term is intended to carry not only a sense of working together but also a willingness on the part of the patient to test hypotheses about self and other. Finally, the most distant relationship is the purely *authoritarian alliance*, in which the therapist is directive and the patient is to comply.

Clients tend to favor one role pattern over others. Occasionally they will verbalize their desires or expectations. If allowed sufficient freedom, they will attempt to shape the relationship according to their preconceptions. Therapists willing to accommodate their styles to the initial preferences of their patients may then consider utilizing these role preferences to engage their patients. Reichert (1983) outlined specific techniques for specific role preferences.

1. Medical modelers prefer an authoritarian alliance with little emphasis on a warm, supportive relationship. Instead they simply wish to provide sufficient detail for the therapist to make a wise recommendation. Such patients can be engaged by direct questioning, didactic instruction, normalizing comments, and homework assignments.

2. Problem solvers prefer collaborative empiricism And want therapists to be knowledgeable and experienced but reserve final judgment for themselves. They are practical and do not desire a warm, self-disclosing relationship. Among the more useful engagement techniques for such people are role playing, behavioral rehearsal, analysis of interpersonal transactions, and *in vivo* experiments.

3. Revelationists prefer classical psychoanalytic roles and want therapists to scrutinize their personal memories, feelings, and experiences and to render expert opinion about them. Like the medical modelers, they are less interested in warmth and compassion and more interested in effective intrapsychic analysis. Useful engagement techniques include interpretation, direct questioning, and role reversal.

4. Explorers want an existential alliance and prefer therapists to be supportive, knowledgeable co-workers who function as guides and companions into their psychological inner space. Useful engagement techniques include reflection of feeling and therapist self-disclosure.

Each of these role preferences can represent key character styles in need of psychological change. The "medical modeler" and "revelationist" may each be unwilling to assume sufficient responsibility for their own actions. The revelationist and explorer may avoid applying understanding in a practical way, preferring only to keep searching. As engagement is strengthened, these character styles may become the object of therapeutic scrutiny.

Of course, some patients mix these styles and others do not fit into any of them. The help-rejecting complainer, that person who desperately wants assistance but fears accepting it, is a caricature of many patients and most frustrating for therapists trying to engage them.

CASE 3.6. The highly directive Milton Erickson was attempting to persuade a most obstinate man to pursue a different line of reasoning in his marital relationship. Erickson wished to prove to the man that he was not considering all possibilities, thereby making him more receptive to Erickson's opinion. He wrote "710" on a piece of paper and asked the man to provide him with every conceivable combination. After the man described 107, 701, 170, 071, 017, 71, 17, 10, 07, 01, 70, Erickson again insisted upon every possibility. While again commenting upon the man's inability to look at all perspectives, Erickson turned the paper upside down to show the man the word "OIL." The patient became noticeably more receptive to Erickson's conceptions (Lazarus, 1971, pp. 222–223)

In the following example, I was attempting to define psychotherapy as a collaborative effort in which we look at the painful elements in the patient's life. She did not care to join me in this effort but preferred to remain aloof from my attempts to help her.

CASE 3.7. A 28-year-old woman about to enter medical school refused to discuss her father because it was too painful for her. I said, "If you were examining a patient's abdomen and he or she expressed pain when you pressed on the liver, would you forget about it and press on the shoulder?" She then agreed that her role was to allow us to explore what hurt her.

The following case illustrates the failure to define roles:

CASE 3.8. A 32-year-old, swarthy, bearded, intimidating poet who professed great knowledge of Tarot cards and astrology sought psychotherapy for anxiety attacks from a 34-year-old psychiatrist.* He complained of being afraid to be alone and then began to read his best poem from a vanity press edition of his work. He was filled with energy as his deep voice bellowed across the small room. The therapist was frightened and when the patient asked, "Do you want to hear more?" meekly nodded yes. The poet read until the end of the hour and then asked to borrow a book. Again the therapist meekly complied. The patient never returned the book or himself to therapy.

---

*Patient was seen before the time when panic disorder was a recognized entity responsive to medications. Had this patient been offered medications, engagement probabilities would have increased.

This therapist failed to assume responsibility for encouraging the patient to talk about psychotherapeutic issues.

Managing the Contract

Although role definitions and content varies across the range of practicing therapists, most psychotherapy relationships are characterized by a set length of time for individual sessions, a set fee, and a set frequency. Patients may challenge these simple constants. The therapist's response to these challenges can serve as demonstrations of competence (or incompetence). Firm, clear guidelines serve as messages that the therapist is in control of these basic elements. Patients who ask for discounts in clinics without sliding scales are indirectly asking about the therapist's sense of competence or corruptibility. Patients who want longer or shorter sessions may be asking about the therapist's ability to withstand their distress. Telephone calls, failure to call before missing an appointment, late arrival, early requests for shifts in frequency, each represent challenges to the therapist's conduct of the relationship. Because these maneuvers around contract issues offer valuable information about the manner in which patients conduct their interpersonal relationships, Langs has elevated analysis of them into role definitions for the participants: The therapist is the manager of the frame, carefully observing patient attempts to alter it (see Langs, 1973, vol. 1).

Therapists may have a personal as well as a theoretical bias towards specific role and contract expectations, as indicated by Freud in 1913.

> Before I conclude these remarks on beginning the analytic treatment a word must be said about a certain ceremonial observance regarding the position in which the treatment is carried out. I adhere firmly to the plan of requiring the patient to recline upon a sofa, while one sits behind him out of his sight. This arrangement has an historic meaning; it is the last vestige of the hypnotic method out of which psychoanalysis was evolved; but for many reasons it deserves to be retained. The first is a personal motive, one that others may share with me, however. I *cannot* [emphasis added] bear to be gazed at for eight hours a day (or more). Since, while I listen, I resign myself to the control of my unconscious thoughts I do not wish my expression to give the patient indications which he may interpret or which may influence him in his communications. The patient usually regards being required to take up this position as a hardship and objects to it, especially when scoptophilia plays an important part in the neurosis. I persist in the measure, however, for the intention and result of it are that all imperceptible influence on the patient's associations by the transference may be

avoided, so that the transference may be isolated and clearly outlined when it appears as a resistance. (Freud, 1963, p. 146)

Demonstrating Specialized Knowledge

Training in psychotherapy inevitably introduces to students theories of mental dysfunction. When expressed to clients with specific reference to the etiology of their difficulties, this knowledge may serve as a demonstration of expertness. Clients often conclude from such explanations that the therapist's ability to comprehend their problems in a sensible theoretical context implies that the therapist will then know how to bring relief. The therapist's clear outline of the process of psychotherapeutic change will also encourage this perception, particularly if clients can visualize themselves proceeding through it. Through their ability to stimulate visions of change, therapists instill hope in their clients, a requisite function of the first stage of therapy (Frank, 1976). Following is an excerpt from Wolpe's (1973) recommended short didactic speech to patients seeking treatment for phobias.

> You have realized that fear figures excessively in your life. . . . Let us consider how neurotic fears originate. The process is really what common sense would lead you to expect. Let me illustrate it by the old fashioned example of the burnt child. The child places his hand on the big black, hot coal stove. He quickly withdraws the painful hand, tearful and fearful. His mother comforts him, but later notes that he keeps away from the stove and seems afraid of it. Clearly, the child has developed a beneficial habit of fearing and avoiding an actually harmful object.
>
> But in some cases the experience also has other and less favorable consequences. Suppose in the bedroom there is a large black chest of drawers. The child may have become afraid of this too — purely on the basis of its *physical resemblance* to the stove — a phenomenon known in psychology as generalization. . . . Your own fears were likewise acquired in the course of unpleasant experiences, some of which we touched upon in your history. . . . Now because these reactions could then be produced by particular stimulus triggers as a result of the process of learning, it is possible to eliminate them by the application of the principles of learning. (pp. 54–55)

In this way Wolpe established himself as a competent psychotherapist who understood both the cause and treatment of psychological dysfunction.

When offering explanations of psychological dysfunction and its treatment to a patient, I also elicit the patient's explanatory model. This elicitation of the patient's personal theory of psychological distress (i.e., cause and treatment) is being suggested for use in primary care medicine (Kleinman, Eisenberg, & Good, 1978) but appears not yet to have found its way into psychotherapeutic practice. By asking for this self-perspective therapists may avoid forcing the patient into their own conceptual Procrustean beds and instead open the way for negotiation between the two of them for an explanatory model with which they both can feel comfortable. Lazare, Eisenthal, and Wasserman (1975) described the following example that illustrates the value of asking the reticent patient for an opinion concerning the best course of treatment:

CASE 3.9. A 55-year-old hospital employee who came to the clinic was interviewed by a psychiatric resident in the presence of three other residents and the senior author. The patient said he was upset and depressed. Some mild depressive symptomatology was indeed elicited. He also explained that he was troubled by his wife's recent hospitalization for a recurrent psychotic condition. The resident attempted to understand the depression in terms of his loneliness or his feelings of guilt, or both, but was unable to elicit responses that would support this formulation. The patient's request was not elicited.

The patient was asked to wait outside the office while the residents conferred about possible treatment options. Psychotherapy and pharmacological treatments were considered. It was decided that the request should first be elicited.

In response to the question, "How did you wish we could help?" the patient replied, "I work in the hospital kitchen and bring food up to the psychiatry ward. It's a nice clean place and they treat the patients well. If you have space, would you call the state hospital and have her transferred? I would feel much better." The transfer was arranged and the patient became asymptomatic. (p. 555)

The therapist's willingness to take into consideration the patient's perspective rather than forcing the patient to take on the therapist's theory may serve as an excellent engagement technique through its demonstration of knowledge and support and may also reduce the likelihood of potential stalemates.

Making Effective Suggestions

The offer of a plan, procedure, or substance that produces beneficial effects establishes therapists as effective and increases client hope for future benefit (Beitman, 1979). Relaxation exercises, when properly carried out, usually increase clients' sense of well-being. Biofeedback machines can teach them how to control body functions. Medications for depression, anxiety, or psychosis may not only increase patients' abilities to engage in psychotherapy, but also increase their confidence in their therapists' training and experience whether or not the medication is given by the therapist or by someone to whom the therapist refers the patient. Said one patient after successful treatment with neuroleptics, "The medication was very helpful in organizing my thinking. I want to see if there are more ways you can help me." Medications do not need to be pharmacologically effective in order to engage patients; the prescription and discussion of its effects may provide an interpersonal matrix within which trust may be established (Beitman, 1981). Simple behavioral suggestions may also serve a similar function, as illustrated by the following case from Cashdan (1973).

CASE 3.10. In one of the early therapy sessions, Beth announced that prior to her entry into therapy, she had arranged a meeting with her mother in Washington, D.C. Beth was scheduled to attend a one-day marketing conference in the city and in a letter to her mother had casually mentioned this. Her mother wrote back suggesting they spend the day together and offered to fly to Washington to meet her. Although Beth had agreed to this arrangement, she found herself becoming increasingly anxious about the impending meeting.

The two had agreed to meet in Beth's hotel room, where they felt they could talk to one another undisturbed. This arrangement in particular made Beth very nervous. Although it was not precisely clear what it was she feared (homosexual impulses toward her mother, acting out angry feelings, etc.) one thing was clear: Beth was terribly apprehensive about meeting her mother within the confines of a small room. I therefore suggested that the two meet at the Lincoln Memorial, and from there go to lunch together; afterwards they could visit the National Art Gallery where they might talk at leisure while viewing the exhibits.

Beth followed my suggestion and returned to the next therapy session in a euphoric mood. The meeting had gone off without a hitch; the two spent a pleasant day together and even arranged a similar rendezvous a few months hence. Beth was delighted with the outcome. (pp. 69–70)*

Direct suggestions, like any other interventions, may have deleterious side effects. Langs (1973) described a case in which the therapist's ap-

*From *Interactional Psychotherapy* by S. Cashdan, 1973, New York: Grune and Stratton. Reprinted by permission.

parently logical behavioral suggestion created a number of negative consequences.

CASE 3.11. The patient was a young man who felt inadequate with women and feared that he would become a homosexual. After a few months, the patient revealed that his mother slept in his bedroom because his father preferred to have the windows open. He felt he was favored by his mother over his father. After a psychotic decompensation on LSD during which his homosexual fears became more pressing, the therapist suggested that he move out of the bedroom with his mother. The therapist had silently reasoned that the homosexual fears were a defense against incestuous wishes.

The patient reacted with fear, distrust, and a sense that the therapist was intruding upon him. He did not move out of the room and began to develop rageful fantasies against the therapist that appeared directly related to this suggestion. (pp. 538–550)

This response indicates that "simple" advice may have complex effects, especially when it is directed to the core of the patient's central problem. The advice offered by Cashdan to Beth penetrated less deeply into her core maladaptive behaviors.

Managing the Termination Variable

Although the average number of sessions per patient across many outpatient clinics tends to range between six and eight (Garfield, 1978), the specific number for any individual patient ranges from one to many hundred. Termination is possible at any time and may often be the best alternative. An evaluation session does not necessarily obligate either person to ongoing therapy. Many therapists set a limit of two to six sessions, after which either person is free to quit. In this way, neither is forced into the relationship without some time to gain familiarity with the other. The freedom to leave increases the depth of engagement.

Many clients quit after one session. A yet-undefined percentage report significant gains from this brief contact. Some may simply be satisfied to know that they are not deeply disturbed and are gratified to be reassured of that fact (Rockwell & Pinkerton, 1982). Others seem poised for change, having defined the outlines of their problem patterns and need but little professional encouragement (Malan, Heath, Bacal, & Balfour, 1975; Rockwell & Pinkerton, 1982).

People in crisis are also likely to be poised for change not because they are aware of the patterns that are creating their difficulty but because these patterns have created an emotional upheaval that has become unbearable. They wish to avoid recurrence and are therefore more accessible to psychological analysis and change. The first few sessions of crisis intervention are focused upon specific practical measures to alleviate the current emotional intensity. When the distress melts away after a suicide attempt, an acute psychotic reaction, severe depressive episode, or domestic violence, patients usually want to seal over the pain and ignore the origins. If the therapist is able to provide the client access to that anguished state of consciousness, this reminder may serve to reengage him or her.

Those who do not enter therapy poised for change or during crisis may be satisfied with short-term psychotherapy (6–20 sessions) during which general patterns of psychological discomfort are uncovered and defined in ways that can lead to change. Therapists who see their upper limit as 20 sessions may be satisfied with the goals of short-term treatment. Those who see the patterns exposed and changed as the products of deeper difficulties will tend to consider their patients for yet further treatment.

The transition from short- to long-term treatment may require a shift in therapist activity and behavior. During crisis intervention and short-term approaches, therapists are more likely to be active and directive. While some continue the same level of activity in long-term treatment, others tend to ease back from the interaction to let it unfold, to give more control to the patient, and to observe carefully the increasingly intense interpersonal distortions that each of them develop toward the other. Patients may need to hear explanations of this shift in roles and its purpose (Amada, 1983). The other long-term alternative is to invite the patient to return if and when further need arises. This form of parting is contraposed to those terminations that are boundary events never again to be recrossed, a kind of death. Instead, patients can be viewed as never "cured" and always susceptible to the developmental crises created by biological and socioeconomic forces. In practice, patients often return to therapists after termination, thereby establishing relationships with intermittent contact (Bennett, 1983). Careful management of termination can strengthen engagement and reengagement. Patients need not be released precipitously or retained without good reason. By appropriate encouragement of separation, therapists set the stage for easy future reengagement. By holding onto a needy but ambivalent patient, therapists can also firm up engagement. Beutler (1983) suggested that termination during the transition from symptom-focused to long-term, broad-band (insight-oriented) therapy increases the likelihood of negative effects. It is better to end firmly or go definitely on than to hesitate and stop (p. 146).

Patients' Attempts to Engage Therapists

An unfortunate consequence of listing of many techniques by which therapists gain influence over their clients is to obscure the attempts by the clients themselves to enlist the therapist's allegiance and commitment. Clients tend to adopt the interpersonal style that has characterized their previous attempts at engaging others in long-term relationships. Among the common patterns are sexual seductiveness, helpless dependency, compliance with expectations, attempts to please, advertising self as superior, warm and friendly Mr. "Nice Guy," and offers of friendship and advice. Each of these techniques is potentially controlling if the therapist is captured by it. On the other hand, the desire to be involved is essential to the therapeutic process.

CASE 3.12. A very attractive, well-dressed, sexually seductive 36-year-old woman presented herself to me as utterly helpless and lost. She quickly spoke of her lover, who was on the board of the hospital and "could have you fired if he wished." She did not know whom to trust and wanted to be certain that he would not hear of the content of our discussion. In one sweep she used a number of engagement techniques, including challenging the potential breach of confidentiality threatened by her lover's position on the hospital board. Her sexiness had to be understood as a ploy for control, her helplessness as a plea for assistance, and her paranoia as a partial product of the uncertainty and terror under which she was conducting her life.

ENGAGEMENT CONTENT

Superficially the content of the engagement stage is usually concerned with problems, psychological pain, and symptoms that may give clues to underlying patterns in need of change. However, until trust is established and the therapist is perceived as competent and capable, underlying themes of distrust and rejection fears will be most critical. In order to pick them up, therapists may need to listen to indirect references to the therapeutic situation, especially those marked by feelings and ideas that involve trust and competency issues. Among one of my more instructive examples was the following case:

CASE 3.13. A 37-year-old mother of two elementary school children had been having panic attacks almost daily for the past 4 weeks when she came for evaluation. I was in the midst of initiating a study of panic disorder in cardiology patients and was using a semistructured interview as part of that study. I also used this format with this woman. I inquired with incisive detail into the nature of her symptoms, ignoring her irritation with my perseverance. At the end of the session she said, "Well, at least you're going to give me a blood test aren't you?" Yes, I was intending to measure her thyroid functioning. When I called her a few days later to tell her the results, she reported that she found my style incompatible for her and had chosen to see a family physician. I was embarrassed. Although I had demonstrated diagnostic and medical competence, she was looking for empathic reception and for some outline of a plan.

In this case, the patient's concerns were evident had I been looking. Sometimes the concerns are more hidden. Patients may make reference to significant others who have rejected them or allude to problems with other help-giving professionals. Perhaps one of the best demonstrations of competence and ability to listen comes with the therapist's acknowledgement of these fears as they emerge in the current therapeutic relationship.

CASE 3.14. A 67-year-old retired academic physician entered his third session with two dream fragments that I had requested. He was moderately depressed and very much wished to resume his avocation as an artist but felt blocked to do so. One of the reasons was a remark by a psychiatrist 30 years previously that his painting was "throwing shit on the world." He felt demeaned by this remark, which left him with a sense of despair about his artwork. The first dream fragment involved his wife, who had told him that he spoke in his sleep. He had asked her to record what he said. In the midst of dream talking one night, she asked him what he had said and he mumbled back, "Oh, nothing, it doesn't matter." She felt hurt by that, but he stated that he usually felt that she never listened to him and that he felt rejected by her. The second dream involved three actors, one of whom was crying. He was one of the actors and his wife and mother were probably the other two. His mother, who was still alive, had joined him and his wife in some unsuccessful real estate deals, and he wondered who was at fault. He had always felt rejected by his mother who never seemed to love anyone, including herself.

Then the patient spoke again of the psychiatrist, Dr. D, who had "peeled him like an onion," had taken away his defenses but not replaced them with anything. He was very angry with psychoanalysts because they just took people apart. I suggested to the patient that he was also frightened by what I might do to him, that he feared that if he opened himself up to me he might be further destroyed. He felt rejected by his wife, his mother, and his psychiatrist. Might he also be likely to feel rejected by me? Of course, he said. I wondered if he would be able to tell me if he felt I was rejecting him. He said he would. I expressed my doubts. He had, after all, continued to see Dr. D for 10 years after his hurtful remark. He said that psychiatrists were always right then, but that things had changed. Would he be willing to bring in more dreams? Perhaps he was frightened with how I might treat them. After all, he said, we've met only three times. We'll give it a chance.

This patient was experienced in talking indirectly about his fears of the psychotherapist and readily accepted translation of these latent messages into terms of the current therapeutic relationship. Sometimes these themes are buried more deeply in the patient's presentations. Patients may unconsciously lie about their outside-the-office behavior to challenge the therapist's ability to catch them. They may exaggerate horrible events in their lives to challenge the therapist's commitment to work with them. They may test the therapist's ability to endure them by repeated criticism, complaints, or demands. Each one of these often unnerving challenges may be approached by considering the engagement context in which they are being offered.

THE THERAPIST'S DECISIONS REGARDING ENGAGEMENT

While engaging a potential client, each therapist is also gauging his or her suitability for psychotherapy: Is this person in need of psychological help at all or is the purpose of the consultation to confirm lack of need? Does a biomedical cause explain the presenting symptoms? Is this person better treated with psychoactive medication alone or with medication in combination with psychotherapy? Is individual psychotherapy best, or should marital, group, or family therapy be considered? How long will psychotherapy take; what are some of its predictable side effects and likely difficulties? Which goals are within reach?

After eliciting the presenting complaint, therapists choose from a wide array of questions and procedures by which to gather information to answer the content questions of the engagement stage. Some remain silent in order to let patients unfold at their own pace; some ask that standardized questionnaires be completed (MMPI, depression and anxiety scales, social and behavioral analysis); some refer for or perform screening physical and laboratory tests. Certain data appear to be required for optimal clinical care: Biomedical and psychopharmacologically responsive syndromes should be considered. History of the presenting complaint in its social, characterological, and biological context should also be elicited in order to provide some estimate of future course. Previous patterns of psychotherapy treatment should also be noted to estimate the possible course of another such attempt. In summary, any data that offers the possibility of predicting and controlling the course of treatment should be gathered. Unfortunately, researchers have gathered little information about patient characteristics that usefully predict the course of treatment. So far, the best predictors involve the patient's early assessment of the patient–therapist relationship (Gurman, 1977).

Is Psychotherapy Necessary?

Some patients appear to represent themselves as patients wishing psychotherapeutic treatment when, in fact, they wish something else (as did the depressed janitor with the hospitalized wife; see Case 3.9). Some may ask for psychotherapy and yet not want it or require it.

CASE 3.15. A 28-year-old lawyer requested psychotherapy because he was falling in love with a woman and wanted to marry her. Although she appeared to care for him, he was afraid that she would reject him. Shortly after he started treatment, his parents were to visit him from his hometown 3,000 miles away. His woman friend's parents had arranged a dinner with them and planned to introduce them to their other relatives. This planning strongly suggested that her parents thought they were about to become his in-laws. The patient could not believe this possibility. Therapy, however, dragged very slowly; he had little to talk about. He did mention that he had entered therapy because his mother had insisted upon it, although the reasons appeared unclear. I confronted him on his lack of involvement and he admitted that he did not feel he needed therapy. We terminated. A few months later, the patient returned for one session, again irrationally anxious about his fiance's commitment to him. They were married shortly thereafter.

The patient had offered much psychological data for analysis, yet, he was not deeply motivated for therapy, and I estimated that for a large cost in time and in money his gains might not be great. Finally, two years after his marriage, he returned once again with similar symptoms, ready to change.

A Biomedical Explanation?

While more than 50% of the mentally ill in the United States seek help for their difficulties from internists, family practitioners, and general practitioners (Regier, Goldberg, & Taube, 1975), some people with true medical illness present themselves to psychotherapists for help. The percentage of such people appearing in outpatient psychotherapy offices may not be very high; patients in state hospital psychiatric units are more likely to have undiagnosed medical illness. Nevertheless, thyroid dysfunction, hematological abnormalities, and drug abuse should be considered among possible explanations for presenting psychological symptoms.

Better Treated with Psychoactive Medications?

Psychopharmacological research is uncovering increasingly more precise indications for each of the four major classes of psychiatric medications: antidepressants, neuroleptics, lithium, and anxiolotics. Often, a medication alone will bring excellent symptom relief for a lesser expense. Psychotherapists who are not able to recognize vegetative signs of depression, thought disorder, manic-depressive symptoms, and panic attacks, are depriving their clients of effective treatment alternatives.

However, medications alone and psychotherapy alone are proving, in some cases, not as effective as the combination. For example, cognitive therapy of depression may be as effective as antidepressant medication; each helps 70% of a selected depressed population. The combination helps 90% (Hollon, 1983). These statistics suggest that of each group, 20% not helped by one treatment is helped by the other treatment, or that there is some synergistic effect of the combination in some of them. In the treatment of schizophrenia, family therapy seems to improve outcome when coupled with neuroleptic medication and may help to reduce the required neuroleptic dose (Goldstein, 1984). In the treatment of manic-depressive illness, psychotherapy is often a useful adjunct, although physicians do not see this possibility as frequently as patients do (Jamison & Goodwin, 1983). For anorexia, (Eckert & Halmi, 1984) and agoraphobia (Mavissakalian, 1984), a judicious combination of both psychotherapy and psychopharmacology may prove to be more useful than either alone.

Individual, Marital, Family, or Group Therapy?

No clear guidelines have been developed to distinguish those circumstances under which therapists should choose a specific therapeutic constellation into which to place a given patient. Training, experience, and personal predisposition appear to have greater influence on a therapist's choice of a treatment constellation than objective indicators. Perhaps, as is being suggested by those who contrast Weissman's interpersonal therapy with Beck's cognitive therapy in the treatment of depression (Hollon, 1983) as well as by those doing overviews of psychotherapy outcome studies (Luborsky *et al.*, 1975; Smith *et al.*, 1980), different numerical constellations, like different schools of therapy, may have relatively equivalent outcomes. Therefore, the therapist's preferred mode and manner is likely the better option since self-confidence probably aids therapeutic efficacy.

However, there may be a few guidelines for a rational choice:

1. Family therapy of many different styles appears to be very helpful for acute and perhaps chronic schizophrenics who are living at home. If parents and other relatives are able to reduce their levels of expressed emotion, then schizophrenic children appear less likely to relapse and more likely to improve (Goldstein, 1984).

2. When one member of a couple is deeply disturbed by the behavior of the other, then marital therapy should be considered. Often the partner will not come for an appointment. If the partner does appear, brief evaluation may indicate that one or both do not trust the other sufficiently to talk directly with each other about their mutual difficulties. One or both may not be committed enough to the continuation of the marriage to attempt to reestablish the trust necessary for communication. If one member of the couple is begun in individual psychotherapy, a likely side effect of successful treatment is divorce. By not coming for marital therapy the reluctant spouse is indicating a resistance to the change requested by the spouse in treatment. If, on the other hand, the partner in therapy does not want the other to enter couples therapy, divorce is also a likely outcome. I believe that these predictions should be offered and discussed during the engagement stage.

3. When patients' social context is intimately connected with their identities and presenting problems, patients' difficulties may be considered to be symptomatic of dysfunction in the marriage or family. Then the social context must be considered for change. However, when the patient's problem is separation from family during late adolescence, and the patient has shown some potential for independence, then individual therapy should be considered in order to aid the separation–individuation process. In such cases, therapists should not be surprised to find that successful psychotherapy may lead to parental divorce, since the patient's difficulties may have obscured marital discord that, upon the patient's release from the family, became more evident. (For example, the mother may be so enmeshed in an adolescence's problems that an affair is unlikely until the adolescent no longer needs her.)

4. Group therapy studies offer guidelines only about those who should be excluded (brain damaged, paranoid, extremely narcissistic, hypochondriacal, suicidal, addicted to drugs or alcohol, acute psychotic or sociopathic) (Yalom, 1970, pp. 157–158) although there are groups for some of these specific clusters. Inclusion criteria have not been developed and, therefore, the decision to use group psychotherapy is largely a clinical estimate of its potential efficacy in defining and altering interpersonal patterns.

5. Among the indications for selecting a specific individual psychotherapy approach, only phobias have shown a clearly better prognosis when psychotherapy includes exposure to the feared stimulus. Exposure may be rapid or slow, in imagination or in real life (Barlow & Beck, 1984).

6. Rational choice is but one of the many factors influencing the therapist's choice of treatment form. Intense desire to retain interpersonal connections can lead family members to insist on family therapy. Denial and projection can lead one family member to insist that another be treated individually as the patient (Sander, 1984). Certainly the therapist's own comfort, training, and experience with the modalities also influence the choice. Therapy groups are often difficult to establish and may therefore be excluded as an option unless the therapist is willing to turn away potential income through referral. Since there is no agreed-upon nosology of family dysfunction, insurance reimbursement is primarily for individual treatment, thus biasing this option.

Goals and Prognosis

At first glance, the goals of psychotherapy seem simple enough: to help the patient to feel better and to cope more effectively. However, the seeker for clearer definitions of therapeutic objectives stumbles through a morass of conflicting ideals and perspectives strongly influenced by the subjective values of the persons judging outcome. Prognosis refers to the course of the current difficulty with and without therapeutic intervention. Using a medical example, the course of pneumococcal pneumonia without penicillin usually spirals through increasing devastation of lung tissue, while with penicillin treatment this deleterious course is usually averted. Can parallel statements be made for borderline personality? Not yet. The questions must be better asked first. Despite limited information, therapists often attempt to make predictions about what would happen to this person without psychotherapy. The answer to this question is entwined with the definition of goals.

GOALS

For the psychoanalyst Wallerstein (in Wolberg, 1967, p. 835), "goalless-ness is a procedural stance essential to analytic work" although others (e.g., McGlashan & Miller, 1982) have listed extensive analytic objectives. Who is to define the goals of therapy? If the patient alone defines them, then the reduction of anxiety about sex or people may be gained simply by avoidance of sex or people. On the other hand, patients may have unrealistic expectations, including a complete revamping of personali-ty, an increase in IQ, or finding a someone who will provide them with cherished ideals of wealth and a happy marriage. If others are to judge outcome goals, new value conflicts emerge. A spouse might wish for greater tolerance of his or her shortcomings. A family might wish for com-pliance rather than challenge to their authority. A totalitarian culture might also wish for submission to the wishes of the state. Insurance com-panies might simply want return to premorbid functioning without em-phasis upon personal growth or increased coping abilities. If the therapist is to formulate the goals, then this list might become an outline of the therapist's picture of emotional and psychological perfection. Each pa-tient would represent psychological clay to be molded by the therapist into a reflection of the therapist's ideals. Are therapist and patient to negotiate goals as suggested by Sullivan (1954)?

After reviewing these conflicting perspectives, the psychodynamic hypnotherapist, Lewis Wolberg (1967, p. 838), stated his own notion of the goals of therapy: "The achievement by the patient of optimal func-tioning within the limitations of his financial circumstances, his existing motivations, his ego resources and the reality situation." This relativistic definition allows much to be read into the term "optimal functioning." For example, is this goal too "selfish?" Are psychotherapists unintentional-ly teaching people to avoid social responsibility in the service of the self (Wallach & Wallach, 1983)? Should altruism be a psychotherapeutic goal?

Goals may also be defined in terms of cost (time and money), side effects, and desired outcome. Neuroleptics, for example, provide a very inexpensive way to control the symptoms of schizophrenia. Family ther-apy is more costly, but in combination with neuroleptics may reduce the required dose, thereby probably decreasing the possibility of the long-term side effect of tardive dyskinesia (Goldstein, 1984). Antidepressant medication is very inexpensive compared to cognitive therapy in the treat-ment of depression. But cognitive therapy may prevent relapse without maintenance medication and also increase adaptive functioning. How does one determine the optimal allocation of the resource of psychotherapy? For example, is society better served by the intensive psychotherapy for chronic moderate unhappiness in a medical student with good work and interpersonal relationships or a borderline adolescent who functions poorly in school and relationships?

Statements about the course of a specific psychological problem without treatment are difficult to make. Environmental richness and unplanned coincidence may provide certain nonpatients with experiences that have tremendous psychotherapeutic effect. Bloch (1979) has summarized the research in psychodynamic therapy that has attempted to correlate initial patient characteristics with outcome criteria. He covered four general areas: (1) factors related to illness (diagnosis, symptom severity, course of illness, initial affect – particularly anxiety and depression), and response to previous therapy; (2) personal factors related to treatment – motivation, expectations of improvement and of the therapeutic process; (3) personal factors not directly associated with the illness – age, sex, marital status, socioeconomic status, educational attainment, intelligence, habitual patterns of defense and coping with stress, previous sexual adjustment, previous social adjustment, and nature of interpersonal relationships; (4) current life circumstances – financial state, marital and/or family situation, and any accidental crisis such as an acute physical illness. Among Bloch's more interesting conclusions were: (a) patients without fresh symptoms appeared to have uniformly low rates of improvement; (b) patients with a high level of felt disturbance and low level of behavioral disturbance have the better therapeutic outcome; (c) socioeconomic class, age, and education do not predict outcome variance.

Diagnosis appears to provide some exclusion criteria (e.g., organic brain syndrome) for some types of therapy and may also predict treatment course. Although variously defined, the term "borderline personality" is used to indicate difficult patients. Perhaps the label may serve as a self-fulfilling prophecy, yet objectively, patients receiving this label are often profoundly disturbed in their interpersonal relationships. Malan (1979, p. 255) listed Hildebrand's exclusion criteria for long-term psychoanalysis done by trainees. While this list does not by any means indicate that psychotherapy should not be attempted, it highlights factors that, if present, are likely to predict a difficult therapeutic course:

- Serious suicide attempts
- Chronic alcoholism or drug addiction
- Long-term psychiatric hospitalization

- More than one course of ECT
- A confirmed homosexual asking to be made heterosexual
- Chronically incapacitating obsessional symptoms
- Gross destructive or self-destructive behavior

Two other categories of clinical data appear helpful in predicting the course of treatment. If the patient has been in psychotherapy before, the manner in which the patient responded to the previous relationship is likely to be repeated again. If therapy went well before, what seemed useful to the patient? If the current therapist is able to pinpoint the circumstances of a stalemate that led to disruption of the previous relationship, he or she may be able to predict its recurrence, as suggested by the following failure.

CASE 3.16. A 48-year-old artist had been in psychotherapy with 10 different therapists and pharmacotherapists for more than 24 years. His first psychotherapy relationship began when he was a graduate student. His therapist had agreed to work with him for 6 months and then announced during their third appointment that this would be their last session. He had felt betrayed by most subsequent therapists as well. When he entered therapy with me, I thought I could help to avoid this impasse, but he managed to patch together a few of my behaviors into a plot to betray him that was not accessible to our discussion.

A final category of predictive data involves the current social network. To whom is the patient currently relating and how are they affecting him or her? Some of these people may be very resistant to change and may also be paying the bills.

ENGAGEMENT DISTORTIONS

Through the relative neutrality of his psychoanalytic method, Freud discovered three interrelated processes common to all psychotherapeutic relationships. When he urged patients to associate freely or to talk about their early experiences, they often remained silent or spoke about something else (resistance). Not uncommonly these resistances were related to their feelings about him and about what he might think of them (transference). Finally, he noticed that he seemed to react in unexpected and irrational ways to the words and behaviors of his patients (countertransference). For much of Freud's life, attention to resistance and transference defined psychoanalytic treatment. Perhaps this definition of psychoanalysis kept other schools of therapy from incorporating these concepts into their treatment strategies, since Freud declared that anyone who uses resistance and transference is practicing psychoanalysis (Fine, 1973). Some cognitive–behavioral therapists recognize resistance as "counterwill" (Wachtel, 1982). Transference does not receive much attention outside psychoanalysis although it is ubiquitous. Countertransference tends to be given less attention than transference within psychoanalysis and is accorded very little concern outside psychoanalysis despite the obvious fact that therapists can be deeply affected by their patients. These blocks or distortions deserve attention during each psychotherapy stage.

Resistance is the paradoxical attempt by the patient to fight the process of change while also wanting to change. Freud and then his daughter Anna (1971) related resistance to defense by suggesting that the manner in which the patient resisted the progress of therapy indicated the types of defenses often used outside of therapy.

CASE 3.17. A 26-year-old graduate student sought counseling because she felt overburdened by her work load and child care. She believed something should change. After the first interview, the counselor realized that her client appeared to create extra activity and extra responsibility. Before the counselor was able to utilize this understanding, the patient called to cancel her next and future appointments because she was "too busy."

The notion that each patient demonstrates in the office the pathological, maladaptive patterns characterizing their lives outside the office is a major treatment assumption in psychoanalysis. Freud and his followers could believe that they had activated crucial patterns in the here and now of the consulting room. Therefore these patterns could be studied as if they were being observed outside the office and in the patient's distant past. Under this assumption, Freud and his followers constructed their theories of psychopathology from their consulting room observations. Transference was a royal road to the psychoanalytic unconscious and to psychoanalytic theory.

Freud was attempting to build a theory of personality from his psychoanalytic method. Research was more important than treatment (Freud, 1963). His assumptions may have been too broad, his conclusions placed upon a tenuous foundation. Nevertheless, his notion that resistance and transference reflect basic patterns of the patient's outside-the-office experience remains an extremely valuable psychotherapeutic assumption. This principle may be stated in many ways, but simply said is, What you see is what they've got. Said with a poetic term, it is: Resistance and transference are synechodochies (the part represents the whole); with a technological analogy: Resistance and transference are a part of a hologram (for which a section contains the information of the whole); and behaviorally: People have a limited number of coping and interpersonal styles, some of which will inevitably be introduced into the threatening interpersonal situation that is psychotherapy.

Resistance may also be created by the patient's social system — people who are invested in the patient's maladaptive behavior. Therapists may unknowingly promote resistance through faulty or misapplied technique (e.g., Basch, 1982). To look to the patient as the only source of resistance and transference is to burden the patient with undue responsibility.

Engagement Resistances

"Resistance" refers to the patient's tendency to subvert the work of therapy. During engagement, resistances occur around issues of trust, belief in the therapist's competence, role definition, and contract agreements. They deserve immediate attention or engagement may be lost. The exact form of attention varies with the therapist's theoretical orientation. Psychodynamic therapists advocate insight and understanding although straightforward behavior may be effective as well, as illustrated in a case described by Goldfried and Davison (1976).

CASE 3.18. A 35-year-old woman in behavioral therapy began to skip sessions early in therapy. First the therapist urged her to rearrange her other commitments. Although irritated by these missed appointments, the therapist was afraid the client was too unassertive to make the necessary arrangements. During the next session, the therapist decided that she actually had become sufficiently assertive and therefore announced that he would bill her for future missed appointments. There were no further missed appointments (pp. 252–253).

The most common easily observed resistances are those that take place over the therapeutic contract. Failure to appear for an appointment, especially without prior notification, because the patient "forgot," often indicates a nonverbal statement about the therapeutic relationship. Requests for reduced fee or time and frequency shifts may hide attempts by the patient to test the therapist's "flexibility" and willingness to accommodate and give. Deeper still, these maneuvers may conceal attempts to probe the therapist's weakness, to undermine his or her ability to manage and maintain the therapeutic contract. How "paranoid" should a therapist be in responding to these and other alterations in the therapeutic contract? Langs (1973) insisted that a wide variety of minor variations in the contract, including touching patients and bringing in significant others were extremely dangerous, and yet other therapists blithely do both without apparent harm. I attempt to steer a moderate course that includes continuous attention to threats to the therapeutic contract especially as therapy progresses, since contract issues often assume greater importance for more intense relationships. Therapists choose many different grounds on which to conduct their battles against each patient's tendency to engage in maladaptive behavior. The discussion of the contract and its limitations provides a clear, discernible, easily identified demarcation observable by both participants. Sometimes the contract lines must be crossed during crisis and under other compelling conditions. Patients must sometimes be seen in hospitals, make contact by telephone, miss appointments, fail to pay bills promptly, or stop treatment at times that therapists may describe as premature. Each of these breaches in the orthodox contract may have meaning worthy of discussion. Nevertheless, overriding reality concerns can take precedence. The setting, types of patients, and theoretical–personal orientations determine the degree of rigidity of the therapist's contract management.

Therapists have four general alternatives when they notice that patients are fighting the contract or their expected rules: (1) simply encourage (or cajole) the person to do what is expected, (2) explain the reason for the request, (3) confront and/or interpret the behavior, and (4) paradoxically accept the potential breach and "go with it."

Encouragement and cajoling represent the authoritarian approach to contract difficulty. If the patient does not take a medication or go for a specific test or request a needed consultation, physicians often rely on their roles as authorities to gain leverage over the patient's reluctance to follow expectations. Physicians may also use explanation, a technique that implies that the patient is equal to him or her and is able to use information to make the best decision, rather than blindly accepting the authoritarian statement. In the following example, the patient was referred to me by a primary care physician and a collaborative approach seemed to be a useful alternative:

CASE 3.19. A 40-year-old isolated single woman living alone in her parents' house had been in psychotherapy with three different therapists over the past 20 years but had found none of the experiences sufficiently helpful. She believed that she was being given toxic substances in her drinking water and felt that her body was deteriorating. I saw her with her primary care physician. Subsequently, she asked that I might see her alone. She also insisted on paying the full fee although her funds were limited. After a few meetings called by her at sporadic intervals, I suggested that we meet regularly within the limits of her ability to pay. Thirty minutes, once per month seemed a proper balance. I explained to her that with this arrangement we would both know we were going to see each other again and therefore could think about what had happened and what might then be said. I silently believed this explanation was particularly important since each of her parents was dying of chronic illness and she appeared to need to know that some relationship would survive. She readily agreed.

Confrontation is the verbal "holding up a mirror" to the client's actions. Reinforcing the contract by stating that missed appointments will be billed is a direct form of confrontation. "Interpretation" is a multiply defined word that generally means finding cause or meaning for a certain behavior pattern. Occasionally, confrontation will lead to interpretation by the patient, as illustrated in the following psychoanalytic example.

CASE 3.20. A woman patient was talking quickly, almost breathlessly, and I detected a tremor in her voice. She appeared to be trying desperately to fill up every moment of the analytic hour. There were no pauses, no moments of reflection, just an outpouring of disconnected fragments of memories. In the preliminary interviews I felt quite certain the young woman was essentially a neurotically depressed person. There was no evidence of a psychotic or borderline condition. I also knew she had been "in analysis" with a reputable analyst in another city who considered her an analyzable patient.

I interrupted the patient and told her she seemed to be frightened, she seemed to be trying to fill up every second of the hour, as though she were afraid of being silent for a moment [the confrontation]. The patient replied quite timorously that she was afraid I would criticize her for having a resistance if she were to keep still. I answered quizzically: "Criticize you for having a resistance?" The young woman then responded by telling me that she felt her previous analyst acted as if it was a failing of hers to have a resistance. He seemed very strict and disapproving and she felt he considered her basically unworthy of psychoanalysis. This reminded her of her father who had a violent temper and often shouted at her as a child that she was "no damned good." (Greenson, 1967, pp. 94–95)*

*From *The Technique and Practice of Psychotherapy* (Vol. I) by R. R. Greenson, 1967, New York: International Universities Press. Reprinted by permission.

On the other hand, therapists may appear to avoid the potential breach in contract as suggested by this example:

CASE 3.21. An attractive, wealthy, 28-year-old woman entered therapy with a 30-year-old woman for reasons that the patient could not explain but that the therapist readily grasped. The patient did not need to work because she had income from investments. She spent most of her day polishing her nails and shopping. She had brief exciting affairs with married and famous men and was unable to sustain any heterosexual relationship. She believed that all she needed to do was to project the right image, and then she would be able to catch a husband, and her dreams would come true. As the therapist delved deeper, the patient skipped an appointment. During the next session, their fifth meeting, the patient declared that she would miss the following session because she was going to Chicago the following day and needed to pack. The therapist left this obvious contradiction alone. Of course she could have taken time from the day before she left town for a therapy session. She had no other obligations. Instead the therapist "let the session proceed without confronting the issue." At the end, the patient described her underlying emptiness in her life and said she would be able to make that appointment. Upon examining the session in supervision, the therapist noted that she had emphasized the patient's ability to choose at many points in the conversation. By not forcing the contract issue and thereby not implying criticism and expectation (as do most confrontations and interpretations), the therapist indicated that the choice of returning for the next session was the patient's also.

This case illustrates a very subtle way to give a patient the experience of making her own choice while gently prodding her to realize what she can and should do.

Engagement Transference

Resistance and transference are not easily distinguished but rather fall on a continuum of distortions of the person of the therapist on the one hand (transference) and distortions of the process of therapy on the other. Transference serves to distort the process of therapy as well.

During engagement, clients often react to the surface appearance of the therapist. Therefore each therapist should know his or her interpersonal stimulus value: How do people normally react to seeing him or her? Young-looking therapists may be greeted with questions of sufficient experience. Attractive women may be perceived by traditional males as a sexual object rather than a competent helper. Black or Asian therapists may be disregarded by patients who do not trust people outside their own race and culture. Blacks may distrust blacks under the assumption that no member of their minority could be successful in a white-dominated culture (Griffith, 1977). Therapists with accents may be discounted or idealized. Therapists with powerful reputations may elicit passive or challenging responses from their new clients.

Clients may also perceive their new therapists in terms of prior conceptions and experiences of psychotherapy as suggested by the woman who would not stop talking (see Case 3.20). They may also have formulated their notions of what therapy would be as suggested by the following case of a psychology graduate student.

CASE 3.22. A 35-year-old unmarried graduate student presented for therapy because he was unable to finish his thesis work. Procrastination characterized much of his school efforts earlier as well. He would play the guitar, eat, and go for walks without completing the tasks that he had set himself for that evening. He was becoming frustrated with his inability to handle himself. He carefully watched me as I interviewed him and then lectured me about the various benefits of different forms of psychotherapy. Finally, I asked him how he wanted to be treated. He suggested that the only way to conduct his therapy was through operant conditioning. He was to be given homework assignments that, if he carried them out, were to bring him some kind of reward. He would not accept, he said, any of the psychodynamic approaches. I pointed out to him that he was attempting to arrange his therapy to fail since he was clearly unable to carry out homework assignments for his thesis. He was transferring that maladaptive pattern into his expectation for therapy. Startled, he agreed.

Many of each new patient's responses to therapy will be at least partially concerned with whether the therapist is competent and whether therapy will help. As they are deciding, each person will show aspects of the manner in which they approach and avoid intimate dependent relationships. Therapy is threatening because potential patients must open themselves up to the influence of another. They want to be liked and accepted, yet they also want some measure of control. These dual purposes characterize their entrance into all ongoing relationships. The patient's struggle to accomplish them begins as they become involved in therapy.

Common interactive styles that achieve in the short run the dual goals of acceptance and control include sexual seductiveness, helpless dependency, idealization, and compliance to therapist expectations. Others include obsessive rumination about cause and effect, excessive self-blame, emotional volatility, self-aggrandizement, paranoid ruminations, and intellectual power. Each one of these ploys is intended to evoke from the therapist a complementary response that fits the style. Since the patient is expert in managing these roles as a result of years of experience in conducting them, these interaction patterns are intended to give each patient a sense of mastery over the relationship as well as a feeling of acceptance. Very often, these patterns represent a major therapeutic focus. For example, seductiveness is intended to elicit desire that can be manipulated; helplessness elicits paradoxical control by allowing the other to think he or she is in control; idealization evokes a sense of being wonderful and the accompanying desire to hold onto the person who stimulates that feeling; compliance usually evokes a feeling of power and control in the therapist.

Engagement Countertransference

Therapists may not notice these character styles and may find themselves reacting with sexual desire or feelings of power or importance. Any inappropriate response to a patient should initiate the search for countertransference responses. But before looking to the patient as a possible trigger of these reactions, therapists must examine their own contributions. Countertransference distortions, whether they manifest themselves as odd behavior, strange feelings, or inappropriate thoughts, are usually the product of forces from both the therapist and patient. In order to isolate the influence of the patient, each therapist must remove the factors contributed by his or her own psyche. The more precise countertransference question is not, "Is it the patient or me?" but rather "what percentage is being contributed by me and what percentage is being contributed by the patient?" (Beitman, 1983b).

The model offered by cognitive therapists (e.g., Beck *et al.*, 1979; Ellis, 1973b; Meichenbaum, 1977) for approaching distorted cognitions is useful here. The dysphoric emotion, fantasy, or dream signals the need to search for cognitions that are not reality-based. They must be challenged by testing them as hypotheses about patient–therapist reality rather than by accepting them as absolute facts. Coupled with the psychodynamic notion that many of these thoughts, feelings, and fantasies may operate as part of a defensive response to other unwanted thoughts and/or feelings, therapists may be better equipped for self-examination. Reflecting upon feelings and thoughts by allowing them to run freely may help to reveal the origins of the distortions. Discussion with a trusted colleague is often very useful when self-scrutiny is insufficient.

Freud (1910) introduced the concept of countertransference to refer to the "analyst's transference to the patient's transference." To him and to many analysts who hold the "classical" position about countertransference (e.g., Reich, 1951), the cause was to be found in the therapist's past. Solution to the problem required self-analysis or return to therapy. Some countertransference reactions are certainly produced by the therapist's past experience. One of the most common is illustrated by the following case.

CASE 3.23. A 32-year-old internist refused to see any patients with a history of alcoholism. She also refused to inquire about alcoholic history in any of her patients. Her father had been an alcoholic, had beaten her mother, and left them when she was 15.

The therapist's contribution to distorted reactions may also be caused by events in the near present as well. Marriage, divorce, pregnancy, the birth of a child, death of a loved one, may each influence therapists' responses to patients.

Just as the appearance of the therapist may influence the patient's reaction to him or her, so may the patient's appearance influence the therapist's response.

CASE 3.24. A very beautiful 25-year-old woman entered therapy with a 30-year-old single psychiatrist who prided himself on his own good looks and his taste for the finer things in life. He was struck by her appearance and despite ethical prohibitions to the contrary, followed his impulse during the first session to end therapy and ask her to dinner. She accepted and in a few months they were married. Within 6 months the marriage ended in divorce and she required psychiatric hospitalization. When I met her socially, she was extremely angry with psychiatrists.

Other appearances that may trigger maladaptive therapist responses include diagnosis (e.g., borderline personality), social and/or economic status (Very Important Person), referral source (e.g., friend or superior), and similarity to previous disturbing patients.

Additional influences on therapists' initial responses to their patients include: training status (beginners fear failure and incompetence), supervision (what will my superior say?), commitment to being a therapist (I don't really care if I do this well), number of psychotherapy patients (full schedule may decrease investment), type of therapy most valued (prefers long-term but patient wants short therapy), and other commitments (does writing academic papers to gain promotion reduce therapeutic skill?).

Once the therapist's contribution to countertransference problems is cleared away, the patient's contribution may be examined. As mentioned in the section on transference, patients often attempt to elicit certain responses from their therapists. If these twinges are examined rapidly, therapists may gain additional information about their patients. In describing borderline patients early in therapy, Kernberg has noted that they will often induce rather odd and disturbing reactions in their therapists and that these reactions may aid in understanding and treatment. By "borderline," most writers mean people who tend to blur self–other boundaries and attempt to fuse with the therapist. In doing so, therapists also tend to lose their own self-definitions and experience some of the disorganized thinking characteristic of these clients. Because the patients evoke old, hidden fears in their therapists, they may become the objects of anger and of the desire to control. These issues were brought home to me in the following case.

CASE 3.25. A 28-year-old divorced woman who had made multiple suicide attempts and had poor self–other boundaries presented in a very helpless manner, wanting me to see her more often than she could afford or I had time. After the first session, I had the following dream: I am having sex without penetration with an adolescent girl; I want to put on a rubber but I don't want to penetrate; I will feel guilty about my wife if I do; there is noise of upset men talking; one rushes off to settle a contract dispute; I believe it is her father; she follows him; I am somewhat relieved but try to follow her; I wake up. My interpretation was: I am becoming intensely involved with this patient but we have not worked out a contract to our mutual satisfaction. We were both experiencing intense intimacy and the desire to run away from it. This dream predicted future difficulties.

I continued to have trouble sleeping because I thought of the patient often and felt quite anxious when I did. I worried about her suicide potential and became convinced that my actions predetermined her degree of risk, thereby reflecting a loss of self–other boundaries. I was reminded of anxious feelings I had had about my mother that were accompanied by a sense that I could not do enough for her in order to make her happy. I made no adequate responses to the patient's interpretations of my behavior as deliberately malicious. As my feelings for both the patient and my mother began to fuse, I felt increasingly helpless and agitated. I was afraid to follow the rules of the contract (time, place, fee, telephone calls) although I knew I should have. I was afraid to withhold from her during therapy as well. I attempted to control her by indirect expressions of anger and further attempts to pacify her. Finally, when we seemed to reach some sense of compromise, she made a suicide gesture with medications other than the ones I had given her. During her subsequent hospitalization, I met with her, her sister-in-law, and her brother. The sister-in-law expressed concerns almost identical with mine: She feared that without her proper behavior, the patient would kill herself. She also felt trapped by these implicit threats and was no longer able to handle her own agitation and anger about the situation. The sister-in-law's response confirmed that I was experiencing a patient-induced countertransference. Unfortunately, I was unable to understand or utilize my responses to help the patient more effectively because of my own neurotic contributions. She called to terminate our relationship and noted the tone of relief evident in my voice.

In this instance, countertransference blocked my helping potential. As will be shown by later examples, countertransference reactions can be an excellent source of information about patients.

4. *Pattern-Search Content*

The goal of the pattern search is to define patterns of thought, feeling, and/or behavior that are within the client's ability to influence and that, if changed, would lead toward a desirable outcome. Useful patterns exist in many different approaches and vary widely in emphasis, terminology, and theory. This chapter will examine reasons for this variability and will describe commonly used "visual data filters" for organizing patient information. Critical background variables and ways of conceptualizing patients' psychological functioning will be examined also. The sometimes arbitrary nature of psychological labels and the potential value of the notion of reciprocal causation to the understanding of psychological dysfunction will be the final considerations of the chapter.

PATTERN VARIABILITY

The causes to which humans attribute their psychological miseries are extremely varied. The astrological positioning of planets against their zodiacal background, the failure of gratitude toward ancestors and parents, the deleterious effect of psychologically disturbed mothers, and the failure to be true to oneself are among the many competing beliefs about the causes of emotional distress (Beitman, 1983a).

The reasons for this wide variation are to be found in cultural forces. Psychological systems appear to be the product of religious, economic, and social pressures that shape the personal conception of the self. Freud's emphasis upon sexual regression was in part a response to Victorian sexual restraint. Behavior therapy grew out of American pragmatism and the burgeoning power of laboratory science. Perls's Gestalt therapy with its antiintellectual rebellion against established treatments was nurtured by the antiwar, drug-taking, self-experiential pressures of the Vietnam era. Furthermore, each therapist's personal ideology is the product of differing degrees of religious, political, economic, and social forces, thereby creating variations within psychotherapeutic ideologies. My own interest in the structure underlying the psychotherapies arose as a result of a belief in unifying principles acquired through my father's religion; a liberal arts education emphasizing the contributions of past thinkers; and the turmoil of the Vietnam era, which impelled me to seek a solution to the ideological warfare in my chosen profession. In the early 1980s, I found myself meeting a wave of interest by others in psychotherapy integration that suggested that cultural forces are moving some of my colleagues in a similar direction.

Consensus among psychotherapists on the content of the pattern search will be most difficult to reach. We no longer live in a simple cause-and-effect universe. Rarely does a single trauma lead to all neurosis as suggested, for example, by Rank (1929/1973) when he declared that the birth trauma explained all subsequent difficulty. Rarely is a single set of reinforcers responsible for a specific maladaptive behavior, as radical behavior therapists hoped to discover. Instead we live in a universe of differential probabilities, where multiple influences seem to be responsible for a specific result. How are we to determine the major and minor influences? How do we determine which major influence must be redirected in order to achieve change efficiently and effectively? These questions are very difficult to answer.

Further confounding attempts toward consensus is the relative nature of the psychotherapeutic interaction. Unlike the cardiac surgeon who each day confronts the same anatomical structures with very small variations from patient to patient, psychotherapists are faced with far greater relative variations when examining the minds of their patients. Like therapists, patients are uniquely influenced by many cultural forces. Their causal attributions, the words they speak, the data they present are far more varied than the hearts the cardiac surgeon attempts to heal. Therapists must therefore adjust their models of mind to the patient's verbal productions and the underlying personal theories. Because the personal experience of each therapist and patient varies considerably, consensus on the content of the pattern search is yet more difficult to reach.

Psychological words are themselves another source of difficulty. They are like spotlights in a dark territory illuminating unknown areas of the human mind. Unfortunately, different charismatic leaders have illuminated overlapping territories and insisted upon different terms. While the terms often highlight distinctions, they fail to acknowledge the common ground. For example, "defenses" (psychodynamic) are closely related to "processing errors" and "automatic thoughts" (cognitive) although the terms are embedded in different psychopathological ideologies. Within psychoanalysis, "splitting" and "grandiose self" refer to similar clinical phenomena although the theoretical assumptions behind the terms are different. Therapists are adept at making words mean what they want them to mean (a probably useful psychotherapeutic skill), yet when it comes to attempts at consensus, old words often stand as rigid barriers.

What can be done with this confusion?

First, the goal of consensus must be clearly defined. Because of the relative nature of the psychotherapeutic interaction, therapists may have to acknowledge that no dogmatic content is possible. Each participant brings idiosyncratic content predispositions. Second, because cultural forces are inexorably changing, therapists must be flexible enough to shift with these changes. Their patients will show them some of the directions of movement. Flexibility is clearly required for the pattern-search content.

But is there any solid ground?

I think there is. My own review of shamanistic, nonshamanistic, the Morita and Naikan therapies of Japan, as well as the major therapies of the United States suggested that underlying most of the content of the pattern search is concern with the self in the social context (Beitman, 1983a). Some therapies emphasize the self, while others emphasize interpersonal relationships. Psychoanalysis embodies a solipsistic view of human psychology, while behavior therapy emphasizes the environment. Cognitive–behavioral therapy (C–B) (Beck *et al.*, 1979) for depression contrasts with interpersonal therapy (IPT) for depression (Klerman *et al.*, 1984) by emphasizing thoughts while IPT emphasizes social roles. To illustrate the overlap between the intrapsychic emphasis of C–B and the interpersonal elements of IPT, consider the following case:

CASE 4.1. A 43-year-old, married housewife, whose children have left home, has been depressed for 8 years following her only hospitalization for severe depression. She is deeply isolated because she believes that she will be severely criticized by anyone with whom she speaks. A cognitive therapist might evoke her negative self-talk, those automatic thoughts that declare her to be incompetent socially, too fat to be liked by anyone, and unable to change any of her prospects of loneliness. She also might describe to a cognitive therapist the jealous, envious, rageful thoughts and feelings she experiences when she is alone. The cognitive therapist would encourage her to test out these self-statements through experience with others. An interpersonal therapist might instead ask her to describe previous positive relationships to her sisters and to friends in another town. Once the more positive role was established as a model, the IPT therapist might encourage her to explore her role expectations and to find new situations in which to repeat the more satisfactory relationships. Both the intrapsychic and interpersonal approaches encourage the patient to change self-concept and concepts of self-with-others by initiating new interaction patterns and examining them.

Despite avowed distinctions, these and other treatment forms are both interpersonal and intrapsychic. The foundation of the pattern-search content is the self and the self in relationship to others.

What should be selected from this vast arena of information?

This question can be answered by listing major categories of content that must then be mixed and matched to fit the predispositions of both therapist and patient. The need to match well is illustrated in the following case.

CASE 4.2. A psychologist friend of mine who thought highly of Albert Ellis and Rational Emotive Therapy (RET) finally recognized that he was depressed and needed help. He called me for suggestions of psychotherapists. I felt he needed to be listened to very carefully and understood in terms of the dynamics of his relationship to his parents. He did not agree with me, but by a series of decisions began therapy with a psychodynamic therapist who listened to him carefully and permitted him a needed catharsis. However, my friend did not like this therapist's emphasis on the past and sought the services of a disciple of Albert Ellis. After the first meeting, he was very enthusiastic about the relationship and rapidly left his depression behind by attacking the many "shoulds" governing his irrational thoughts. He had selected the content that suited his perceived needs.

Perhaps my friend would have responded well to existential or psychodynamic approaches *if he had wanted to*. Many labels may be used to expose and clarify underlying patterns of psychological dysfunction. What is important for psychotherapeutic change is not whether the terms used to explain the problem according to a warmly embraced theory, but whether or not the client can understand or use the idea behind it. If the client cannot use the idea, it is not psychotherapeutically effective even if the therapist is convinced of its explanatory power. Therefore any of a number of contents are potentially able to lead to desired change. This conclusion implies a vision of the human mind in which there are potentially many different handles by which to grasp a maladaptive pattern and to change it. In the next section, I have gathered seven of the best-known visual data filters to substantiate this perspective.

VISUAL DATA FILTERS

Because pictures often capture more information than many words, psychotherapy theorists have attempted to present their perspectives on psychopathology through diagrams, formulas, and acronyms. Figures 2 through 7 contain seven visual slogans that outline mental processes for psychotherapy exploration. Each of these fulfills the same basic function: The data emitted by the patient is filtered according to the outline suggested by the perceptual aid. Without these transparent patterns to fit over observed reality, each psychotherapy patient would appear to be an undifferentiated, unintelligible homogeneity (Kelly, 1955, pp. 8–9). Is there a best way to filter the patient's data? Which ones are best for which patients (and for which therapists)? Can they sometimes be fit together?

In order to illustrate the use of these data filters, I will utilize the following case.

CASE 4.3. Eric, a 34-year-old married man's presenting complaint was "I go to pornographic movies too often, and I have fantasies of women in bondage. These fantasies disturb me and give me pleasure."

As suggested earlier, there are many different handles on the human mind by which change may take place. The presentation of this case from seven different perspectives should illustrate this point.

Stimulus → Organism → Response

All therapists use the formula diagrammed in Figure 2, often without thinking about it (Driscoll, 1984; Hart, 1983). The "response" is the target symptom(s) that in the case of Eric are images of women in bondage and trips to pornographic movies. Therapists then seek the stimuli for these responses and the thought–feeling internal states correlated with the stimuli. Because the environment is stimulus rich, and internal states are also full of possibilities, the stimulus → organism → response formula is a first general organizing principle.

The cognitive therapists Ellis (1962) and Beck (1976) have modified this formula into the A→B→C sequence. A is the *activating event*; B is *belief*; and C is the *consequence*. This narrowing of the terms is intended to highlight the cognitive bias toward thinking and its influence on consequence. For Eric, the activating events were sexual arousal, usually

Figure 2. Cognitive-behavioral therapy.

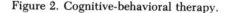

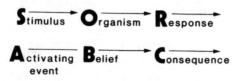

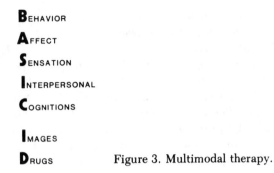

Behavior

Affect

Sensation

Interpersonal

Cognitions

Images

Drugs   Figure 3. Multimodal therapy.

after not having had sex with his wife for a few weeks, and a reduced work load that permitted him time for thinking about other activities. The bondage fantasies represented his own "internal porno house." He then went to the movies in the hope of finding some dominance–submission theme. Among his thoughts associated with going to the movies were: "I am studying the sexual underbelly of the United States — a kind of sexual sociology" and "I wonder if anyone will catch me down here."

BASIC I.D.

The BASIC I.D. acronym (Figure 3) is Arnold Lazarus's (1976, 1985) compromise between ideal behavioral analysis and clinical reality. Ideal behavioral analysis is based upon the experimental investigation of the single case by which the behavioral therapist asks the "right" questions about each client's symptoms and devises procedures to answer them. According to Baer, Wolf, and Risley, "an experimenter has achieved an analysis of behavior when he can exercise control over it" (quoted in Yates, 1975, p. 46). This idealistic approach is very difficult to match in clinical practice because it requires therapists to see each patient as a new experimental challenge. Instead, behavioral clinicians, like their psychodynamic counterparts, search for standard techniques that can be applied in standard ways to standard clients (Yates, 1975). Lazarus has responded to this need by devising a perceptual filter with characteristics compatible with the behavioral–scientific ethos. BASIC I.D. encompasses seven categories of data, each of which has standard questions likely to produce quantifiable answers that may be used as measures of improvement.

The content of the seven categories includes, with Eric's illustrations:

> Behavior: Which behaviors do you wish to increase and which ones do you wish to decrease? Specific questions about each

behavior include: what?, where?, how?, when?, and who?, but not why? and should be characterized by frequency, intensity, and duration measures.

Eric — pornographic movies, once per month, alone when I have nothing to do.

Affect: What negative feelings would you like to reduce or eliminate, and what positive feelings would you like to increase or amplify? Feelings should be associated with behaviors, rated in degree of pleasantness or unpleasantness and the types of emotions (anxiety, joy, anger, and/or depression) clearly defined.

Eric — feeling guilty, dirty afterward as well as estranged from my wife.

Sensation: Among your five senses, what particular kinds of reactions would you like to reduce or magnify? Review sensations (vision, touch, taste, hearing, smell) and rate in degrees of pleasant or unpleasant and levels of under- or overawareness (for example, amplifying somatic sensation).

Eric — increase sexual comfort with my wife.

Images: What "mental pictures" or images are bothersome and which ones would you like to bring into sharper focus? Standard imagery motifs include return to childhood home, and going to a special safe place.

Eric — bondage fantasies.

Cognitions: Which thoughts, values, attitudes, or beliefs get in the way of your happiness? "Shoulds" and "perfectionism" are common examples.

Eric — I should go to the porno movies because I feel like it.

Interpersonal: In your dealings with other people, what gets in the way of close personal, loving, and mutually satisfying interactions.

Eric — I feel guilty, like I'm hiding something. I can't be myself.

Drugs: Under what conditions do you use drugs (including alcohol, coffee, and tobacco)? Also include psychological complaints, health maintenance efforts, physical appearance, and the possible role of psychotropic medications.

Eric — I smoke cigarettes only at porno movies.

In defending the necessity to review all modalities, Lazarus insisted that "it is easy to isolate any one modality and argue that it is the key area of assessment and therapy. . . . From a multimodal perspective, however, it is therapeutically deleterious to aggrandize any particular modality — they are all important" (Lazarus, 1976, p. 41).

Spirals

The wave pattern in Figure 4 represents a basic tenet of communication theory and an integral part of many couples and family therapy approaches. Watzlawick, Beavin, & Jackson, (1967, p. 56) proposed the following example: "Suppose a couple has a marital problem in which he contributes passive withdrawal 50 per cent of the time while her 50 per cent is nagging criticism. In explaining their frustration, the husband will state that withdrawal is his only defense against her nagging, while she will label this explanation as a gross and willful distortion of what 'really' happens in their marriage: namely, that she is critical of him because of his passivity. Stripped of all ephemeral and fortuitous elements, their fights consist of a monotonous exchange of the messages: 'I withdraw because you nag' and 'I nag because you withdraw.'" The wave pattern then represents an arbitrary slice through an infinite oscillating series, each contributor to which perceives the other as causing the misery. In order to break the paranoid deadlock in which each feels the victim of the other, therapists must grasp the general pattern. This observation leads to a general axiom about interpersonal relations: If two people are involved in a chronically maladaptive interaction, one must first hypothesize that each is contributing equally to the mutual dysphoria. Their "solu-

Figure 4. Communication analysis. Reproduced from *Pragmatics of Human Communication* (p. 57) by Paul Watzlawick, Ph.D., Janet Hemlick Beavin, A. B., and Don D. Jackson, M.D., by permission of W.W. Norton & Company, Inc. Copyright © 1967 by W.W. Norton & Company, Inc.

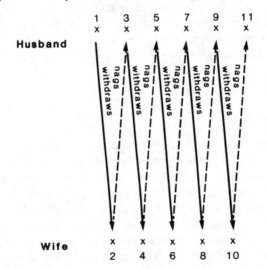

tions" to the problem (e.g., nagging and withdrawal) then become the therapeutic focus.

When placed vertically instead of horizontally, the infinite oscillating series resembles a vicious (or virtuous) cycle that may become tighter and more dangerous. The arms race exemplifies the pattern applied to international politics, as described by Joad in 1939.

> If, as they maintain, the best way to preserve peace is to prepare for war, it is not altogether clear why all nations should regard the armaments of other nations as a menace to peace. However, they do so regard them, and are accordingly stimulated to increase their armaments to overtop the armaments by which they conceive themselves to be threatened. . . . These increased arms being in their turn regarded as a menace by nation A whose allegedly defensive armaments have provoked them, are used by nation A as a pretext for accumulating yet greater armaments wherewith to defend itself against the menace. Yet these greater armaments are in turn interpreted by neighboring nations as constituting a menace to themselves and so on." (Quoted in Watzlawick *et al.*, 1967, p. 58)

Eric and his wife had established a sexual interaction in which neither of them could initiate sex. Each blamed the other for the difficulty. During their early courtship, he blamed her for being "too aggressive" and then she blamed him for "being too cold and distant." Neither was able to take the refusal of a sexual invitation without feeling deeply hurt. Each could not acknowledge the possibility that the other might not have been interested or needed some encouragement to be interested. Furthermore, his wife was disgusted with his pornographic movie excursions and was irritated by his attempts to have her accompany him. She had early on refused his attempts to engage her in bondage games. They had reached a stalemate in which each blamed the other and felt victim to the other.

Parent–Adult–Child

In transactional analysis (Figure 5), the personality is represented by three circles set vertically. These separate "ego states" bear some resemblance to Freud's superego–ego–id (Berne, 1961). This diagram may be considered to be a popularized transformation similar to the conversion by cognitive therapists of stimulus→organism→response into activating event→belief→consequence. The "parent" state is said to be the product of unquestioned beliefs imposed on the child by external sources, usually the parents. The "child" state is the product of internal responses (usually feelings) to external events, usually mother and father. The "adult" state

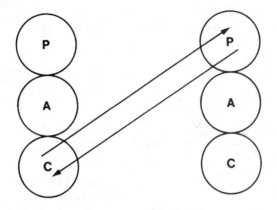

Figure 5. Transactional analysis (after Berne, 1961, & Harris, 1967).

develops from exploration and testing of external reality and is repeatedly updated by new decisions, experiences, and probability estimates (Harris, 1967).

Elements of the personality may come into conflict, often the "child" rebels against the "parent." For Eric, this conflict took the following form: He wanted to do something that violated cultural norms. His mother had often flirted with him. She hated his involvement with his high school girlfriends. Going to the pornographic movies was like having dates with girls his mother did not like.

In transactional analysis, two personality diagrams are often juxtaposed and lines are drawn between elements to illustrate a specific ego state of one person interacting with a specific ego state of another. Adult–adult transactions are usually ideal. In Eric's marriage, he appeared to be acting out the role of "child" rebelling against his mother's incestuous behavior but not quite breaking away from her by having a true affair. His wife was the disapproving parent who tolerated his misdeeds in order to keep him at home. Further analysis also suggested that the wife was acting out the role of the mistreated, abused child that she had felt herself to be during her childhood, and that Eric was acting as the neglecting parent who preferred other women to her.

Psychodynamic Triangles

The two triangles in Figure 6 represent, according to Malan (1979), almost every intervention that a (psychodynamic) therapist makes. The first may be called "triangle of conflict" and consists of defense, anxiety, and hidden feeling or impulse. The second is called "triangle of person,"

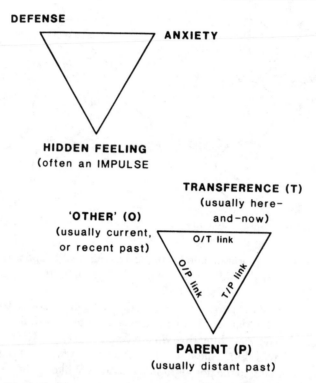

Figure 6. Psychodynamic triangles. From *Individual Psychotherapy and the Science of Psychodynamics* (p. 80) by D. H. Malan, 1979, London: Butterworths. Reprinted by permission.

namely other (O), parent (P), and transference (T). The two triangles are related by the observation that the hidden feeling or impulse is directed toward one or more categories of the triangle of person. They are drawn standing on each apex because the hidden feeling and the parent can be regarded as "lying underneath" the other two, more deeply in the unconscious.

For Eric, the triangle of conflict could be drawn as the conflict between his internal "parent" and internal "child." But as is so often suggested by psychodynamic therapists, the analysis of one conflict uncovers other more deeply embedded conflicts. Eric's use of pornographic movies and bondage fantasies were defenses against the anxiety created by his deeply felt rage (impulse, emotion) at women or anyone who tried to control him. His mother had controlled him by her seductiveness and her threats of emotional abandonment; and he was afraid that unless he had total control over a woman, he would hurt her or be terribly vulnerable to her. However, his therapist (T) was a man. Eric tended to react to me as he had to his father. His father had surrendered child care to his mother and thereby had abandoned him to her. He therefore felt that his therapist also was not going to help him but rather would let him drift into continually more emotional danger. His response to male employers (O) was similar in that he wished to get to know them as people but avoided at all costs coming under their control or influence. The movie trips and bondage fantasies served to keep distance between himself and his wife (O) thereby protecting himself from her control, his rage at the potential harm she might cause him, and his fear of vulnerability to her.

Existentialists may also use the triangle of conflict. Yalom (1980) replaced the feared impulse or emotion with feared awareness of an "ultimate concern" (death, responsibility, isolation, and meaning of life). He represented it linearly: Ultimate concern→Anxiety→Defense. Eric could consider the possibility that his bondage fantasies helped to bind his anxieties about being out of control, at the mercy of someone else, a vulnerability that echoed his fears of annihilation and death.

Parts of the Self

The "self-nuclei" diagram in Figure 7 represents a variation on a common theme. The "self" is often described as composed of many different parts. The psychopathological model for many selves, the multiple personality, has served for Bandler and Grinder (1979) and Beahrs (1982) as a useful way to understand many less disturbed personalities. Beahrs, for example, likened the human mind to a symphony orchestra:

> Like the overall self, it is a complex whole with a personality of its own, but it is composed of many component parts. Each orchestra member has its own sense of identity and unique personality, but they all function together in a coordinated collaborative endeavor to the advantage of the whole and of each one. The music is made by the composite of parts but transcends being mere algebraic sum; it is held together and organized by the leadership of an executive, the conductor. The conductor makes none of the actual music but is in charge. . . . (p. 65)

During the psychotherapeutic interview, these different states of mind emerge as observable recurrent patterns of behavior that have both

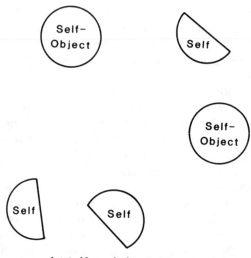

Figure 7. Disparate nuclei (self psychology). From *Models of the Mind* (p. 68) by J. Gedo and A. Goldberg, 1973, Chicago: University of Chicago Press. Reprinted by permission.

verbal and nonverbal components. A specific state is characterized by clusters of elements composed of:

> facial expression, posture, intonation, and inflection in speech, focus and content of verbal reports, degree of self-reflective awareness, general arousal, shifts in degree and nature of empathy, and other communicative qualities. The change in states of a person in psychotherapy is recognizable in the same way as the change in atmosphere in a drama, from cheerful sunlight to thunder and lightning, or the shifts in musical work, of the sounds of rhythm, harmony, timbre, and tonality. (Marmar, Wilmer, & Horowitz, 1984, p. 195)

For Jung the term "archetypes" served to describe some of the more prominent states of mind. The "primordial images" that appear with great variation among many peoples without losing their basic pattern, are sometimes the forms in which the personality presents itself. Eric, for example, was enacting the archetype of the dominant man attempting to capture and cage women for his own pleasure without regard for them. Intrapsychically, Eric may also have been described as attempting to tame the "anima," the female element in the male unconscious. According to Jung, Eric was required to liberate his anima from the devouring aspect of his internalized mother image (since she, in his mind, held tightly the feelings he could give to another woman) (Jung, 1964, p. 125).

Beck (Beck & Emery, 1985) used the term "mode" to describe a superordinate organizing principle of the cognitive structure that persists over diverse situations. The mode is a subsystem of the cognitive organization designed for certain adaptive purposes such as self-enhancement, breeding, and survival. Thus there is a narcissistic mode, an erotic mode, a hostility mode, and a depressive mode. The mode evoked is dependent on the customary linkage between a set of schemas and that type of situation (p. 59).

In terms of self psychology, from which the diagram in Figure 7 is directly drawn, the psychologically disturbed person has not gained a clear sense of self but instead relies upon other persons to maintain self-concept. Ideally, the self is complete unto itself and is surrounded by a constellation of others with whom the self relates as a separate self. In this diagram taken from Gedo and Goldberg (1973, p. 68), the complete circles represent "self objects" by which the authors mean self-concepts that require another person (an object) in order to be functional. The other, instead of being appreciated as separate, serves a specific set of functions to maintain a sense of self. Eric was not psychologically separate from his wife. She served to regulate his day by structuring his behavior, by defining limits of his behavior, by listening to his fears about work, and by repeatedly soothing his anxiety about being worthless. He could barely recognize her own individuality outside of his needs for her.

The partial circles simply labeled "self" are intended to depict partial aspects of the self that coexist without integration. They are self images without another to support their existence. Eric, for example, had been a reasonably successful athlete in high school and had gained some acclaim through his exploits. He continued to have a self-image as "hero" but failed to find anyone to support this image of himself. It, therefore, remained alive but unintegrated. He often tried to have his wife acknowledge this side of himself; he enjoyed describing his exploits to other men. His bondage fantasies may have served to nurture the sense of power he had achieved as an athlete but had since lost.

During termination, as Eric looked back on his treatment he commented upon the ideas that had been presented to him during the pattern search. He found the anima-within idea compelling because he could define his struggle against the dominance of his internal image of his mother. The stalemated struggle between him and his wife, which resembled the arms race, appealed to his political interests. Calling himself a child with his wife as the parent did not seem like a great revelation and was, therefore, not helpful. What he found most useful was to think of the bondage and pornographic movie trips as a way to keep himself from being controlled by his wife. During his therapy, each time he thought of going to the movies or having bondage fantasies he considered this defensive purpose. Did he really need to fear control by his wife?

Couldn't he initiate sex himself? What's so bad about being turned down? Then the ball is in her court. This intrapsychic shift reduced his fantasy time and decreased the frequency of his movie excursions. A psychodynamic therapist might say that the defense had been correctly interpreted. A cognitive therapist would claim that he had replaced maladaptive thinking with adaptive thinking. An interpersonal therapist would claim that he had redefined the rules of his marital relationship. Each explanation highlights a limited aspect of the multifaceted process by which human psychological change may be labeled.

During a follow-up appointment 3 years after termination, Eric reported to me that the fantasies and movie trips had become yet less compelling. The birth of his child had reduced this interest yet further.

BACKGROUND VARIABLES

In this section, I will outline a word-based description of the background or contextual variables of the psychotherapy patient's mind and describe several major variables encompassing the person functioning in his or her environment — patterns of emotional expression, expectations, major interpersonal styles, intrapsychic conflict, self–other boundary weakness, and the deep unconscious. Systematic eclectic psychotherapy requires a number of clear principles and variables that are adaptable and moldable to the requirements of each psychotherapy dyad (Beutler, 1983). These latter patterns and the cultural and developmental contexts in which they are embedded together form a pragmatic outline of the psychotherapy patient's mind. The chapter ends with a discussion of deviation amplifying feedback and with the presentation of evidence that there are many different patterns that may be useful for change.

Culture

Human groups of all sizes and longevity are characterized by distinct patterns of behavior and thought. Each family has its own distinct ideas and values that at once distinguish it from other families while also identifying it with larger religious, political, socioeconomic, and/or ethnic groups. Each family member is a carrier of cultural tradition, of historically derived ideas to be transmitted to future generations. Parents, teachers, political and religious leaders, mass media, and other communicators (psychotherapists included) convey both explicitly and implicitly the values that characterize the culture within which they are embedded. "Cultural systems may, on the one hand, be considered as products of action, on the other as conditioning elements of further action" (Kroeber & Kluckhohn, quoted in Favazza & Oman, 1978, p. 293).

Because we are immersed in our culture, we have difficulty stepping outside of it. We are metaphorical tadpoles immersed in water, who can appreciate our aquatic surroundings only when we become land-hopping frogs. To appreciate the influence of culture on the presentation of psychological problems, one must step outside of his or her own culture to notice how ethnocentric one's own view can be.

For example, Malinowski reported in the 1920s that in the Trobriand Islands, male children developed a hatred toward their mother's brother rather than toward their father. Some critics claimed that this evidence shattered the universal applicability of the oedipal conflict, while others suggested that the boy's feelings were displaced from the father to the uncle. The latter argument is patently ethnocentric in its implication that the Viennese complex was primary; the former criticism ignores the primacy of the family romance and its bitter antagonisms and fails to allow for cultural variations of these themes (Favazza & Oman, 1978).

For psychotherapists, cultural awareness may be of great assistance in predicting recurrent patterns of concern among different patients as well as in enriching one's understanding of one's origins. Parents may be blamed for certain behaviors, but they are often agents of prevailing cultural prescriptions for proper parental behaviors. For example, during the age of women's liberation, many men look back upon their relationship to their fathers with feelings of anger and despair. "He hardly spent any time with me. I never got to know him. I realize he provided for the family but he never told me about himself." Many of these fathers were instructed to leave the raising of the children to their wives. Some of the next generation of men are receiving conflicting messages about more active participation in child rearing. These crosscurrents of cultural values may be resolved in future generations, or perhaps in the future, men may complain that their fathers spent too much time with them, thereby preventing them from playing with their mothers.

Culture also predictably influences people's interpretations and responses to major inevitable developmental shifts in their biological aging. From the riddle of the Sphinx (what walks on four legs in the morning, two legs in the afternoon, and three legs in the evening), through Shakespeare's ages of man, and Erik Erikson's (1963) identity and the life cycle, increasing attention has been paid to "biochronology" and the self. Therapists can predict from the patient's age and culture the likely conflicts facing him or her.

Biocultural Aging

In all cultures, developmental milestones of children and adults are correlated with certain specific cultural expectations. Colarusso and Nemiroff (1981) have summarized much of the work of American researchers that attempts to define age-specific biopsychological hurdles. Perhaps the most important conclusion to this research is that each age has its difficulties and that no age is free from biocultural challenges. The differences among people are not whether they face challenges, since they all do, but rather the manner in which they attempt to surmount them. We are all on a one-way journey toward biological death. The unstoppable flow of this irrepressible river of time carries us through change and loss. Each age predicts its own specific changes, thereby making each patient's age an excellent predictor of current challenges to his or her psychological resources. Some have failed to meet the challenge of one developmental stage, thereby altering the content of future developmental milestones. The person who, for example, never leaves home, staying forever with a parent, without dating or marrying, is still swept along in time but faces challenges different from those who do leave.

Any statements about age-specific losses and changes are simply generalizations and approximations. Following is a brief summary of the stages of aging in Western culture.

ADOLESCENCE (13–19)

With the rush of physical changes comes ejaculation and menstruation, infatuation and masturbation. Physical and social pressures push the growing child yet another step away from parents and now firmly toward his or her peer group. The work self is also being dreamed. Separation from parents during late adolescence is the common psychological task.

EARLY ADULTHOOD (20–40)

Sexual conflicts and the desire for intimate, ongoing relationships lead to commitment to one sexual partner, with marriage and children the most common consequence. Each of these elements is easily the focus of difficulty. Sexuality may be excessive or inhibited, intimacy may be distancing, and commitment may be feared. Children may seem like a solution to all of the foregoing difficulties yet only mask them and create more difficulties. Western culture is highly supportive of divorce, thereby providing an easy way out of a difficult problem but often causing yet more problems. Western culture also aggrandizes early adulthood and especially the female and male body of the late teens and early 20s. The loss of these youthful features in middle adulthood marks a painful loss that many do not take easily.

MIDDLE ADULTHOOD (40–60)

Children grow toward independence; the body shows more wrinkles and gray; dreams of success cannot be totally realized; limitations become clearer and death becomes more believable. Caught in the middle between children and parents, the middle-aged adult watches parents die and becomes an in-law and then a grandparent, marking three quick steps along the march to death. Any of these changes may trigger psychological reactions requiring external assistance.

LATE ADULTHOOD (60 YEARS AND UP)

Illness strikes close to home; friends (perhaps spouse) die; much less life time lies ahead than has already passed. Death is clearly coming; losses are more permanent; energy is decreasing. Each new limitation is a partial death that must be mourned. The children are becoming the caretakers and the grandchildren are reaching for independence. What is the meaning of each day?

Childhood

A great deal of what we are is created in the cauldron of our family. Early life relationships often seem to set the patterns for later adult relationships. If therapists choose to do so, careful analogical listening will reveal outlines of the distant past in each patient's description of current key interpersonal relationships. Freud used the term "repetition compulsion" to describe what he thought was an innate drive to recreate in the present the relationships of the past. There are many alternative explanations. Perhaps some patients need to recreate the old interpersonal dynamics in order to master them. For example, the woman whose father was an alcoholic and who marries alcoholic after alcoholic may simply be trying to cure her father in the guise of each new marital challenge. Perhaps she is repeating this pattern because of a desire to relieve herself of the guilt she felt for having not stopped him from drinking in the first place. Could she also be recreating this style of intimate interaction because it is the only style she knows? From the social learning perspective, her parents modeled marital interaction. They may have reinforced her for participating with them. While therapists usually view the repetition compulsion as pathological, the desire to recreate family relationships can also be fostered by the pleasant, loving element of those early interactions and the desire to carry forward the culture, rituals, and behaviors of one's parents. Sons and daughters often find themselves acting like their own fathers and mothers to their children. These crucial parenting models are difficult to deny. Going to the opposite extreme (e.g., strictly raised child becomes permissive parent) indirectly continues the influence.

No matter how a specific therapist weighs the importance of the past, some patients will insist upon discussing it. Whether in psychoanalysis or not, some will talk about early sexual experiences; fecal and urinary themes may predominate. Some need to recount early traumas, particularly rape and incest, now more easily discussed. In addition to early parental insults, experiences with siblings may be of greater importance than is usually considered (Bank & Kahn, 1982). The birth of a sibling can rob a tenuously adapted child of already limited parental nurturing. The death of a sibling can evoke prolonged guilt and grief. Rivalry and incestuous longings may carry forth into the present.

THE PERSON-IN-THE-ENVIRONMENT

The influences of the past, culture, and the aging body are felt only in the here and now. Surrounding each patient are layers of contexts molding responses "right now." During the Vietnam era, radical therapists drew attention to the vast influence of political, social, and economic ideologies on the mental–emotional states of Americans (Agel, 1971). Through their gradual awakening to the political process, many women have come to realize that they belong to an oppressed group, and that psychological change could be achieved not through adaptation to the status quo but through fundamental alteration of attitudes and behaviors that contribute to their oppression. Radical therapists have also highlighted the influence of economic values on the conduct of United States citizens by pointing to the corrupting influence of greed nurtured by raw capitalistic ideals. The acceptance of war as a means to settle international disputes has psychopathological reverberations (Lipton, 1985).

The interpersonal context is more regularly addressed by psychotherapists because change initiated by the individual is more likely to bear fruit in this context. We are interpersonal creatures, dependent upon the approval, and acceptance of others. Our self-expression is often held in check by the expectations of others. For some patients, individual psychotherapy is too weak a means by which patients may change their environment. If so, the critical others holding such patients in check must be addressed as well.

Attention must also be placed upon the less animate current environment. The presence of excessive food, drugs (including alcohol and tobacco), firearms, television violence, and other potentially harmful psychological toxins may also need to be addressed directly.

As mentioned in Chapter 3 (Engagement), the current biological context also must be considered as a contributor to psychological dysfunction. Dietary abnormalities (starvation), biochemical shifts (depression, mania, panic attacks), and other physical illnesses (endocrine or blood disorders) may each strongly influence the presenting problems.

Presenting Problems

Patients usually present painful problems to be solved through psychotherapy, while therapists usually try to understand the problems in terms that facilitate change. The achievement of this objective often requires that the presenting problem be transformed into a different language or replaced by less obvious but more changeable problems. If presenting problems are construed as symptoms of conflict, the therapist searches for opposing dualities. If they are construed as defenses, the feared impulses, feelings, or thoughts become the goals of the therapist search. If the symptom is thought to be a marker for interpersonal difficulty, therapists attempt to define the interaction correlated with the symptom. If the presenting complaint is considered by the therapist to be a signal for maladaptive cognitions, the patient will be instructed to help uncover such thoughts.

The presenting symptom may often undergo a variety of transformations until the therapist alights upon the most changeable element. Goldfried and Davidson (1976) described a client whose marriage "is faltering due to the frequent arguments he has with his wife. In carrying out the behavioral analysis, it may be revealed that the arguments typically occur when he has been drinking. When does he drink? Whenever he's had a hard day at work. What contributes to the pressure at work? The excessively high standards he imposes upon his own performance" (pp. 22–23). Rather than focus on the fighting behavior itself, the therapist may choose to examine the husband's unrealistic standards for self-evaluation.

All therapists seem to believe in their ability to find a causative or explanatory element that will increase change potential. They differ in their chosen directions. Some go laterally in the near present to other behaviors and cognitions as did Goldfried and Davidson in the previous paragraph. Some go into the preconscious and shallow unconscious searching for underlying conflicts and defenses. Some plunge more deeply, searching for childhood experiences and other unconscious forces. Some use emotion as the guide to uncover difficulty.

Useful patterns are available in different approaches. There is no reason that all useful general patterns should not be used. Among the useful ones are: patterns of emotional expression, expectations, major interpersonal styles, intrapsychic conflict, self–other boundary weaknesses, and deep unconscious states.

Patterns of Emotional Expression

Emotion is like a wild card in the game of psychotherapy; it can be used in countless ways depending upon its context. Behavior is observable; thoughts are captured reasonably well by words; but emotion is very slippery. To attempt to grasp the concept of emotion is like trying to hold water in one's hand. Most of it slips through one's fingers leaving only a moist, wet reminder of its presence. Emotion is very difficult to define (Lazarus, 1976).

Painful emotions like depression and anxiety are common presenting problems. Clients often know that they are feeling the "wrong" feelings but have no clues about what to do. Emotions may serve as markers for key thoughts and behaviors. Emotional shifts during interviews often serve as triggers for increased therapist attention. A tear, a trembling voice, a shift in position, a grimace are but a few of the signals alerting therapists to important psychological areas. Cognitive therapists use this clinical fact systematically by instructing their patients to record situations outside the office when they feel negative emotions that may signal dysfunctional thoughts. One side benefit of this cognitive homework is to encourage patients to increase their attention to their own emotions. Lack of emotional awareness is a common difficulty for many people and this exercise fosters change in this direction. Many patients mislabel their emotions; calling anger, depression, or anxiety, hunger. Children learn their emotions as they learn the alphabet. A caretaker describes to them the label for the heightened affective state — "you're angry." If the state is not labeled correctly or if the model mislabels or does not name his or her own emotional states, the child does not acquire an accurate vocabulary for internal states (Peake & Egli, 1982). Bruch (1974) offered the following example.

CASE 4.4. Nathan, a thirteen-year-old Jewish boy showed rapid changes in behavior following his bar mitzvah. Until then he had been the bright hope of his family. He became preoccupied with guilt, feeling an urgent need for atonement of his sins. This overshadowed his thinking and he developed a whole series of rituals; he explained whatever he did or did not do as being motivated by fear of guilt. No progress was made in therapy until attention was paid to the broad area of feeling tones which he never mentioned and which he said, when asked, he did not experience. Nathan had grown up in a family in which "not giving trouble" and "taking it" were praised virtues. It was gradually worked out that the sensation he called "guilt" was aroused whenever there was the slightest manifestation of any other feeling in him for which the appropriate term might have been "anger," "anxiety," "bodily discomfort," or "demands" based on them. (p. 97)

Emotion both internally felt and expressed may be used to defend against unwanted other feelings. Anger is commonly used to hide fears of vulnerability. Depression is often used to hide from hurt and to evoke caretaking. Shallow, shifting emotion may be used to screen the experiencer's awareness of more frightening feelings.

CASE 4.5. A 30-year-old graduate student was often hysterical because the woman he wanted to love him was still seeing other men. He could not sleep, pleaded with her everytime he saw her, and was filled with anxiety and need. These shallow intense emotions served to shield himself from experiencing his fear of being isolated.

Emotions served for this man and serve for many others as a way to make decisions. Rather than being able to weigh pros and cons, he would think of alternatives and register the emotion correlated with visualizing each possibility. Just as one can place too much emphasis upon rationality in decision making, one can overemphasize "what feels right" as well. In the question of decision making, emotion and that yet more vague human function, intuition, seem to overlap. Psychotherapists are often required to respond to their patients by emotional–intuitive means although this decision-making mechanism is difficult to study. Yet when therapists encourage their clients to rely on their own abilities, one of these abilities is this poorly understood contribution to decision making.

Perhaps the most difficult emotion to understand is love. It is also the most precious. Poets and musicians attempt to capture it but psychotherapists often seem more comfortable with anger. Do therapists only try to clear away the impediments to loving or do they teach some form of loving by their example?

Expectations

Not only are we molded by what is past, and are living permanently in the present, but we are also shaped by our anticipated self–other interactions. The influence of the future on present behavior is mediated through past experiences by which each of us gains some estimate of what might happen.

George Kelly (1955) attempted to formalize this notion by stating as a postulate that "a person's processes are psychologically channelized by the way he anticipates events" (p. 46). The term "operant," which may be defined as an event probabilistically linked to the occurrence of prior events, first appeared to be unrelated to expectations. Then behavioral researchers were forced to assume that rats learned to anticipate connections between operants and target behaviors (like lever pulling) (Murray & Jacobson, 1978). This human ability to anticipate the future may be used to understand unconscious motivation as well. If, for example, a person causes another person emotional pain without intending to do so, therapists may hypothesize that perhaps the unintended outcome was unconsciously sought. Stated as a rubric: Outcome is motivation.

Cognitive therapists (Beck *et al.*, 1979) use the terms "automatic thoughts" and "cognitive schemata" to refer to ways of processing information that lead to a prediction of what is to happen next. Depressed or anxious people generally predict the worst and respond with feelings and behaviors that reflect the predicted negative consequences.

Bandura coined the term "self-efficacy" to describe one's own estimate of the probability of successfully carrying out a stated objective. The notions of "demoralization" (Frank, 1974) and "hopelessness" refer to similar presenting problems of people who do not believe that their efforts will bear fruit or who lack the sense of mastery.

For those of us who are able to settle physiological needs (hunger, sleep, protection from the environment), the self-evolving-toward-the-future is confronted with the need to construct the broader context called "purpose" or "meaning" in life. The ultimate solution to this problem is probably that it is best to ignore it (Yalom, 1980). Yet the desire to comprehend the purpose of one's present-day activities drives some to work for years on books like this simply so that they can have some growing entity into which they can place their energies and hope to see the cumulative result. The alternatives in Western society are many. One may choose the self-centered aims of accumulating money, gaining power, or achieving fame. The altruistic desire to help others is less rewarded though still practiced in Western cultures, as are variants of selfish altruism.

Major Interpersonal Styles

Among the hypotheses concerning the development of one's major interpersonal style is the following suggested by Kopp (1977).

> Such styles are protective attitudes developed early in life as necessary ar-
> mor against an emotionally destructive environment. At first they served
> to keep the patient from the surrounding dangers. . . . Now in adult life
> these attitudes are self-maintaining. In limiting the patient's experience of
> anxiety, they restrict the possibilities of new experience. Ironically, in this
> way they prevent the realization that the original danger is past. As with
> all avoidant defenses, these have been set up to hold off catastrophe. Unex-
> pected experiences and risky behaviors are limited. . . . Thus, every bit
> of avoidant behavior is reinforced by the absence of consequent catastrophe.
> (pp. 130–131)

Jung (1964) used to term "persona" to describe the protective cover
or mask that an individual presents to the world. He suggested that it had
two purposes: first to make a specific impression on other people; second,
to conceal the individual's inner self from their prying eyes (p. 287). Kopp
and others would insist that the persona or character style also defends
the individual against awareness of inner conflicts and memories.

Using behavioral terms and perspectives, Cashdan (1973) suggested
that ongoing interpersonal relationships are based upon implicit and/or
explicit "contracts" that are meant to satisfy personal demands and needs.
"Where two people negotiate for the use of each other, strategies function as interpersonal chips, behavioral devices used to reduce the risk of
being cheated. They represent each person's idiosyncratic attempt to maximize gain and minimize cost (avoid pain and disappointment) in relationships where long-term commitment is at stake" (pp. 51–52). For
Cashdan the term "strategy" overlaps with "persona" and "character
style."

Character strategies take place in an interpersonal context. Not only does one style seem to characterize a specific client, but significant
others seem also to respond in stereotyped ways. The more enduring the
relationship, the more likely that the interaction is characterized by
predictable patterns. Each partner seems to shape the behavior of the
other in order to achieve a mutually acceptable fit.

In summary, character strategies are probably adaptive reactions to
early experiences used to hide the pain of internal conflict and memories,
to control others while minimizing emotional vulnerability, to achieve
certain desired responses (approval, acceptance, noncriticism) from oth-

ers, and to establish predictable, safe, useful patterns in permanent relationships.

Therapists may focus on different links in this chain and still be
able to achieve psychotherapeutic change. This observation suggests
that psychological shifts may require only the alteration of one or a few
aspects of a specific complex, an observation that has important implications for models of the change process. If alteration of only a few discrete
elements is necessary for successful change, then therapists should strive
to determine the most accessible link rather than force most patients to
fit into one predetermined to be the "best."

Many other terms have been used for this important area of psychotherapeutic attention. Each is embedded in its own theoretical structure.
Each highlights (and de-emphasizes) different areas of interpersonal functioning: coping, defenses, security operations, meta-communication, operants, and games. The proliferation of terms simply highlights the importance of interpersonal functioning to psychotherapists.

What are some of these interpersonal strategies? They may be observed in the engagement stage of every psychotherapy encounter, and
they are no doubt partially determined by Western culture as well as by
early family influences. They have been described in immense detail with
confusing overlapping terms. Cashdan (1973), for example, described the
sexual, martyr, and dependent strategies. In the sexual strategy, sex is the
medium of exchange. It is the solution to problems, the promise of the
future, and the reason to stay together. The self-effacing, self-sacrificing
martyr attempts to convince the target that the other cannot survive
without him or her, while the dependent strategist plays the other side
of the helper–helpee duality by attempting to convince the target that
without help he or she will not survive. These strategies may be enacted
in many variations, some of which have been described by Eric Berne
(1967). The game called Alcoholic, for example, often has four players
but can be managed by two. The alcoholic is *it* and requires a *rescuer*
(often the friendly physician but it could be the spouse), a *persecutor* who
judges and blames (often the spouse), and sometimes the kindly *patsy* who
supplies money and drink. Often the spouse plays all three roles to achieve
a sense of being needed (pp. 73–76). Satir (1967) described marriage relationships in which one partner is the "blamer" and the other is the "placator." These roles may shift. The "placator" is a mix of martyr and dependent strategies while the "blamer" is the omniscient one.

Other common characteristic strategies include power ploy, passive–compliant, paranoid–needy, and,honesty–equality. In power ploy,
the player projects an image of strength in categories targeted to be im-

portant to the listener. Variations include: Look how much money I have; look how important I am in the community; look at how tough I can be; look how intelligent and knowledgeable I am; and look what I can do for you. The passive–compliant strategists attempt to gain their control without intimacy by gauging the expectations of their targets and attempting to fulfill them effectively. They never have to reveal themselves but feel chronically unacknowledged. The paranoid–needy strategist presents self as terribly afraid of being hurt again, yet indicates the potential for immense love if the other person is able to tap the frightened exterior. The honesty–equality ploy may approach an ideal but may be also used as a mask of an ideal. Open and honest people may hide significant aspects of themselves. Honesty may be used to challenge the listener's willingness to persevere. Honesty may become a brutal weapon to disparage and distance others while following the often-preached idea "honesty is the best policy." This homily does not indicate under what conditions honesty is the best policy. It is doubtful that any single interpersonal "policy" is useful at all times.

Character strategies may be clarified by reference to the processing errors noted by Beck *et al.* (1979) (personalization, exaggeration, minimization, selective inattention, arbitrary inferences). For many cognitive therapists, processing errors seem to arise within the organism as biological givens. Yet each of these ways of misconstruing sensory input can be used as part of a character strategy. For example, "exaggeration" (sometimes called "catastrophizing") refers to the tendency to take a small bit of negative information to mean that one's world is breaking. The catastrophizing person communicates intense helplessness likely to trigger a rescue response in a predisposed other, leading to a possible dependent strategy. "Personalization" refers to the tendency to impute self-referential meaning to random events. The most extreme example is the psychotic's belief that television personalities are talking to him or her, but in less extreme cases, personalization may lead to overblown or deflated self-opinion. The overblown self-opinion may lead to the presentation of self as powerful, beautiful, and brilliant, thereby hooking susceptible targets looking for an ultimate rescuer to which to cling.

Intrapsychic Conflict

Intrapsychic conflict often pits "shoulds" against "wants," individual desires against the internalized expectations of others. Intrapsychic conflict has been rediscovered by many different therapists and has, therefore, received many different labels. Among them are: angel versus devil, superego versus id, parent versus child, topdog versus underdog, internal dialogue, and tyranny of the "shoulds." "Defenses" refers to the compromise reached between the conflicting elements as a way of binding the associated anxiety. "Ambivalence" is a form of intrapsychic conflict more often describing difficulty in choosing between two apparently equally good (or bad) alternatives.

Once the poles of a conflict have been outlined, therapists tend to flesh out the details. This fleshing-out process often leads to new and more basic conflicts present in other realms of the patient's life. These underlying conflicts have also received different labels. "Cognitive schemata" refers to fundamental data-processing templates that filter information and organize responses in regular patterns. "Nuclear unconscious conflicts" refers to fundamental opposing dualities formed in childhood that shape each patient's construction of current conflicts. These terms are related in that schemata are rules derived from earlier conflicts. The differences are more in the way therapists construe the source. Psychoanalysts prefer to define childhood memories from which visual–emotional analogies may be drawn, while cognitive therapists prefer to isolate word-based rules (e.g., I should be liked by everyone or else I am worthless). These points are illustrated in the following example:

CASE 4.6. A 32-year-old accountant entered therapy because he had multiple physical complaints that had no apparent biomedical sources. He quickly described his tendency to procrastinate, particularly when success loomed close. He berated himself viciously about what he should do — clean his bathroom, finish his books, call prospective clients, enter a company contest — he did nothing. As therapy progressed, he admitted his problem with premature ejaculation. He was so afraid of failing at sex that he often preferred to masturbate without telling his partner. He then felt guilty for not being interested in sex. He soon related his fear of failure at sex to his fear of failure at work, which was maintained by his procrastination.

In this case, the tension between the "shoulds" to succeed and the "wants" to just sit and be cared for produced the physical symptoms (somatization, a form of defense or coping). Further discussion uncovered the patient's premature ejaculation, another manifestation of fear of failure, in part relieved by masturbation. The underlying schemata for these conflicts was the self-statement: Do not try to succeed on your own because you will be unable to manage by yourself. He received this idea from his overprotective mother. For much of his school life, he was easily hurt by peers, required intermittent psychiatric treatment, and generated much concern in her about whether or not he could survive on his own. His father also appeared highly dependent upon his mother, and his very earliest memories suggested difficulties in separation. Any sexual or work success meant that he was separated from his mother and implied that he would not be able to function on his own.

The nuclear unconscious conflict could be conceptualized as the tension between his own desire to individuate and his internalized mother image who feared his separation. In cognitive terms, these early experiences developed the cognitive schemata—"I can't succeed on my own, so don't try, even though I should." Therapists of different schools can probably select either image or word targets with equal success over large numbers of patients. However, visually oriented patients could likely respond more quickly to parent–child analogies while digital–word-oriented people might respond more quickly to the cognitive approach.

Self–Other Boundary Weakness

Self-conception is developed in an interpersonal context. Misunderstanding of the self and its relationship to others is central to most psychotherapeutic investigations. Through their self-observers, patients report their self-conceptions, which are also revealed by the manner in which they relate to the therapist.

The evolving self may be visualized as a dotted-line circle developing toward a solid-line circle. The more solid the line, the less permeable the self. The entirely dotted-line person is poorly formed, easily molded by external forces, continuously changing, and thereby confusing to the self-observer. People who describe voices outside of themselves talking into their brains, or feel as if they are the universe filled with intense spirals of force penetrating through them, are describing metaphorical holes in their self–other boundaries. With a few more metaphorical solid lines, the self becomes either all good or all bad, characteristics that mark concepts of others as well. These polarities have received different names because they are embedded in different theories. "Splitting" describes the tendency to shift the conception of the same person from one extreme to the other depending upon the circumstances (Kernberg, 1975). "Grandiose self" and "idealized parental imago" describe relationships in which the self is either aggrandized or depreciated (Kohut, 1968). "Supplicant" and "special self" describe the same self concepts against the background of death anxiety and isolation. By becoming a supplicant searching for an ultimate rescuer, the patient is placing him- or herself within the protecting mantle of an all-powerful other to avoid death anxiety. By becoming special, grandiose, or all-powerful, the person avoids self-conception as an ordinary mortal (Yalom, 1980).

Although many patients appear to be set in one or the other state, therapists may hypothesize that under the grandiose self, there lurks a depreciated self and vice versa. The grandiose self is often a defensive presentation for a weak, poorly defined and poorly regarded self. Once an underlying permeable self is threatened with exposure, deep, felt rage is likely to emerge. The rage may be considered a protective device against the fear of annihilation sometimes accompanying the vulnerability caused by exposure.

Grandiose and depreciated selves tend to seek out their complements. They form relationships that confirm their self-conceptions or tend to adjust to relationships that fulfill their expectations of self-definition. By creating supplicant–ultimate rescuer pairs, patients avoid confrontation with their underlying weak self-definitions and the feared vulnerability accompanying that awareness and reality. Sometimes the term "fusion" is best applied to pairs in which the identity of one or both is lost in the other. The experience of falling in love is a temporary altered state of consciousness in which the self becomes totally absorbed in a misconception of the other. The pathological state is more chronic; without the other, the self does not have complete boundaries and metaphorically "bleeds psychic contents." In one example, the separation from his wife drove a 28-year-old man to suicidal ideation and great irritability because he no longer knew who he was.

In psychotherapy, many dotted-line selves (borderline patients) move up the individuation continuum through the partial-dotted-line self (narcissistic self) through to the more integrated self (neurotic and normal) (Adler, 1981). The more integrated selves may then be approached as having intrapsychic conflict. Therapists need to adjust their concepts as their patients move toward better integration.

The Deep Unconscious

Conventional psychotherapies tend to stay with the near present. Nevertheless, sometimes patients erupt with reports of strange memory traces. Dreams are the most standard entry into the far reaches of human consciousness, but current life experiences and certain drug experiences may also evoke deep unconscious reactions. Much more is recorded in our brains than is conventionally thought. While memories associated with the first 5 years of life are relatively easy to accept, thanks to Freud's clear and persistent encouragement to search for them, other, more time-encrusted levels are less accepted. How accessible are the preverbal experiences of the young infant, of the birth experience, of life in the uterus? Grof's experiments (1975) with LSD have added to the perception that these experiences are accessible to all of us and sometimes important. Jung's (1964) finding of similar symbols in vastly different cultures implies yet a deeper layer of convergence among all humans. The individual relationship to the spiritual dimension is buried deeply within most humans. For some psychotherapists and for some clients, theological and spiritual concerns provide useful avenues to psychotherapeutic change.

LABELS FOR PATTERNS: THE ARBITRARY RELATIONSHIP BETWEEN SIGNIFIER AND SIGNIFIED

I assume that each perspective on pattern-search content survives because each has some practical value to practitioners and to clients. I assume that each viable perspective highlights some portion of psychological reality and that different terms sometimes have overlapping meaning for similar psychological territory. Many psychotherapists seem to have become distracted by their attachment to particular words, and, like people whose cultures are defined by their language, are reluctant to reach compromises with psychotherapists using other words.

Why should compromises be sought? Conflicting ideologies obscure the underlying realities described by their words. If, instead, psychotherapists compare their descriptions of psychological territory observed from different perspectives, they increase the likelihood that triangulation will sharpen knowledge. In this way, the mind may be more sharply comprehended.

The labels therapists apply in their search for patterns bear an arbitrary relationship to psychological reality. There are probably many different ways to grasp a mutable pattern. In fact, therapists may need to address only parts of key patterns to achieve change. Attention to thoughts instead of emotions, transference instead of spouse, childhood memories instead of future self-image may simply represent emphasis on different parts of the same pattern. Furthermore, attention to one element does not preclude attention to the other. Talk of emotions usually includes thoughts; transference is often related to current intrapersonal relationships; and childhood memories shape visions of the self in the future.

Some research evidence suggests that there are many different handles by which psychotherapeutic change can be initiated:

1. The general finding from overviews of psychotherapy research indicates that no one form is clearly superior to any others (Luborsky *et al.*, 1975; Smith *et al.*, 1980).

2. Evidence from studies of short-term therapy of depression indicates that many different forms may be useful: Interpersonal (Klerman *et al.*, 1984), cognitive (Murphy *et al.*, 1984), social skills, and psychodynamics (Hersen *et al.*, 1984).

3. Evidence from one study comparing cognitive therapy and drug therapy for depression suggests that positive change seems to proceed along the same lines with both treatment forms (Simons, Garfield, & Murphy, 1984).

4. Evidence from one study comparing cognitive therapy and supportive–expressive psychoanalytic psychotherapy, each with drug counseling, and drug counseling alone suggests that the closer therapists stayed to their psychotherapy manuals, the better the outcome (Luborsky & Auerbach, 1985).

The generally accepted idea that exposure is the underlying principle governing the treatment of most phobias (Marks, 1976) holds promise for the discovery of other change mechanisms for other problems. The efficacy of drug therapy as well as various psychotherapies in the treatment of depression suggests that there are many ways in which change may be instigated. The suggestion that holding to the manual is more critical than the type of therapy implies that psychotherapy requires a specified focus within a systematic procedure rather than a specific content. Frank (1976) insisted that a common ingredient for all psychotherapies was the therapist's belief in a certain set of techniques and a theory for applying them. Not only does this belief give therapists confidence but it forces them to pursue specific problem areas in specific ways. The human intrapsychic–interpersonal system is in a complex equilibrium. Successful psychotherapy seems to require the introduction of a carefully placed deviation or set of deviations into that system. These changes are then amplified by their effects to achieve a more desired homeostasis. It appears to be less important that therapists introduce one specific deviation than one of a limited range of deviations. If true, outlining the limits of the range of alternatives for specific patients working with specific therapists would become a psychotherapy research objective.

ALTERNATIVES TO CAUSE AND EFFECT:
HOMEOSTASIS AND DEVIATION-AMPLIFYING FEEDBACK

Therapists tend to assume that their patients' symptoms can be explained. However, 20th-century science has provided us with more than one way to explain naturally occurring phenomena. The cause-and-effect model has served scientific and technological advance exceedingly well by helping to isolate variables related by time. According to Maruyama, "'effect' can be predicted from the 'cause' with some probability, and the 'cause' can be inferred from the 'effect' with some probability" (quoted in Pentony, 1981, p. 142). The search for childhood causes of adult psychopathology, for the behavioral contingencies of symptomatic behavior, and for the cognitions maintaining depression are among the many examples of cause-and-effect thinking among psychotherapists.

"Effect" flows from "cause" unidirectionally. The relationship between the cause–effect events is nonreciprocal since in this form of explanation, effect does not influence cause (for example, therapist influences patient, but patient does not influence therapist). Beginning in the 1940s, scientists developed models of reciprocal causation operating through feedback loops. An example of reciprocal causation is temperature regulation by the body or by thermostats through which any deviation is countered by feedback to the controls that adjust the system in the opposite direction. In deviation-countering feedback systems, a fixed pattern comes to characterize its functioning regardless of the initial conditions under which it was formed. These are homeostatic systems, geared to maintain set functioning against the pressure of external forces. In psychotherapy, this model describes the "neurotic equilibrium" by which patients tend to maintain set patterns of thinking and behavior despite clear evidence against this course, and to the tendency of families to act to counter threats of change to their interaction patterns.

Certain change introduced into a homeostatic system can overcome the homeostasis to produce a "snowballing" effect by which the deviation is amplified. Examples of these processes include the growth of an organism, the rise and fall of a culture, the accumulation of capital in an industry, the growth of a city, the evolution of living organisms, the growth of friendship or hatred, and the interpersonal processes leading to mental illness or recovery. This model appears to be growing in influence (Pentony, 1981).

Each model has its own utility and validity. Physical and biological scientists are moving away from the nonreciprocal models, and perhaps psychotherapists might consider expanding their range of selection as well.

Reciprocal causation is a "process configuration" that is relatively free of content when compared to the sections of human psychological functioning just described. Reciprocal causation refers to the relationship between interrelated psychological elements rather than to the nature of the elements of themselves. Patterns of emotional expression may feed intrapsychic conflict that may feed major interpersonal styles that may influence self–other boundary stability that may influence patterns of emotional expression. Elements may feed forward or feed back on each other, resulting in stable but dysphoric equilibria. Therapists attempt to intervene in the system by promoting a deviation or series of deviations from the current norm that will break the current homeostasis and shift the equilibrium in a more desired direction. Therapists seem to encourage their clients to alter some aspect of their intrapsychic and/or interpersonal equilibrium in the hope that it will bring significant change. If therapists are able to conceptualize the multiple interacting forces both maintaining the current equilibrium and also most likely to be amplified if changed, then greater efficiency in intervention becomes possible. Perhaps the spouse is the critical link, as is often true in the treatment of agoraphobia. Perhaps emotional awareness or conflict resolution are essential. In complex cases, the first critical variable may be replaced by new critical variables. An alteration in self-expression leading to a changed interpersonal style may lead to marital discord or uncover a maladaptive pattern in a child. Reciprocal causation appears to offer a way to understand how systems maintain themselves and how they may be altered.

5. *Pattern-Search Methods*

In the preceding chapter, I outlined mental areas crucial to psychotherapeutic investigation. Patterns of emotional expression, expectations, major interpersonal styles, intrapsychic conflicts, self–other boundary weakness, and the deep unconscious may each be relevant to understanding the problems with which patient's present their therapists. They are not totally distinct since each one may be characterized in terms of others in the list. For example, intrapsychic conflict is often carried out in interpersonal relationships. Expectations and patterns of emotional expression may be revealed in both intrapsychic and interpersonal terms. Yet each stands relatively separate as well.

This chapter is concerned with how to look, how to examine the person/patient for the much-needed information required for change. While notions of causes of human psychological dysfunctioning are numerous, the methods by which psychological information may be gathered are more limited. Some approaches are generally applicable; for example, listening and asking good questions. Others are better designed for specific target areas. For example, taking a future history is an excellent way to specify expectations (Melges, 1982).

The question of how the data should be organized is more complex. How does the therapist pick from the list of visual data filters presented in the first part of Chapter 4? When are the therapeutic triangles from psychodynamic therapy the most efficient means for pattern definition? What about interpersonal spirals, parent–adult–child, psychodynamic triangle, BASIC I.D., multiple selves, and A→B→C? What about other models of psychopathology not listed here? Therapists seem to enter psychotherapeutic relationships with their own theories of psychological dysfunction, their own favorite areas in which to look, and their own predispositions toward techniques for gathering information. These three aspects of the pattern search reciprocally influence each other, narrowing options while specifying certain patterns. For example, a therapist convinced of the simple beauty of the A→B→C approach to thoughts and emotions, may ignore self–other boundary weaknesses, thereby losing sight of a critical variable. Each model of psychopathology, each technique for investigating the psyche, aids in specificity while losing the general picture. Therapists must be able to judge instances when they have plumbed the depth of a model of psychopathology with a related investigatory tool and come up empty. One value of systematic eclecticism is its provision for backing out of unfruitful depths and being able to enter another organizing system with different techniques. To understand some patients effectively requires being able to alternate models, to link content areas with each other while varying technique.

The first section of this chapter describes general approaches to pattern-search methods: the use of questionnaires, various forms of listening, and questions. In the next section, I have attempted to link types of inquiry with types of content. The connections are not 1 : 1 correlations since some methods are more specific, for example, for uncovering emotions than they are for uncovering intrapsychic conflict. The final section reemphasizes the importance of the pragmatic–functionalist $S \rightarrow O \rightarrow R$ and the reciprocal causation concepts.

QUESTIONNAIRES

Paper-and-pencil tests to be completed by patients at home or before coming into therapy sessions are being increasingly used. Not only do many questionnaires offer rough quantitative measures of difficulty and baseline measures for change but they also provide information that might otherwise not have been found. Since they are often used in the first few sessions, they also serve as engagement techniques since they usually imply therapist thoroughness.

There are innumerable questionnaires. The shorter ones tend to be easy to take and to score but do not reveal subtle forms of data that the more time-consuming ones can. Some, such as the Minnesota Multiphasic Personality Inventory (MMPI) and the Symptom Check List-90 (SCL-90) (Derogatis, 1977), offer global assessment through the use of many different scales. Others are specific for mood — for example, depression (Beck *et al.*, 1979) or anxiety (Zung, 1979). Some pick up phobias (Marks & Mathews, 1979), others look for strengths of social network (Weissman & Bothwell, 1976). Packages of questionnaires that can be used by outpatient psychotherapists and that serve clinically useful functions while providing standard, reliable outcome data by which success or failure may be measured have yet to be devised. Nevertheless, the advent of computerized psychometric testing is rapidly pointing toward cost-effective ways of gathering large amounts of significant information that may be useful for the practice and measurement of outpatient psychotherapy.

Among the broadly useful paper-and-pencil assignments is the daily activity homework assignment. It fails as a measure of psychopathology but serves as an efficient window into the client's daily life. It simply requires that the daily activities be recorded on an hourly basis. If certain behaviors (drug taking, sex, snacking) are targets, then these may be emphasized. If certain moods are to be monitored (depression or anxiety) then their severity may be rated at each hour and/or during significant events. The diary may then be further structured around target symptoms (Beck *et al.*, 1979).

LISTENING

The study of language is generally broken into three divisions: semantics, syntax (grammar), and pragmatics. "Semantics" refers to the meaning of language and "pragmatics" refers to its effects. Three different philosophical positions about the meaning of human speech characterize three ways of listening to patients. This section is concerned with these three meaning filters for human speech. A later section on metacommunication will address some of the pragmatics of human communication.

Patients may be thought to speak in metaphors, allegories, symbols, or other modes requiring interpretation. This position is espoused by psychoanalysts and those other therapists interested in translating the language of everyday life into hidden meanings.

Patients may be thought to speak as scientists, as reporters, as witnesses, or as objective observers of the phenomena of their lives. This position is espoused by cognitive and behavioral therapists and those other therapists who take the patient's words at face value. These therapists usually assume that some data is missing but that once it is described, it too is to be taken at face value.

Patients may also be thought of as communicators of existential experiences. They are people attempting to let another person know what it is like to be who they are. They are points of conscious experience trying to find other points of such experience. This perspective is espoused by existential and humanistic psychotherapists.

These three positions are not mutually exclusive. Some therapists are comfortable switching among and between them. Some patients speak more from one perspective than another. Often the same patient shifts from mode to mode. They also may be shifted by therapist responses. When therapists should shift their own perspectives and when they should consider shifting their patients are unanswered questions.

Symbolic Speech

Freud's *The Interpretation of Dreams* (1900/1938) brought the search for symbolic meaning into modern medicine although allegory, metaphor, and synecdoche have played roles in healing systems for as long as humans have tried to cure others of disease and discomfort. Through the examination of his own dreams and the dreams of others, Freud developed a way to translate these natural symbols. Jung followed, as did many others, each adding his or her own notion of how these symbols could be understood. The search for objects of interpretation spilled past dreams into Freud's consultation room (transference, free association) and then into everyday life. The world became rich with allegory, a place where slips of the tongue, parenthetical laughter, and simple choices of words became the subject of intense scrutiny. The search for symbolic meaning has remained the cornerstone of the practice of many therapists. The patient is viewed as a kind of everyday poet who is forced by fears of direct expression and ignorance of his or her own mind to compromise direct self-expression through the approximations offered by symbols.

Langs (1973) criticized colleagues who fail to appreciate the meaning of patient expression in terms of their unconscious conflicts and fantasies. He insisted that "real" problems be subordinated to the search for the hidden, unconscious fantasies through attempts to interpret the patient's associations.

> Real problems are often used as a defensive covering for neurotic ones and this is a defense that the therapist should not participate in. Therapists who prefer to focus on real conflicts tend to stick to manifest content and the surface material of sessions. They ask direct questions regarding these issues and encourage conscious, reality-oriented thought in the patient. Their own interventions are similarly reality-oriented and direct, rather than interpretive. In contrast, therapists who are interested in intrapsychic conflicts value indirect associations as the "royal road" to repressed fantasy material. When the main neurotic problem or its precipitate is not clear, such a therapist will listen to the patient's associations in the hope of discovering these vital clues. His questions will not be reality focused, but will be directed toward the search for derivatives of the repressed. (p. 292)

Metaphors may be simple and direct. For example, Malan (1979) used the following vignette to show the activity of unconscious expression:

CASE 5.1. A university student in biology at last overcame his intense shyness to the point of being able to ask a girl to come out with him. It was summer, and after dining out together they went for a walk in the country. During the evening the tension of shyness between them had gradually eased, and as they walked through a field he was able to turn to her and risk saying, "It's nice here." She replied warmly, "Yes, it is," and there was a short silence. Suddenly, apparently apropos of nothing, she said, "We've a dog called Sandra, and one day she ran off for a long time, and a few weeks later we discovered that she was going to have puppies," and the conversation continued, naturally and easily, on the subject of what the puppies were like, and the kinds of home that had been found for them. (p. 18)

Malan implied that there are clear sexual innuendos in that abrupt turn of the conversation. It was a statement both of her wishes and of her fears of the consequences, expressed as a compromise through the story of the pregnant Sandra. A more aggressive student of psychology, interested in decoding this message for his own benefit, may have been surprised by the likely rebuke of any sexual advances because he may have been reading but half the message. Besides desiring sexual intercourse, the girl might also have been saying that she needed to be assured of adequate placement of potential progeny (e.g., through marriage) before she would enter a sexual relationship. For a therapist, the simple story of Sandra would represent an unconscious conflict about sexual relationships.

Sandra's story is, for the meaning-seeking therapist, like a dream sequence. It becomes a set of symbols that can be translated into more basic ideas. Unfortunately, the rules for transforming symbols into basic meaning are far from clear. One definite factor is the context within which the symbols are presented. Because the story of Sandra took place on a date between two people who might be likely to share sexual attraction, the Sandra story may be viewed as an expression of sexual conflict. Were the story told to a girlfriend, one could also read sexual overtones had there been a hint of lesbian attraction but the feared consequence of pregnancy would not fit. If the story were being told to a parent, then one might wonder if the teller was not already pregnant and was indirectly asking for advice about what to do with the child.

The elusive nature of context is illustrated by the following vignette:

CASE 5.2. Mrs. A. H., a young, married woman, began this session with a dream. She is in a hospital bed, asleep; then she awakens within the dream and sees a nurse and a doctor. They have a wheel and are going to gas her. They do it twice and then she actually awoke. In the session, she went on to talk about death, funerals, and being embalmed. She had had severe abdominal cramps the night of the dream and they were worse after the dream. She was having problems with her son's poor eating habits and her daughter's lying. She had been furious with them and screamed at them; she had also quarreled with her husband. The dream reminded her of the death of her father; had Heaven placed her in the hospital that day to show her that he died in peace or to punish her? She had worn the shoes that she had put on for his funeral for several weeks after. The gas was like the Rubin's test, in which the doctor had put air into her some years back, in order to see if she had any diseases of her reproductive organs which could account for her infertility at that time. (Langs, 1973, p. 312)

What is the context for this session? What is the central problem, the current adaptive task for this person? Langs listed three alternatives:

1. The patient was in the process of terminating therapy. She was indirectly describing being harmed (gassed) by the doctor. She wanted the doctor to impregnate her (put air into her) and was reacting to the desire for impregnation with guilt and the need to flee. The abdominal cramps represented contractions associated with the fantasied birth.

2. The patient was considering divorce because of her husband's cruelty. Because of her rage at her husband, she is longing for her father and for a sexual relationship with her therapist. Her rage at the children is also displaced anger at her husband.

3. In fact, her father had recently died and there was little question that this was the central problem for her and the main theme of the session.

According to Langs, the correct interpretation of this sessions is as follows:

> In her manifest dream Mrs. A. H. puts herself in her father's place and suffers from his symptoms. Her subsequent associations (as well as those of the previous session) reveal latent content of the dream and the intra-psychic conflicts and unconscious fantasies with which the patient is struggling. Thus she longs to be with her father and undo his loss, to die with him as he did. She is also angry with him, and this is reflected in the displacement of her rage onto her husband and children." (pp. 313–314)

In addition to the variety of patient contexts from which to choose, therapists bring to the translation process a variety of schemes for making symbolic transformations. Like those who interpret great works of art, poetry, theatre, and film, viewers of the context of therapy sessions often differ widely on the meaning of the work. Interpretation can be arbitrary and capricious. In the preceding case, Langs knew the "correct" interpretation. But what is the measure of a good decoding of patient symbols? Some would argue that correctness is measured by closeness of fit to a specific analytical theory. Effectiveness, usefulness to the patient, is, no doubt, the better measure of "correctness" for interpretations (Applebaum, 1975).

Objective Speech

Although according to Chessick (1982a), Langs represents therapists who believe that any deviation from symbolic speech suggests a resistance to therapy, many therapists assume that their clients are telling them the "truth." Truth is veiled in many shadows and ultimately is arbitrarily determined by the viewer's perspective. Nevertheless, the scientific method has proceeded rather successfully under the assumption that elements of reality could be observed and measured; from the data collected in this way, technology and understanding have expanded astonishingly during the 20th century. Many therapists make their clients into research assistants who venture out into their worlds to collect the data essential for psychotherapeutic investigation. Ideally, the therapist would become an invisible form with 360-degree vision perched on each patient's shoulder, recording events from that perspective. Unfortunately, this ideal would create an information glut requiring further processing, and the time expenditure would become prohibitive. Reliance upon the patient as an objective observer is limited by the fact that events are filtered and misconstrued in ways that often are at the root cause of the person's applying for assistance in the first place. Therapists who listen for objective speech like those listening for symbolic speech must keep in mind alternate ways of explaining what is being described. What is being left out? What is not being said? What are the alternate ways of understanding these events?

Therapists who listen for objective speech are seeking audiovisual maps of each patient's reality. What is going on? Who is there? How are they interacting? What is the setting? What is not being reported? What other details are relevant to comprehending these interactions?

Experiential Speech

People are also points of consciousness through which experience flows. Experience is registered in shifts of feeling states. These transitional states mark our existence. To listen for latent content is to put distance between listener and speaker. That distance is created by the therapist's need to search for some way of translating what is being said. The need to interpret objectifies the speaker. To listen for objective speech is to label, categorize, and to type human functioning, thereby removing the listener from the speaker's ongoing experience. Rather than categorize or interpret, therapists may choose to climb up the client's stream of verbal productions into his or her ongoing experience. In order to do so, therapists must let go of preconceptions and focus their attention on the existential being of the person speaking. This task requires relinquishing the common filters we must use to navigate our ways through the potential mine fields of human interaction, laying aside fears, and turning away from one's own concerns. The therapist's previous experiences aid in tuning into the experience of the other. The purpose is the creation of a community of mood in which both seem to be sharing the same experience. This, according to Buber, is "imagining the real," swinging boldly into the life of the other (quoted in Havens, 1975). It can be treacherous because the listener to experiential speech can lose his or her own boundaries and float into the unchartered waters of another's world. One may stay too long and become too completely identified with the other. The shock of this experience may then hurtle the therapist away from this and future immersions in the world of the other.

There are lesser ways. To listen empathically is to be objective about the other person's subjective experience without necessarily entering into his or her life. To record the inner speech of the other, to understand his or her ways of processing events, is to be objective about inner experiences.

QUESTIONS

Of the four types of statements available to psychotherapists (declarative, interrogative, exclamatory, and imperative) the interrogative is probably the most frequently used by psychotherapists. Nevertheless, the most effective and efficient use of questions has yet to be experimentally determined. Some psychodynamic therapists speak strongly against the regular use of questions. Weiner (1975) argued that the inquisitive interview style has a number of major disadvantages: (1) it sets a question-and-answer model for the interview process, thereby implying that all the patient has to do is answer the therapist's questions; (2) it implies that the therapist will determine the content of the hour; (3) it suggests that after the patient has answered all the questions, the therapist will then respond with an answer to the patient's problems (p. 101). Weiner suggested that questions be rephrased into declarative sentences. For example, "How did you feel about that?" could be phrased: "I wonder what feelings you may have had about that" (p. 102).

This attention to the potential impact of a sentence type on client behavior is characteristic of the psychodynamic therapists' sensitivity to their own behavior. They do not want to disrupt the flow of symbolic speech with therapist-imposed directives, but to allow the patient to associate as free of the therapist's direct influence as possible. Cognitive–behavioral therapists, on the other hand, are pursuers of facts, of events, of transactions, of potential influencers of behavior. How-what-where-when-who questions constitute much of their utterances. The psychoanalytical Langs (1973) suggested that each session should contain no more than three or four questions (p. 393). He even accused users of these questions of having strong fears of unconscious and primitive fantasies, for he believed that frequent questions will often keep the material to more superficial descriptions (p. 400).

Different times in therapy seem to require different approaches. Sometimes therapists want to stay with the surface, with reality factors, because there is much to learn and change at this level. Sometimes the more restrained use of questions will be necessary in order to promote deeper, more symbolic speech. If therapists do find themselves asking more questions than seems useful, they should wonder about their motivation and the patient's influence. On the other hand, the failure to ask questions may be a countertransference-based reaction to the client's reality needs (Basch, 1982).

Questions may appear to be simple requests for information but, as illustrated by the following case, they can be veiled directives.

CASE 5.3. A 25-year-old unassertive man was in therapy in part because he could not counter the requests of his immediate supervisors. After a few sessions, he was confronted with a request from one of his supervisors to arrange a dinner meeting ouside of office hours for an out-of-town visitor. When the patient told his therapist that he had failed to say "no," his therapist replied with an apparent question: "What made you comply with his request?" This apparently relevant question camouflaged the instruction "You should have said 'no.'" (Strupp, 1973, pp. 306–307)

Questions are but one of many indirect ways that therapists convey their own values and opinions to their patients (see Chapter 9 for other means).

Indirect Questions

There are many indirect ways of promoting client exploration of content areas in which the therapist is interested. Rogerian empathic reflections (active listening) illustrate the manner in which interventions may appear to have one function but also have another. As summary statements of client here-and-now emotional experience, empathic reflections are intended to confirm the client's experience by helping him or her know more precisely what it is and to make it more acceptable. Therapists using this technique cannot reflect all client emotion and therefore must be selective. By responding to certain content and not to others, therapists are encouraging clients to continue in the manner that has elicited the therapist's responses. If the function of questions is to direct client attention to certain content areas, then empathic reflections seem to perform a similar function. In an analysis of audiotaped sessions by Carl Rogers, Truax (1966) confirmed this hypothesis. He found that Rogers responded differently to five of nine client behaviors (speech patterns) under study and that the rate of emission of these behaviors increased during therapy.

Nonverbal signals may also function to reinforce or discourage patient expression of certain content. Increased attention, leaning forward in the chair, turning away, frowning, coughing uncomfortably, are each examples of potentially influential communication. In psychoanalysis, in which therapist silence is the rule and the patient cannot see him or her, auditory signals may assume greater significance. Blowing the nose, swallowing, stomach grumbling, the movement of note paper, or squeaks of the chair may alter patient speech. If done consistently, they may function as nonverbal questions by cuing the patient to reflect upon what he or she just said.

Therapist silence may serve many functions, depending upon its context. Under the right circumstances, it functions as an excellent way to encourage the client to continue talking about the current subject. For example, if the client has just stumbled into an emotionally laden content area and is going deeper into neglected feelings or thoughts but then stops, therapists are predisposed to rush into the uncomfortable silence with a question or comment that pulls the client out of the inner experience toward the therapist's reality. A tactical silence may be quite useful under these conditions, for it permits the client to continue talking about it. A question or comment is more likely to discourage continuation. If the patient pulls away from the content, then a question may be used to reevoke the subject.

LINKING CONTENT TO INTERVENTIONS

Certain techniques increase the likelihood of bringing forth certain content. Although different patients may interpret the same instructions in different ways, therapists seem able to circumscribe chosen areas of psychological interest.

Patterns of Emotional Expression

Direct observation of the patient in the office is the most straightforward way in which to monitor patterns of emotional expression. How readily does an emotional subject bring out changes in facial expression, voice inflection, tears, body movements? How readily does the patient catch him- or herself in such expression? Perls (1969) tracked these nonverbal signals with great intensity and developed a number of techniques to bring out emotion lurking beneath the surface. One often-used technique he called "exaggeration." If the patient expressed a flicker of feeling, for example, through the clenching of a fist, the therapist urged the patient to exaggerate that motion by clenching and then pounding. Often the original clenching signaled contact with a large, out-of-awareness feeling.

Emotions can serve as markers of key interpersonal and situational experiences. Homework assignments that require clients to record their emotions are useful in developing patterns of emotional expression. The triple-column technique of cognitive therapy (Beck *et al.*, 1979), for example, requires that patients record their thoughts at times that they experience negative emotions. Although the assignment is directed toward highlighting thought processes, it also requires patients to observe and record their feelings. For patients who are not aware of their feelings, this assignment may increase their understanding of when and how they feel.

Dream diaries can be useful in uncovering or defining emotion. For particularly rigid, intellectual deniers of their emotional selves, dream analysis can provide ready access to emotions screened off by ordinary consciousness.

CASE 5.4. A 62-year-old logician presented with multiple somatic complaints. These symptoms resolved after she was able to recognize that her pains were the result of repetitive emotional hurts suffered at the hands of her spiteful younger daughter and neglectful husband. She was rigidly overcontrolled in her emotional expression, and could not discover how deeply she felt about much at all. Since she was a very orderly person, she readily followed directions to record her dreams, which were filled with sexual triangles of many forms. Sometimes representatives of her father and her husband were sexually involved with her; sometimes two women and one man filled the scene. Usually the fear of being displaced by someone else was easily discernible. The patient could accept that these productions were the responsibility of no one else but her and that they indicated how deeply she felt about the triangle she was maintaining with her husband and daughter.

Expectations

The triple-column technique of cognitive therapy is well suited for the exploration of maladaptive cognitions that lead to predictions of probably negative consequences. Take, for example, a 45-year-old business man who feels acutely depressed at 10:00 A.M. and at 5:30 P.M. on the way home from work each day. Is there any link between these two temporal events? Yes, he says. At 10:00 A.M., his wife usually calls him at work and at 5:30 P.M. he is thinking about seeing her at dinner. His thoughts then could merit further scrutiny.

The first of three columns of this diary form contains the situations under which the dysphoric events are taking place. The second describes the type and intensity of the emotion associated with each event. Consequences other than negative emotions may also be included here (screaming, walking out, hitting, crying). The third column is to contain the "automatic thoughts" that link the situation to the consequence. For example, the unhappy 45-year-old businessman may be thinking: "I never should have married her in the first place. She'll never understand me."*

The "triple-column" technique should lead to the definition of recurrent themes in the automatic thoughts (e.g., nobody can ever understand me) — a thought that may be presumed to be the source of negative emotion under a number of circumstances. These underlying themes may

---

*I wonder if sometimes cognitive therapy may construct automatic thoughts rather than always "discover" them. Some patients have great difficulty finding them. If therapists tell them what these thoughts are to be then such patients can report them "spontaneously."

be elicited by viewing the automatic thought record longitudinally and also by in-depth questioning of a specific event. Following is a brief outline for the in-depth approach to a specific event (from Hollon, 1982).

1. Ask for the specific example and then ask the following questions: (a) What were you thinking? (b) What were you feeling? (c) What did you do? These questions encourage the patient to verbalize the details of the situation described in the triple-column diary. "I wished I wouldn't have to go home. I felt anxious and depressed. I stopped in a bar first and when I arrived at home I started yelling at her."

2. Then ask: What does that mean to you? Much like asking the patient to associate freely to a dream element, this question is intended to elicit the underlying thoughts contributing to this sequence of events. "She has never understood me. Whenever I tried to explain to her how I felt or what I wanted, she always turned away. I should never have married her. She just won't try." The therapist may check the completeness of these associations by asking him- or herself whether or not he or she would feel this way if believing these thoughts. If not, search, for more thoughts and feelings.

3. Once an underlying belief is discovered, ask the patient for evidence to substantiate it. Absolute words like "always" and "never" are among the easiest to challenge (e.g., She *never* understands me).

4. Ask for alternative ways of construing the other person's response (e.g., Perhaps she did understand but not in the way you wanted. Perhaps she was occupied with other concerns. Early in therapy, the therapist may generate alternative views, but as treatment progresses, the responsibility shifts to the patient.

5. Ask for the real implications of the situation. Or put more bluntly, "so what?" "What is so important about her always understanding you?"

6. A fourth column may be added to the other three. The patient is asked to record acceptable alternatives to the maladaptive automatic thoughts. "It would be nice if she understood me each time I spoke with her, but to expect that is unreasonable." The fourth column may then contain more adaptive replacements for the original maladaptive thoughts.

Visual imagery exercises may provide an avenue for the exploration of the anticipated future. Melges (1972, 1982) suggested that the therapist might take a "future history." Rather than ask about the near or distant past, Melges asked many of his patients to tell them about an event that was to happen some 3 months in the future. For example: "Think about the next time your entire family will be getting together. Tell me what you think will be happening as you interact with the important others in your life. Describe it as if it were happening now." The patient is then asked to talk out loud about how he or she would like to feel, act, and think under the same circumstances. Patients often have difficulty imagining themselves acting in their desired ways. These blocks to carrying out the ideals in fantasy help to flesh out maladaptive patterns.

Major Interpersonal Styles

Much psychotherapy involves the study of the client's interpersonal processes. Therapists may assume that certain interpersonal styles characterize client's behavior in important relationships since most of us develop a narrow range of alternatives. There are a number of ways in which to elicit and examine these basic interpersonal patterns.

TRANSFERENCE

Most patients bring to psychotherapy characteristic ways of attempting to control significant interpersonal relationships. These patterns may be observed in most psychotherapeutic interactions. The psychoanalytic approach is particularly designed to highlight these patterns as well as to make them the subject of discussion. Through the following maneuvers, psychoanalytical therapists induce their patients to act toward them as if they were highly significant others:

1. personal anonymity through suspension of manifestations of real self;
2. relative neutrality toward the patient's behavior and words;
3. active interest in transference phenomena (thereby encouraging its development);
4. interpretation of resistances to transference (indirect criticism of the lack of its development);
5. regular prolonged and frequent scheduling of meetings;
6. therapist's acceptance of distortions without anxiety and need to correct them (quoted from Dewald, 1976).

INSTRUCTION TO "BE ALONE" IN THERAPY

A standard part of psychoanalytic treatment is the placement of the patient in a "closed space," removed from the interaction with the therapist. The patient is asked to be alone in the presence of the evenly hovering attention of the quiet, observing therapist. This instruction may be useful in nonpsychoanalytic therapies as well. For example, the beginning of a therapeutic relationship is often characterized by crisis intervention, focus upon here-and-now symptoms and behaviors. As these problems resolve, patients leave or use the success of these early sessions for further exploration of themselves in order to prevent a repetition. The once-helpful, supportive therapist may consider withdrawing from the therapeutic field, however, first instructing the patient: "Next session, I will not be so active in helping you. I've rushed in to aid you during our first sessions but you do not need that help now. I will simply sit and listen."

CASE 5.5. After receiving this role realignment instruction, a 28-year-old mother of one child returned to therapy and described her attempt to go swimming the previous evening. She did not go through with it because the last time she went swimming she almost drowned. Further exploration of this failed plan uncovered her fear of being alone in therapy, of having to swim in her own thoughts. She very much depended upon other people to define her role for her. Now she was afraid she would drown in ill-defined role expectations. Her struggle for self-expression became transformed into anger at her therapist for not responding, for not telling her what to do. When asked with whom she had felt this way before, she replied, "My parents, especially my mother." As she saw how much she was still being controlled by them and their lack of response to her, she defiantly searched for self-expression first in therapy and then with her husband. Soon she was able to talk with her husband and parents without fear of not fulfilling their role expectations.

METACOMMUNICATION

In addition to having at least three different forms of meaning, human speech is also pragmatic — it is intended to have an effect on the listener. One pragmatic function of speech is as a tool, used by the speaker in his or her attempt to define the roles by which the dialogue is to take place. Human communication seems to involve attempts by the communicator to define the nature of the interpersonal relationship and thereby control it. Watzlawick, Beavin, and Jackson (1967) used the term "metacommunication" (communicating about the communication) to refer to the speaker's attempt to define the rules of the conversation/relationship.

Therapists, for example, attempt to induce their patients to take certain roles with them. Sometimes the rules are explicitly defined, more often they are implicitly defined. Patients, too, attempt to impose their structure on the relationships. One of the ways in which these maneuvers register in therapists is through countertransference reactions. If the therapist feels that he or she is being switched into a way of being that feels unnatural, foreign, and uncomfortable, the patient's subtle attempt to transform the rules of the relationship may be at work.

These pragmatics may also be observed in patient reports of interpersonal patterns. No matter what the content, the effect on the listener becomes the critical focus. For example, the overly polite person is encouraging the listener to follow the rules associated with a certain form of interpersonal decorum. The "totally honest" person is attempting to form a conversation based on this interpersonal form. The excessive questioner appears to be interested in the life of the interviewee but also is controlling the interpersonal flow by directing content. The effect of client speech on a listener adds vital information about client metacommunication.

CASE 5.6. A 31-year-old businesswoman was suffering through the trial period of her first job placement since finishing business school. She was not doing well. Her interpersonal life was isolated, she had only her dogs. She was overly polite, self-effacing, and guarded in therapy. She reported the following interchange:

SUPERVISOR: You look good today.

PATIENT: Thank you. That really makes me feel good to have you say that.

SUPERVISOR: You hurt my feelings by saying that.

What prompted this odd response? What did the patient leave out? Her ingratiating excessive politeness may have been mistaken for a hidden anger that said: "You have been treating me poorly for many months. I expect you to continue to do so. This compliment does not fit in with your previous behavior."

ROLE-PLAYING

By encouraging clients to enact interpersonal experiences, therapists may both see and hear the phenomena in question and therefore comprehend them more directly. A patient who reports that she once again did try to speak to her withdrawn husband without success may convey during role-playing how her timidity sprinkled with sarcasm might have encouraged his withdrawal. Her verbal report might never have indicated so clearly her own role in the final result.

Interpersonal role-playing can be used in assertiveness training as a test for the client's current adaptive abilities under circumstances requiring assertiveness (Brady, 1984). As in the construction of the starting point for an imagery exercise, a detailed immersion into the sights, sounds, feelings, and movements associated with the situation to be enacted is helpful in anchoring the client to the situation. Resistance to role-playing of any kind is not uncommon, often because clients claim that it seems too artificial. Therapists may exhort balking clients to proceed by extolling the value of direct information from direct observation. On the other hand, Wachtel (1977) noted that rather than being too artificial, role-playing turns out to be all too real. The client is stripped of pretense, left only to enact what actually happened and what actually is felt.

Interpersonal role-playing may be arranged in a number of ways. The client may be asked to respond to a standard tape recorded situation requiring standard behavior (like assertiveness). Clients may simply play themselves in critical scenes while the therapist plays the significant other. Role reversal may also be quite helpful. Therapists play their clients while the clients play the other person. In this way, therapists learn firsthand what it is like to be the client and clients learn what it is like to be that often inscrutable other.

ENVIRONMENTAL OBSERVATION

The difficulties bringing people into psychotherapy take place outside the consulting room. Much psychotherapeutic energy is spent describing in the office the patient's problems outside the office, using many of the pattern-search techniques described in this chapter. Another alternative is to physically shift into the patient's environment.

The most direct approach is to enter the client's home or work place. Another approach is to create an environment that might resemble the patient's social system. Inpatient psychiatric units are hardly typical examples of the workplace and home, but, nevertheless, offer a rough approximation in which patient behaviors with staff and others can be observed. Group therapy is yet another controlled approximation of a social system, in which individuals enact their typical social behaviors under controlled conditions.

In outpatient practice, a simple way to approximate the patient's interpersonal environment is to invite a significant other into the office. Although the psychoanalyst Langs has claimed that this action may have serious detrimental effects (1973, p. 195), the procedure is commonly used and often useful. Sometimes patients themselves do not report the critical information easily gained from a third party.

CASE 5.7. A 24-year-old man with chronic schizophrenia was quite reluctant to describe his activities in his once-weekly sessions. The therapist wanted to respect his right to confidentiality but moved slowly to bring the patient's parents into treatment because he was concerned about the man's life outside the office. The session after the parents finally came, the patient committed suicide by overdose. While the one explanation for the suicide could have been the parents entrance into the office, they offered much evidence to suggest that he had been morose for months and had been storing his medications for at least 2 months. Instead of attributing the patient's suicide to the parents coming to the office (although the temporal correlation is compelling), a more likely cause was the therapist's failure to act more quickly to get them involved.

Research in the treatment of schizophrenia is strongly indicating the value of family therapy (Goldstein, 1984).

Third parties may be enlisted as "research associates" who gather data in specified ways or answer interview questions. They also may be asked to observe and record data in regard to specific behaviors and their antecedents and consequences. For the therapist who suspects a contributory role of another who considers him- or herself uninvolved with the patient's problem, this assignment may gather evidence to demonstrate the manner in which that person is contributing. For example, a husband may be asked to describe the antecedents and consequences of his wife's angry outbursts and in doing so may define more clearly his role in precipitating them.

Third parties may be asked to be themselves in a role-playing scene, thereby recreating the typical interpersonal problems between them. Often with a little discussion of a central emotional difficulty, the pair will reenact their difficulties and demonstrate patterns the primary patient could not have reported verbally.

CASE 5.8. A 44-year-old husband demonstrated in his relationship to the therapist and by his own description that he avoided confrontations with his wife and everyone else. The manner in which he avoided was unclear until his wife came into the office and they began to talk with each other. He managed to stop any form of disagreement with her by agreeing with her, despite the fact that he held an opposite view. This pattern of agreement in order to avoid confrontation then became the subject of therapeutic scrutiny.

NEW BEHAVIOR OUTSIDE THE OFFICE

Behavior change is a clear psychotherapeutic objective. New behaviors may induce a variety of effects on others that are critical for psychotherapeutic investigation. The very act of coming to therapy sessions may cause significant interpersonal reverberations and may require analysis to avoid premature termination. Psychoanalysts describe the "transference neurosis" by which most of the patient's neurotic difficulties become focused on the analytic relationship and are reduced in outside-the-office interactions. This reduction in patient-initiated neurotic behavior may disturb the interpersonal equilibria of those others who commonly anticipate the patient's neurotic behavior. The accomplishment of the behavior-change goals of psychotherapy may also create responses by others requiring further pattern analysis. For example, changes in the assertiveness levels of a spouse may elicit declarations of intention to divorce or may uncover psychological difficulties masked by the identified patient's more obvious problems. A husband of an agoraphobic, for example, may find his sexual impotence or alcoholism the focus of his wife's inquiry when she becomes less afraid to leave the house.

Clients may be instructed to ask questions of others that challenge their own beliefs about those people's intentions. For paranoid patients particularly, this exercise is invaluable in confronting irrational concepts about the meaning of the behavior of others.

CASE 5.9. A 24-year-old medical student was convinced that the resident under whom he was working did not like him and wanted to make the service time difficult for him. Evidence for this conclusion came from the grumpy manner in which the resident said "hello" to him and the minimal interest he gave to the student's write-ups. The student was asked to generate further alternatives about the possible source of this behavior. He could not, but did agree to ask other people their opinions of the resident's behavior. While talking to another medical student and a nurse, he asked directly for their opinions of the resident's behavior and they each said he was in the midst of a divorce that was weighing on him greatly. The success of this effort led the patient to ask questions in other circumstances, and this further helped him to reduce his tendency to see other people's negative behavior as directed against himself.

Many patients are also prescribed medications while in psychotherapy (Beitman, 1984). The manner in which these medications are taken or not taken may also reveal additional information about patients.

CASE 5.10. A 45-year-old family practitioner was prescribed antidepressants during psychotherapy following his divorce. Shortly after beginning the medication, he went on a 2-week vacation during which he experienced painful urinary retention secondary to the antidepressant. He did not, however, stop taking it. When asked later by his psychiatrist

what he would have told one of his patients with this side effect, he replied
that he would have suggested stopping it. When asked why he did not
stop it, he replied that he preferred to "tough it out." He seemed to have
a similar reaction to the problems of his marriage. Rather than correct
difficulties, he preferred to tough them out as well.

Intrapsychic Conflict

The identification of the warring intrapsychic factions may be made in
a variety of ways. Fundamental to characterizing them is the assumption
of their existence, for without that belief they could not be elicited.
Transference reactions, contradictions, and incongruities between speech
and nonverbal behavior provide methods by which to identify conflicting
intrapsychic agencies.

TRANSFERENCE

In Case 5.10 the previous section, a family practitioner failed to discontinue a medication that was causing him discomfort through common side
effects. He would have told his own patients to discontinue the medication
but chose for himself to "tough it out." These actions suggest not only that
he preferred to tough out problems in his marriage but also that he preferred to force himself through unnecessarily painful situations. One may
assume that his two major intrapsychic agencies repeatedly fight over
pleasure versus accomplishment, compassion for himself versus intense
self-discipline. His wife (or his therapist), caught within his interpersonal
sphere, might come to represent to him one side of this duality. The wife
might respond with frustration at being told to forget the problems, just
keep going. The therapist might, it is to be hoped, not become caught
up in the patient's attempt to induce him or her to play the complementary role but, instead, might note the nature of this relationship for possible interpretation. Psychoanalysts might tend to identify the parts in
terms of superego and id and relate them to parent–child relationships.
These analogues may be useful to some patients. Others might just as well
prefer topdog–underdog or parent–child or the tyranny of the shoulds.

CONTRADICTIONS

Careful attention to client words will usually reveal contradictions. "I
want to go with her" may be followed sometime later with "I want to
let her go and be rid of her." "I want to keep this job" may be followed
by "There is no future here for me." "I love her and want to stay married

to her" may be followed by lists of reasons never to see her again. These dualities, often characterized as ambivalence, represent expressions of intrapsychic conflict.

Latent content may be a rich source of dualities. Hidden beneath overly kind and respectful attitudes may be rage. Behind expressions of concern may be the desire to abandon. A set of symbols may represent a compromise between two psychic agencies (see section on symbolic speech above).

INCONGRUITIES

The term "contradiction" suggests speaking against oneself. The term "incongruity" is used to describe a lack of fit between the verbal and nonverbal modes of expression. While congruence between verbal and nonverbal speech tends to reinforce both to make the final message clearer and more forceful, incongruent and conflicting messages tend to confuse the final meaning (Watters, Bellissimo, & Rubenstein, 1982). By separating out the strands of incongruent messages, therapists can identify signals from two conflicting psychic agencies.

CASE 5.11. A 30-year-old man entered his 15th session saying, "I'm glad to be here." His mouth was in a frown, his eyes were frightened, and he slinked into the chair. During the previous session, they had agreed that the therapist would say little but instead allow the patient to speak without prompting and direction. The patient appeared to be expressing his ambivalence about the arrangement. He wanted help but feared being hurt by it. Intrapsychically, he described himself as being composed of a gnarled, ugly little gnome who bears the brunt of everyone's misery, and a rational agency that observed others in order to protect the gnome. The rational agency covered its hate for the gnome in gracious attempts to be useful.

Self–Other Boundaries Distortions

Listening to the manner in which patients describe themselves and observing one's own reactions to patients are two primary ways of noting self–other boundary weakness. Extremes of black-and-white thinking: "He's totally no good and she's absolutely the most marvelous always," may sometimes be significant statements. When patients actually seem to see no gray but only pure good or bad in many relationships, then their views of others are highly imperfect. This imperfection suggests a distorted notion of the self (Kernberg, 1975).

Patients may describe themselves as excessively dependent upon certain others, or extremely fearful of being hurt by others. These descriptions imply interpersonal fragility suggesting weak self–other boundaries. Close relationships may be highly dangerous, may explode self-definitions and lead to extreme psychological pain.

CASE 5.12. A 30-year-old graduate student in English had been married for 11 years. His wife mirrored his every mood. He believed that they felt together emotionally most of the time. Their life seemed like a minuet, each dancing gracefully, joyously to a tune only they heard. Then she announced that she was leaving him for another man. Her affair had been ongoing for a few years. He became suicidal. Without her as part of himself, he did not know who he was. He felt disembodied from reality and could feel nothing but a vast emptiness. He had been cut loose from his moorings. Apparently he had demanded that his wife reflect his every mood and she had agreed. The sudden rupture in her behavior temporarily broke the integrity of his self-concept, which had depended upon her. He was metaphorically bleeding his intrapsychic contents out of the rupture in his self-boundary.

Patients tend to cast their therapists in roles that complement their self-concepts. When therapists feel totally bored, evil, omniscient, or empty of feeling, they may be receiving clues that the patient's self–other boundary weaknesses are closing around the therapist.

THE DEEP UNCONSCIOUS

Visual imagery provides access to many aspects of psychic life (Singer & Pope, 1978) and is particularly useful for exploring the deeper layers of the unconscious.

For Freud and his followers, dreams were a royal road to the unconscious, because their expression was relatively unhampered by the censorship of ordinary consciousness. When patient and therapist met almost daily, written records of dreams seemed unnecessary and perhaps distorting. Jung also took great interest in dreams but asked his patients to record them soon after awakening, since details tend to be lost as ordinary reality intercedes. These recordings became dream books and allowed Jung and his patients to observe sequential changes in dream symbols and their meanings to the patient's life progression. Many other therapists have turned to dreams as a means to grasp the inner life of their clients, each molding these nocturnal productions into shapes fitting their theoretical predispositions. Despite the variety of theories into which dreams have been fit, a consistent approach to their analysis has emerged

(Beebe & Rosenbaum, 1975). The degree of emphasis given each step will vary with patient, therapist, and context.

1. Get a verbatim report of the entire dream (either by having the patient record it or by taking notes as the patient describes it).

2. Ask if any additional parts of the dream come to mind during or after the report.

3. Ask the patient to think about the dream, letting one thought lead to another while reporting the thought chain.

4. Select elements that stand out and ask the patient to associate freely to these emotions, symbols, and interactions. By so doing, the patient may capture the experiential richness of the dream and be able to report emotions that were not evident in the first report. These fresh emotions are likely to clarify the meaning of the associated dream elements. Perls (1969) requested his clients to pretend that they were each a dream element and to describe themselves as that element using the first person. In this way he evoked emotions associated with each element.

5. Attempt to define the events of the preceding day that seemed to trigger some of the dream symbols (day residue). Find elements of the dream that are also evident in the day event.

6. Ask the patient to interpret the meaning of the dream. "What do you think of all this? What does it mean to you?"

7. Offer some of the therapist's ideas about the dream — thoughts that came to mind as the patient was struggling to describe and understand it. Therapists should restrain the often compelling urge to report their associations since they may be based on too little information.

Perhaps the simplest instruction for gaining access to symbolic imagery is to ask for recurrent waking fantasies — those images that are part of the patient's daily mental life. Not only do people have repetitive nocturnal dreams but they may also have repetitive images while masturbating, daydreaming, or engaging in sexual intercourse. These fantasies may be analyzed as if they were dreams and may be followed over time to reflect changes in the patient's psyche, as illustrated by the following case.

CASE 5.13. One woman gained intense sexual pleasure from masturbation fantasies in which she was captured, tied with rope, sexually teased, and finally released to have intercourse. Gradually she became the person to dominate the other in her fantasies and later still, eliminated most of the power struggle except briefly during foreplay. This transformation reflected a growing sense of self-confidence and self-definition.

When Jung found his patients unable to report vivid, symbol-filled dreams, he suggested that they construct a scene from which to build imagery. He used the term "active imagination" because it "means that the images have a life of their own and that symbolic events develop according to their own logic — that is, of course, if your conscious reason does not interfere" (Jung, 1968, p. 192). He continued, "When we are careful not to interrupt the natural flow of events, our unconscious will produce a series of images which make a complete story" (p. 193).

"Active imagination" has been further developed through the invention of a variety of starting points for an imaginary sequence. As a group, they resemble Rorschach's inkblot tests, in that each starting point provides a stimulus into which each patient may project partial contents of his or her mind.

Schorr (1978) developed a series of images for investigating self-concept while Leuner (1978) developed a series of standard motifs or images designed to explore relatively deep layers of unconscious activity.

LINKING METHODS AND CONTENT
TO VISUAL DATA FILTERS

The major objective of the pattern search is to capture patterns with precision sufficient to define some set of thoughts and/or behaviors that if changed would lead to positive, desired resuls. The various types of listening, questions, homework, and role-playing assignments provide the raw data for this objective. These data are usually organized for presentation to the client. (I say "usually," because some therapists [e.g., Erickson, Rossi, & Rossi, 1976] do not present the patterns but simply prescribe ways around them. Under these conditions, the therapist alone is the one requiring a clear grasp of the set of thoughts and behaviors that if changed may lead to the desired results.)

Theories of psychopathology have provided many therapists with ways to organize their understanding of their clients' lives. Unfortunately, the conflicting terminologies, philosophies of existence, and deeply entrenched beliefs associated with many theories has made compromise difficult to reach. The ideological conflicts also indicate the uncertainty of our concepts of ourselves.

Two of the visual data filters described in Chapter 4 seem to stand out from the ideological and semantic confusion to offer psychotherapists useful, generic ways of organizing their data for presentation to their patients. S→O→R and DAF spirals are relatively free of ideology and appear to offer practical, universal, and flexible meta-patterns by which to organize other visual data filters and content areas.

The S→O→R template serves many different theories of psychopathology because much psychotherapeutic data is collected by asking questions linking a dysphoric emotion or maladaptive behavior to its immediate environmental–temporal correlates. Generally speaking it is fundamental to a functionalist (Hart, 1983) or pragmatic (Driscoll, 1984) approach. The BASIC I.D. directs therapists to fill in blanks along seven dimensions, each of which is linked to environmental antecedents and consequences. The cognitive therapy $A \rightarrow B \rightarrow C$ is a simplified variation on the theme through which Beliefs (automatic thoughts) are defined by identifying Activating events and their Consequences. The psychodynamic triangles also fit comfortably within the $S \rightarrow O \rightarrow R$ template because both the "current significant other" and the "therapist" legs of the person triangle direct therapist and patient to identify the interpersonal–behavioral consequences and intrapsychic defenses and thoughts triggered by interactions with these two stimuli.

The $S \rightarrow O \rightarrow R$ concept is but a slice through time, a photograph of an ongoing interaction between the self and the environment. In reality, each response or consequence acts as a stimulus for the next event leading often to a chain of reciprocal causation (see Figure 8). Each response may trigger either interpersonal or intrapsychic events that lead to further responses. Patients may not need to see the entire sequence. For therapists, multiple reciprocal causation may also be quite difficult to grasp. Patients appear to require from their therapists knowledge with sufficient detail to permit the confident application of effort leading to the possibility of desired change.

Sometimes patients and therapists get in each other's way as they approach this objective. The next chapter is concerned with these blocks.

Figure 8. An interaction spiral.

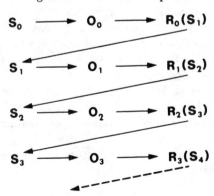

6. *Resistance to Pattern Identification*

Therapists usually bring to the therapeutic encounter some expectations of client behavior, but often, clients do not follow these expectations. Some of the common clashes between therapist expectations and client behavior during the pattern search will be outlined in this chapter.

The terms "resistance," "transference," and "countertransference" are psychoanalytic words that are central to psychoanalytic clinical theory. "Transference," particularly, has been accorded a great deal of psychoanalytic attention because it is the fulcrum around which the interpretative method turns. On the other hand, these terms are granted relatively little attention in the nonpsychodynamic approaches, almost as if the phenomena encompassed by them do not exist in nonpsychodynamic therapies. I take the moderate position between these two extremes. I assume that in conventional psychotherapeutic practice, patients bring to the therapeutic relationship interaction patterns characterizing their responses to intense, threatening, and/or provocative situations. These patterns have a variety of sources and may be triggered and shaped by a variety of forces. They appear as distortions to the therapeutic process because the patient appears to be failing to meet therapeutic expectations. These distortions, resistances, and blocks can be exceedingly useful to the conduct of therapy, especially for the pattern search, because they provide in-the-office, directly observable examples of some key behavior patterns.

One can conduct therapy with strict attention to distortions as samples of behavior, or one can conduct therapy thinking of distortions as nuisances that must be circumvented. To be able to do both requires recognizing when a resistance or transference reaction can be woven into the central aim of therapy and when it is so peripheral as to warrant being ignored.

In addition to blocking engagement-stage objectives, clients may also block pattern-search objectives. They may fail to carry out the specified data-gathering techniques by not doing homework assignments, by remaining silent, or by refusing to follow any of the many possible ways to gather information. They may bring interpersonal behavior patterns that seem completely unnecessary to the therapeutic task. These patterns may be associated with odd, unnerving, and inappropriate therapist emotions and behaviors. These therapist distortions can provide useful avenues of understanding, as suggested in the final section of this chapter.

GENERAL RESISTANCE TO PATTERN IDENTIFICATION

Hypotheses about the cause of a patient's resistances varies with the therapist's constructs about causes of psychological difficulty. If the therapist believes that psychological dysfunction is created by intrapsychic conflict or by automatic thoughts generated from underlying cognitive schemata, then the therapist will conclude that resistances originate within the mind of the patient. If the therapist believes that behavioral disorders are maintained by environmental contingencies, then he or she will conclude that resistances are caused by forces in the patient's environment (including the therapist). Since psychological dysfunction may be attributed to both internal and external influences, both inner and outer reality can be part of the problem. Furthermore, the pattern-search method selected by the therapist may predict whether intrapsychic or environmental causes are more likely. If the data is to be gathered by homework assignment, then environmental forces are more likely to be controlling variables. If the data is to be gathered by free association, then intrapsychic causes are more likely. However, this artificial boundary begins to shred whenever therapists contemplate the interaction between client perceptions of self in relationship to other and the behavior of others toward the client. Each influences the other. Selection of a "cause" simply provides the therapist with a place to start.

Resistances are often very frustrating to therapists, yet they usually represent the patient's best effort toward conforming to the expectations of therapy. This axiom is crucial because it encourages therapists to accept with understanding these often irritating phenomena.

Resistances may be classified into two groups: those related to the therapeutic objectives and those that are not. The division is ultimately dependent upon the therapist's predisposition to translate a resistance into a form correlated with the therapeutic focus. A patient's late arrival may, for some therapists, become the focus of an entire session, while, for others, an apology and its quick acceptance will be the limit of attention paid to it.

Lying on the borderline between goal-relevant and goal-irrelevant resistances are those apparently generated from misunderstandings by the patient of the therapist's expectations. The woman in Case 3.20, talked incessantly to the psychoanalyst Greenson because she was afraid he would criticize her for being silent. She demonstrated a misunderstanding of her role as patient apparently triggered by her previous psychoanalytic relationship. If one were to hypothesize that this misunderstanding fell on a mind ready to grasp it, then the therapist could hypothesize that this resistance indicated the character style of excessive compliance. Patients who refuse to role-play themselves with others or who refuse chair-doubling exercises with complaints of artificiality may misunderstand the purposes of the assignment. However, they may fear these exercises because they are actually too real (Wachtel, 1977). Patients who fail to do cognitive homework often present a technical excuse (I did not have time, I did not know how to answer the situation column). Each of these excuses reflects some underlying motivation to avoid the work of therapy and may be addressed. The person who did not have time may have wished, for example, to avoid showing his roommates that he had to do the exercise. What he meant was that he did not have enough time alone without fear of being discoverd. The person who did not know how to answer the situation column may not want to reveal, for example, those times when she struck her child.

In speaking of in-the-office resistances, Sullivan (1955) said:

> Following the introduction of the threatening subject, things don't go so well or so simply. The patient begins to use all manner of devices to avoid any four-square collision with the disturbing topic, and the instrumentalities available to the human for doing just this are often exceedingly impressive. But it is of such things as these that the practice of psychiatry [psychotherapy] is composed. They can be no more than subject matter for further observation and study. They are data. (p. 219)

This position is an option for all therapists confronted with a resistance. Is this a sample of the patient's behavior critically linked to the problems for which we are seeking solutions or is it simply a smoke screen to be penetrated and forgotten?

Resistance to Ground Rules

The basic ground rules of specified meeting time, length of session, frequency, and fee are potential stimuli for resistances. Any patient (or therapist) failure to follow these rules may often hide motivation relevant to the therapeutic endeavor. However, as one of my patients cleverly noted, rule violations may be too easily interpreted as patient psychopathology: "If you come too early, you're anxious about something. If you're late, you're hiding something. If you come on time, you're compulsive."

CASE 6.1. A 40-year-old divorced mother of two teenagers requested help from a new primary care physician because previous physicians were of no help. The new physician diagnosed panic attacks and started her on a low dose of imipramine. The following week, her symptoms were markedly improved. During the second meeting, they discussed her lack of social involvement. She then contacted old friends and enjoyed herself very much. She also became less focused on her somatic symptoms. During the third meeting, they further defined her social network. She was pleased with these discussions because "I never tell anyone about myself." Although her physician silently thought a month might be sufficient, she requested a return visit the following week. The patient appeared 30 minutes late for her fourth appointment, having previously shown up early. She stated that a friend had asked her for a ride and she could not refuse. The patient described another successful symptom-free week with good social contacts and felt that the next meeting should be in one month. The physician agreed.

The patient's late arrival could have reflected two related character problems. She could not refuse her friend the ride although she would be late. She might also have noticed that her physician did not want her to come back so quickly and feared having offended him. Together these hypotheses suggest a subservient, martyr, go-by-the-expectations-of-others character style that fit with other data. However, symptom remission was the main focus and therefore the analysis of the late arrival was not necessary.

Sometimes buses are late; bosses are demanding; accidents intercede; or children are sick. Reality does influence lateness or failure to arrive. One may become suspicious of the car running out of gas on the day of the appointment by following the sometimes circular reasoning that consequence is motivation (e.g., patient unconsciously did not put gas in the car *in order* to miss the session).

Patients may request changes in appointment times, decreases or increases in frequency or length of session. Each request carries both reality and latent messages. Few issues are as heavily charged as the fee question. Requests for devious arrangements are not uncommon. Arrangements to pay cash at a lower rate to help the therapist avoid income tax reporting while providing the patient still less outlay form part of the "underground economy." Are such requests psychotherapeutically legitimate, or are they tests of the therapist's corruptibility?

CASE 6.2. A 48-year-old man who had been in psychotherapy for 24 years requested that I reduce his fee after we had been meeting weekly for over 6 months. He claimed financial difficulty. I gave in because I felt I had been of little help to him. The patient interpreted my behavior as a statement that I believed I could no longer help him. We terminated shortly thereafter. He was correct.

The meaning of money to the patient is most crucial. Bruch (1974) offered the following two contrasting examples.

CASE 6.3. A young woman . . . was unusually nonserious, even playful about making use of the treatment time. She was a student teacher and her husband a graduate student, both on very low incomes. Accordingly she was charged the lowest fee at that time. . . . Later it was learned that she was the daughter of a very wealthy family. . . . On inquiry it was learned that she gave the doorman [at her parent's apartment] who called a taxi to take her to the clinic, a tip exactly equal to what she paid for her therapy sessions. (p. 14)

CASE 6.4. A foreign student, a displaced person who was without resources whatsoever and who supported himself as a hospital technician [did not make] it clear that this was night work of a few hours only. . . . [The fee] represented about half his income, and he lived at a poverty level but was too proud to mention it. (p. 14)

Gifts, telephone calls, requests for meetings outside the office, referrals by patients of friends or relatives for treatment, and requests for unindicated medications are a few of the many patient maneuvers deserving attention for possible data directly related to the patient's presenting problem (Langs, 1973).

Therapist vacations are sometimes powerful stimuli for patients. Usually, patients are not as disturbed by their own vacations as they are by their therapists' departures. Reactions can be extremely intense, leaving some susceptible people psychotic. For those patients who are deeply attached to their therapists and/or terribly vulnerable to thoughts of separation and loss, therapist vacations can be the source of quick and valuable data regarding the importance of abandonment.

Resistance to Self-Observer Alliance

Implicit in many therapeutic contracts is the assumption that the patient will tell the therapist crucial information and that the patient will organize this information according to the therapist's suggestions. Patients can be engaged in therapy, feel comfortable with the therapist, and yet be unwilling or unable to explore inner states (Dickes, 1975). This self-appraisal capacity has been labeled many ways: metacognition, experiencing versus observing ego, self-monitoring, self-corrective feedback, witnessing and reframing (Goldfried & Padawer, 1982). The failure to communicate about personal experience creates difficulty in the pattern search.

CASE 6.5. A 38-year-old woman had stabilized her mood and organized her life more effectively through the patient listening and understanding of her therapist. However, each time he attempted to comment on her experience, she became emotionally labile. She often ridiculed him, his mannerisms, and his words. These openings for his comment were rare since she skipped quickly from relevant introspection and behavioral reports to puns, jokes, and laughter. Confrontation of these resistances led to different smoke screens. If he suggested that her behavior in the office was similar to her behavior outside the office, she ridiculed the assumption that there was any connection between inside and outside. If he requested details of her interactions with others, she changed the subject. He became increasingly frustrated with her and often discharged his anger at her with quick verbal barbs or passive–aggressive acts (like failure to respond when necessary). He needed to surpass the combined patient-induced and therapist-induced countertransference reaction, to confront gently her fear of communicating with him about her experiences. The meaning of her resistance lay in her fear that any man would penetrate and destroy her if she let him into her psyche.

Resistance to Pattern-Search Methods

Patients often fail to respond to therapists' data-gathering instructions. Unless the instructions have been misunderstood, this failure often provides an opportunity to examine the patient's maladaptive responses. Therapists must be careful not to push too hard but rather to judge their clients' brittleness. Instead of pushing past the resistance, its examination is sometimes the more prudent course, as suggested by the following case.

CASE 6.6. A 20-year-old woman, who was self-supporting while living alone, remained deeply attached to her father. She was in therapy with a transactional analysis–Gestalt therapist who had recognized her reluctance to express negative emotions. He led her through some gestalt awareness exercises that quickly made her aware of the anger within her. But she did not want to experience this anger; nor to acknowledge its existence. She retreated into a "gray space" where she felt more comfortable. The therapist pressured her to get her in touch with her feelings. She touched upon that anger, became frightened, and left the session in tears. Shortly thereafter, she took an overdose of aspirin and was hospitalized. In the hospital, she described a sense of being tricked into experiencing her feelings. More importantly, she revealed her fear that she would lose control if she became angry, her fear of anger in other people, especially her father, and ultimately her fear of insanity. For these reasons, whenever she approached negative feelings, she became very anxious. Instead of pushing further with very effective awareness techniques, the therapist would better have shifted to increasing the patient's awareness of her fear of anger.

To shift from a data-gathering technique to examining the resistance as data requires nimble-mindedness. To accept the resistance as the patient's best compromise between internal and perceived external reality requires nonjudgmental acceptance, and the paradoxical belief that allowing the resistance to emerge into the forefront will likely aid in its solution.

NOT ALLOWING THE THERAPIST TO SPEAK

Sometimes patients will not allow their therapist to speak, as demonstrated in the following case.

CASE 6.7. A 28-year-old man was depressed about his marriage and his failure to complete his PhD thesis. Although he appeared insightful, he spoke incessantly and became very irritated whenever the therapist interrupted him. When he was confronted with his use of speech as a barrier to communication, he felt reproached. He became frightened that he might never be able to speak again. He revealed that his mother and maternal grandmother had used words to fight with others. Any disagreement carried the threat that one person might be annihilated. If he lost, he would become a non-person, but if he won, then the other person would be extinguished. He became immobilized with this unsolvable dilemma and simply kept talking to the therapist to avoid disagreements that might extinguish one or the other of them. (Bruch, 1974, pp. 136–137)

This resistance may also be called a transference reaction because the patient was transferring onto the therapist behavior and thought patterns characteristic of interactions with previous significant others. It might also be called a coping strategy, a character pattern, a security operation, or a role distortion.

REFUSING TO DO COGNITIVE HOMEWORK

Some patients are unable to carry out cognitive homework because they are unable to identify the emotions required to fill in the blanks of the triple column (Chapter 4). Others do not want the therapist to know certain weekly activities. Some simply do not want to think about the fact that they are in therapy while they are out of the office. They prefer to have the therapist do the work with little outside cooperation from them.

REFUSING ROLE PLAYING

Role playing may not only be too much like reality but also may evoke uncomfortable thoughts and emotions. The refusal to participate in these often useful exercises sometimes reflects fears of being controlled by the therapist, who usually must direct the proceedings.

ATTACKING THERAPIST'S QUESTIONS AND/OR EMPATHIC STATEMENTS

Both questions and empathic statements are attempts to burrow beneath the surface of the patient's surface presentation. People who repel these efforts are generally very afraid of being hurt, controlled, penetrated, or unduly influenced.

READING THERAPIST'S NONVERBAL RESPONSES
AND IGNORING VERBAL ONES

Patients with poor self boundaries tend to listen to therapist's tone of voice, gestures, and body movements rather than his or her words. This interpersonal focus can be very frustrating for therapists searching for words to help. Many of these patients have been taught by experience to distrust words and to place more reliance on crude interpretations of nonverbal cues. Many also realize how disconcerting this form of interpersonal tracking can be to the speaker.

TAKING ALCOHOL OR DRUGS BEFORE SESSIONS

Mind altering chemicals reduce each patient's ability to report crucial daily events and to remember the content and purpose of therapy. No doubt the patient who uses drugs before a psychotherapy session also uses them under other anxiety-provoking situations. The place of alcohol and drugs in the lives of such patients may be explored to define other anxiety-provoking situations that require chemical mind alteration.

Resistance to Pattern-Search Content

Clients may fail to report classes of personal information relevant to personal change. They may emphasize the past, work, heterosexual relationships, emotions, future plans, or the therapeutic relationship to the exclusion of other areas. Therapists may have to scan content categories to decide what is missing and why. No scanning is required to understand what the silent patient is omitting. These people can frustrate most psychotherapists whose procedure relies so heavily on verbal communication. During my first and only encounter with a completely silent client, I acted out my anger by reading while she sat with me. I failed to simply sit with her and accept her as she was. Rogers described a situation in which the therapist responded differently:

CASE 6.8. The client was a high school student whose words during many sessions could have been recorded on a small piece of paper. The therapist simply attempted to be with her. Nevertheless, teachers and advisors noticed that she had changed markedly since beginning therapy, culminating with her election as "Woman of the Month" by the girls of her high school. The therapist had simply tried to stay with her. (Rogers, 1951, pp. 158–159)

Periods of prolonged silence may have many meanings and often possess great emotional power. According to Winnicott, the patient may need to be "alone in the presence of someone" (quoted in Morgenstern, 1980, p. 251). In the following case reported by Morgenstern, a 30-year-old pediatrics resident remained silent for 25 of 30 sessions.

CASE 6.9. She had sought help to limit the bitterness she felt whenever friends moved away. Most pertinent to her history was the manner of her father's death 2½ years earlier. During the last few days of his life, he enveloped himself in a silent curtain that the patient could not penetrate. At first the therapist accepted her need to be silent, but during sessions 21 to 25, he became anxious to bring therapy "to life." He saw this desire as a recapitulation of the patient's efforts to bring her father back from his dead silence. The patient had induced him to sit with her silence as she had to sit with the silence of her father. The therapist described this role reversal to the patient. A few sessions after the interpretation, the patient agreed. Subsequently, she experienced greater personal independence and was able to commit herself to a heterosexual relationship. (pp. 252–255)

Some patients tend to act rather than use words to describe their situations. Therapists must decide whether the action is a resistance or a good experiment. For example, if a man coming to therapy because of marital discord became frightened about discussing his premature ejaculation, he might precipitously separate from his wife. He might then claim that he had solved his marital difficulty and no longer needed treatment.

In the treatment of severely disturbed patients, therapists may confront the emergence of psychotic thinking. Paranoid delusions and the activation of forgotten but disturbing memories are likely contents. These breakthroughs in the "repression barrier" may be considered resistances but they are also "minipsychotic" episodes characteristic of some borderline patients (Brinkley, Beitman, & Friedel, 1979; Gunderson & Singer, 1975).

CASE 6.10. A 25-year-old prostitute who had made multiple suicide attempts sought therapy for pervasive dysphoria. In the middle of therapy, I asked her parents to come to an interview despite her protests to their coming. For many nights after the family interview, she was plagued with vivid memories of the times her parents had been called to see the school principal because of her bad conduct. She was terrified by her inability to forget these intensely negative experiences. This response greatly impeded the progress of therapy.

This resistance was elicited by a technical change, and, while it had fundamental significance, was triggered by my change of format. Therapists must look for their contributions to treatment blocks.

PATTERN-SEARCH TRANSFERENCE

As he explored the unconscious minds of early psychoanalytic patients, Freud was often perplexed by their tendencies to subvert his explorations with silence or trivia. He gradually concluded that these resistances could often be linked to thoughts and feelings about him. These responses seemed to have evolved from early family relationships and were transferred onto him. In this way "transference" provided Freud and his followers a view of early parent–child relationships in the way that an archaeologist's examination of artifacts provides a view of earlier times. Glover in 1937 illustrated the extreme to which this perspective has been taken: "An adequate conception of the transference must reflect the totality of the individual's development . . . he displaces onto the analyst not merely affect and ideas but all he has even learnt or forgotten throughout his mental development" (quoted in Sandler, Dare, & Holder, 1970a, p. 670).

Freud was less interested in developing a psychotherapy than he was in designing a research procedure by which to explore mental functioning. He was seeking a theory of personality. The psychoanalytic setting and ground rules are exquisitely formulated to foster the emergence of the patient's interpersonal distortions. The almost daily visits make the analyst a regular part of the analysand's life. The out-of-sight listener provides fewer reality checks, because facial expressions and bodily movements are not available for feedback. With minimal verbal emissions from the therapist, the patient lacks another reality check — words and their communicative feeling tones. Lying down reduces the analysand's field of vision and mobility, makes him or her "shorter" than the therapist, and apparently more vulnerable. Encouragement of fantasy and dream reports stimulates the more distorted aspects of the patient's thinking, while reinforcement of reports concerning childhood experiences reactivates the immature feelings associated with earlier periods of development. Transference interpretations highlight the analyst's interest in past–present distortions and define his or her role as an object of future distortions. Some analysts believe that most analysand utterances are in some way statements about the analyst, a belief that places them in a paranoid position (everything he says is about me) and a grandiose position (I'm so important that he is consumed with reactions to me) (Langs, 1973, 1974; Malan, 1979). These analysts probably indirectly communicate this role expectation to their analysands, thereby helping to fulfill the prophecy.

On the other hand, transference reactions may be blunted by a number of techniques: irregular, brief meetings; elicitation of reality-based and problem-oriented content, rapid correcting or ignoring of interpersonal distortions; and clear expression of the therapist's real self and values. Despite these efforts, transference distortions may persist because each psychotherapist represents a powerful stimulus to unconscious yearnings for psychological transformation.* The hope for pain relief, for inti-

---

*This point was brought home to me during the forced terminations created by my leaving Seattle, Washington, for Columbia, Missouri. Of 20 patients being forced to terminate, four required hospitalization within the 4 months between the announcement of my

mate self-revelation, for compassion and concern, for an ultimate rescuer begins in each human mind with the parent archetype into which many therapists are unconsciously fitted. Therefore, the therapist's appearance, behavior, tone of voice, and words are likely to be amplified in the patient's mind, resonating with previous experiences of people offering similar possibilities. The image of the therapist can then become confused with those other images, thereby creating responses that distort the therapist's person and purpose.

Transference distortions may be short- or long-lived and may have many different sources. After engagement, with the establishment of trust in the therapist, patients become increasingly susceptible to using previous interpersonal constructs in interpreting the actions of their therapists. These older attitudes are often misapplied, but are used because they have apparently been effective. They may reflect key intrapsychic and interpersonal problems, some of which reflect deeply disturbed personalities. Some are derived from previous therapy experiences or are triggered by events outside or inside the therapy office. Some are realistic reactions to inappropriate, neurotic behavior of the therapist. To be useful to therapists, these distortions must be anticipated, noted, and described. Some will be directly relevant to the therapeutic task, while others will require little attention. Some will tell therapists a great deal about themselves. Following is a brief catalogue of the many types of blocks to therapeutic progress attributable to the patient's distortion of the therapist during the pattern search.

Key Interpersonal and Intrapsychic Patterns

As the engagement progresses, patients tend to maneuver the therapist into roles that characterize their relationships to others and to themselves. Each therapist's first responsibility is to avoid becoming deeply enmeshed in the patient's role-induction efforts. For the purposes of the pattern search, these efforts are often remarkably revealing about the patient's interpersonal and intrapsychic makeup, but only if the therapist is able to escape their influence and observe the patterns. Countertransference reactions can also impede or aid each therapist's vision. The following case illustrates some of these points.

---

going and my actual departure. Three were being seen less than 30 minutes per month. The fourth had been seen weekly but with long stretches of no visits as well. All four were taking psychoactive medications prescribed by me. Each was grateful for my help and was terrified of relapse with my departure.

CASE 6.11. A 45-year-old manic-depressive woman at first refused to accept lithium treatment until she had been deeply depressed twice more after my initial evaluation. Her character style during the engagement was rapid, flippant, "gamey" sexuality by which she attempted to avoid self-revelation. After numerous confrontations on her "games," she initiated more subtle ones. When she finally accepted lithium treatment some 12 months later, her avoidance manipulations were dramatically reduced. In fact, she felt herself as "empty," with nothing underneath those attractive, socially effective facades. She complained about how her deceased husband had controlled her, how she felt empty and worthless without a man, although she ran her own business reasonably well. She described how at age 16 her father had tried to stop her from marrying, but she persisted in entering the relationship. She was beaten and then deserted. Years later while in psychotherapy, she entered a new relationship that most of her friends told her would be destructive. She cast me in the role of her friends, encouraging me to tell her that she should stay away from the man, who did jilt her. She took an overdose of diazepam (Valium) supplied by her primary care physician. At the time of the overdose, I had not yet seen that I was being placed in the role of her father, who had tried to stop her marrying at age 16. She became involved with another man, who assumed the role of lay therapist for her manic-depressive illness, and induced him to suggest that she stop therapy. My jealousy and competitive feelings signaled again her attempt at repetition of the adolescent triangle.

Interpersonally, the patient was repeating a familiar role, and intrapsychically, she was avoiding responsibility for the effects of her actions. She seemed to prefer that her men be responsible, so that she could blame them for what happened to her. When this formulation was presented to her with direct evidence from her sexual relationships, she perceived quite clearly the pattern needing to be relinquished.

This complementarity between intrapsychic and interpersonal explanations may also be illustrated in the following case:

CASE 6.12. A 20-year-old woman living at home with her parents described long-standing fears of disappointing her mother. She tried desperately to live up to her mother's expectations of her. She also described the many different ways her mother had failed to live up to her (the client's) minimal expectations. She very carefully scrutinized her therapist's behavior to see what she expected from her as well.

From an intrapsychic perspective, the patient could have been denying her own disappointment with her mother and projecting that disappointment onto herself by believing that her mother was disappointed in her. She therefore would feel that she must reduce her mother's disappointment. In other words, the feeling she perceived in her mother was her own feeling. From an interpersonal perspective, the patient could simply have been attempting to fill her mother's expectations. But were they really her mother's expectations? How did she know? And if they were, must she continue to follow them? The end necessity from both perspectives is to examine her mother's expectations very carefully to see how much is her own misperception and how much is accurate reading.

Deeply Disturbed Personalities

Many patients presenting themselves for psychotherapy do not possess clearly definable interpersonal patterns for intimate relationships. Instead, they are adapted to superficial social relationships but become chaotic once interpersonal distance begins to close. Egalitarian therapists are likely to be fooled by many of these superficially intact people and will be surprised and frustrated by the confusion lying beneath the facade. The thinner the facade, the more quickly do the underlying faulty perceptions and intense emotions emerge. These stimuli can prove very disturbing to therapists as illustrated by the borderline patient described in Chapter 3 (see Case 3.25). Rather than becoming a here-and-now representation of a parent, the therapist comes to represent often more sinister and powerful forces. The variations are myriad but the underlying elements are relatively constant. Deeply disturbed persons are often furious at therapists for not caring enough, for not doing enough, and often terrified of their power to annihilate or to heal. They may challenge the therapist's ability to hold onto his or her own self image as therapist and person. They may want to merge with the therapists to be either fully controlled or to control fully. Commonly the therapist is either placed on the pedestal and idealized as the all-good, all-powerful, ultimate rescuer or is depreciated as an incompetent, malicious, or irrelevant leech. The less disturbed the patient, the less intense the extremes.

Deeply disturbed patients say and do many deeply disturbing things. One wrote notes of rage and suicide in her own blood and sent them to her therapist. Some purchase homes near their therapist's office or home. Many ride by their therapist's houses. They may threaten to kill therapist's children, to destroy the therapist's office, to initiate lawsuits for malpractice, to refuse to leave the session. They may rage at the therapist for the entire hour or series of hours, or make obscene phone calls to the therapist's home, or demand to be seen in the middle of the night. They may make sexual advances in the office. They may kill themselves.

The following case illustrates a transference from a patient on the more extreme side of the "deeply disturbed" continuum. Superficially she was well adapted.

CASE 6.13. A 32-year-old divorced mother of four had been hospitalized twice for psychotic episodes and had recently terminated with her previous therapist because "he made sexual advances toward me." In the first session, she accused her male therapist of having a sexual interest in her. She said that she could see he had an erection and that the movement of his hands meant he was ready to enter her. Over the subsequent sessions, she interpreted any movement by him as an indicator of sexual readiness. He decided to hold as still as possible. Then she proclaimed that she had total control over his body and over the next few sessions, stopped talking about his sexual interest. Then she claimed she was pregnant with his baby and during the subsequent months went through labor and delivery in her fantasies. She then became the baby and wanted to be raised by him. During the entire course of treatment, she refused neuroleptic medication and remained superficially adapted in her life. She had, however, told her relatives and the clinic receptionist that she was having sex with her doctor.

This patient's distortions of the person of the therapist could serve as projective tests for therapists of varying theoretical predispositions. Her sexual and aggressive drives were baldly exposed. Her desire to control the other out of fear of being controlled by the other is obvious. The attribution of her own sexual and aggressive strivings to the therapist while denying these feelings and instead reacting to the therapist as if those feelings were his, may be another explanation of the interaction.* She also demonstrated the tendency for deeply disturbed people to dichotomize relationships into either–or, good–bad categories. The less disturbed the patient, the less extreme the dichotomizing, usually because less disturbed people are more able to see themselves as distinct from the therapist.

---

*Although I seriously doubt the possibility, the therapist could have had sex with her. More likely, she interpreted his professional–personal willingness to be involved (which may have had a sexual tinge to it) as sexual desire.

CASE 6.14. A 24-year-old graduate student sought therapy because he had had two homosexual encounters but did not want to enter the homosexual life-style. He felt more sexually attracted to men, enjoyed their bodies more fully, and liked their sexual handling of him. However, society would make life more difficult for him as a homosexual, and he found himself wanting to raise a family. After a few sessions, he reported believing that I was thinking about him most of the time as if I were perched on his shoulder watching his life. During therapy he rambled on about his experiences as if I was there only to listen to him. He had conceptually enveloped my personality into his own and was using me as a part of himself (a self-object).

This patient's self–other boundaries were less disturbed than those of the erection-perceiving woman of Case 6.13. He could at least distinguish my selfness more accurately although he did subsume me under himself. Yet closer to the better functioning end of the continuum are the "twinning" transferences described by Kohut (1968). The patient perceives the therapist as separate yet identical to him or her. Said one patient to me, "I come here and I feel as if I am more alive because you affirm myself by agreeing with me. I know you will affirm me because you and I are very much alike." In the other least disturbed of Kohut's narcissistic transferences, the "mirroring" patient holds the therapist as separate but believes that the therapist exists only to gratify the patient's needs for approval, reward, and recognition.

CASE 6.15. A 35-year-old artist was working feverishly on his sculpting but refused to show it to anyone. Instead he kept waiting until "it was good enough." Nevertheless, he would show his wife partially completed pieces and insist that she acknowledge their potential greatness. His wife was mildly interested in art and found herself unable to evaluate his work with any confidence. The patient became very frustrated with her. He also attempted to enlist his therapist's approval by bringing in photographs of his work and going on at length about the details of his efforts. He quit therapy when he was unable to elicit approving responses from the therapist.

Expectations from Previous Therapists

Experiences with previous therapists socialize people to the role of patient. A man who thought all therapists were deceitful (Case 3.16) was betrayed by his first of 10 therapists. That person had promised him that they would meet regularly for 1 year, but after 3 months told the patient, without explanation, that the next session would be their last. This man brought that expectation, bolstered apparently by his own sense of inner betrayal, unresolved by his long line of therapists, into all subsequent psychotherapy relationships. A young woman entered therapy thinking that I would talk to her about myself during the major part of our time together. Her previous therapist, who had been in the midst of divorce, had found a comforting ear in this person–patient and subverted the therapeutic process for his own benefit. She also preferred to listen rather than to reveal negative aspects of herself. On the other hand, previous therapists may also accelerate the therapeutic process by having properly prepared the person for the role of patient.

Unresolved termination problems in a previous therapy may spill over into the next one. The case of the betrayed man mentioned above is illustrative. Other problems include an idealization of the lost therapist accompanied by depreciation of the present therapist, leading to a resistance to reengagement. Anger at the loss of the previous therapist may be displaced onto the new therapist. Simply adjusting to a difference in style may stagnate the new relationship.

Nonpsychotherapeutic physicians may influence patient expectations of psychotherapists, especially when the patient is referred by a biomedical physician. Some come with the clear belief that "whatever the doctor says, I will do" — an idea that medical practitioners like to have their patients believe but not usually what psychotherapists want. Any previous sexual encounter with helping professionals will also color the following psychotherapy.

Case 6.16. A 32-year-old woman was unable to relax during the first psychotherapy session with her new therapist. After the therapist confronted her anxiety, she recognized the problem. Her previous therapist had hypnotized her and made sexual advances toward her while she was in a trance.

External Circumstances and Events

External circumstances can strongly influence patient responses to therapists. An isolated person is likely to depend more heavily upon the therapist's warmth and kindness than are those with social support. Isolated persons are also more likely to show wider swings in their out-of-office moods and behavior as a function of their perceived criticism or acceptance by the therapist. External changes and losses may force any patient to seek greater support from their therapists. Death of an important person, finalizing a divorce, work or relationship failure, and other similar events may serve to exaggerate dependent transference reactions.

Expectable Events of Therapy

Many of the ordinary, expectable events of therapy may trigger interpersonal distortions or exaggerate them. Emotionally charged therapy experiences, for example, may exaggerate transference reactions.

CASE 6.17. A 50-year-old woman with a history of three psychotic episodes but with periods of excellent functioning during most of her life spoke with me, her third therapist, about the painful thoughts associated with her mother's death. Her chosen profession as a nurse in a kidney dialysis unit was in part an unconscious reaction to her anger at the technological limitations of medicine at the time her mother had died of kidney failure. She had come to recognize that each patient she helped through dialysis, especially those who went on to successful kidney transplants, were brief momentary victories over the forces of death that had claimed her mother. However, whenever she recalled the experiences surrounding her mother's death, she became deeply agitated, tearful, and unable to return to work. She became furious with me for "forcing" her into the grief work she had requested and terminated therapy because I was being "vicious" to her. After another psychotic episode, while her subsequent therapist was on vacation, she called me for medications. I was able to interpret for her the abandonment anger she felt at her therapist's leaving her. I also suggested that her paranoid ideation about a plot between him and me against her was a screen for her continuing anguish about her mother's death. Upon resuming therapy with her therapist, she discussed her mother's death with him. She again called me to tell me that she was "forced" into grief work and that she hated her current therapist for treating her so cruelly. Her rage had many sources. She was angry at her mother for abandoning her; at herself for not saving her mother's life; and at the medical profession that her therapist symbolized. She opted once again to discontinue therapy, only to return again to do battle for her own psychological freedom from the horror of her past.

In a less complicated example, a 26-year-old student who was terribly afraid of exposing his very vulnerable, internal, emotional "child" allowed that part of himself to be exposed and touched in therapy. For the next few weeks, he was in love with me for allowing him to experience this precious part of himself.

Although the therapeutic contract is ideally never altered (Langs, 1973), in actual practice, changes in its details often take place. Any of the following alterations may trigger or enhance transference distortions: raising or lowering the fee, increasing or decreasing meeting frequency or length, shifts in appointment time, telephone interruptions, therapist vacations, or perceived breaches in ethics or confidentiality. Sometimes patients perceive these shifts correctly — as manifestations of countertransference reactions. These realistic triggers to exaggerated patient responses reflect distortion of the therapist's perceptions of the patient rather than the patient's distortions of the therapist.

Transference Triggered by Apparently Insignificant Therapist Behaviors

In the ordinary conduct of their professional activity, therapists may be surprised to witness very intense patient responses to apparently insignificant therapist behaviors. These behaviors may stimulate sensitive psychic areas that lead them to confuse the past and the present. Apparently appropriate silence may trigger quick anger because, upon examination, the patient's father used a similar tactic as punishment. Raising my voice once triggered a patient to cry. She reported that the image of her abusive, loud father had appeared in her mind. Fromm-Reichmann (1961) described a young woman who told her analyst of plans to go to a party. Pleased with this progress, the therapist said "fine." At the next interview the patient reported that she had not gone to the party because the therapist said "fine" exactly the way her mother would say it (p. 103).

Rather than attempting to avoid transference triggers, therapists must anticipate their occurrence and be ready to integrate them into further understanding of the patient's interpersonal distortions.

Countertransference-Induced Transference

Therapists are fallible, imperfect creatures. We make errors; at times we are ignorant of our own interpersonal motivations; sometimes we ignore our feelings; we may blame others for our own difficulties. Therapists sometimes enact their own psychological difficulties on the patient and then blame the patient for his or her odd reaction by calling it transference. The following is an example of a therapist's not so subtle abuse of his patient.

CASE 6.18. A 30-year-old male therapist had seen a 38-year-old, depressed, homosexual man for five sessions. The patient was uncomfortable and irritable during the sixth session; he was talking about termination. The therapist interpreted his desire to leave therapy as a fear of coming too close to another man, despite the patient's claims to the contrary. There were, however, some realistic reasons for the patient's discomfort with the therapist. First, the patient was being charged a fee although he was a member of a health plan permitting him free access to any of the hospital's services. Second, the therapist had quickly asked the patient if he was sexually attracted to him, thereby demonstrating his ignorance of homosexual attractiveness. (The patient had replied, "Are you sexually attracted to all women?") Although the patient did have trouble with intimacy, he was more likely reacting to the therapist's financial exploitation and lack of understanding.

Patients have a greater influence on therapist behavior than is commonly recognized (Singer & Luborsky, 1977). They can elicit from therapists odd behavior that may have little to do with the therapist's own neurotic patterns. If a patient induces a therapist to respond in odd ways that then trigger the patient to respond in yet odder ways, then the patient is introducing a deviation that is amplified by the therapist's responses to which the patient then responds, thereby continuing a vicious cycle. This cycle may then stabilize at a new nontherapeutic interaction pattern, usually becoming a stalemate, sometimes spiraling into tragedy.

The following case illustrates a not uncommon sequence fostered by inexperience. Briefly, a therapist invests him or herself in the successful outcome of therapy with a deeply disturbed person, suddenly finds him or herself enmeshed, and then abruptly tries to break the intense connection.

CASE 6.19. The 18-year-old woman entered therapy with multiple shifting somatic symptoms, uncontrollable laughter and crying, and unremitting abdominal pain, all of which began shortly after she left home to attend college. She was considered a "problem child"; all developmental stages had been stormy. Within the first 3 weeks of therapy with a psychiatric resident, her somatic symptoms disappeared. The transference was very positive, eroticized, and intense. The patient expressed a desire to displace all of the therapist's other patients.

During the first several months, the patient displayed a wide variety of antisocial symptoms, but gradually it became apparent that she genuinely wanted to be "good" in order to gain the love of the therapist. In time she decided that being "good" included having a steady job, not having indiscriminate sex or taking illicit drugs, and only being "appropriately rebellious." During the ensuing months, she looked "as if" she were any other young adult female secretary in a metropolitan office. The transference relationship continued on in an intense, positive, and deeply dependent basis. Gradually she revealed her wish to merge with the therapist through the following fantasy: She wished to be physically attached to the therapist, perhaps with epoxy cement and carried about with him forever.

In part, the therapist's own omnipotent fantasies were coming true. This very disturbed person had made a startling recovery and no overt psychotic thinking or behavior could be observed outside the transference. The therapist decided to encourage the patient to date and offered to ask her friends and family to fix her up with nice men. In retrospect, the therapist was reacting against the deep enmeshment he experienced with the patient.

Although she responded positively to the suggestion, in the next interview she was overtly depressed. She became circumstantial, tangential, and rambling. She then made a suicide gesture and was readmitted to the hospital, at which time she was grossly psychotic. The patient subsequently made it clear that she felt the therapist's discussion about dating was an attempt to get rid of her. She then demanded physical affection from the therapist (to hug her) and when this was not forthcoming, made another suicide attempt in her therapist's office. (Stone, 1971, pp. 22–24)

Recognizing Transference

DIRECT DISTORTIONS

The distortion of the person and purpose of the therapist is sometimes clear, direct, and obvious. Patients may request meetings outside the office, suggest a business deal, hint at sexual liaisons, offer a gift, idealize or depreciate the therapist. They may also report fantasies about the therapist. More commonly, transference distortions are latent in the patient's dreams, speech, and/or actions.

LATENT DISTORTIONS

In order to hear transference references, therapists must have some predisposition toward poetry, toward the metaphorical and analogical. Without this "right brain" way of listening, transference illusions will be lost. Why do patients speak about their therapists as Shakespeare's characters often spoke to each other? Why not speak directly, precisely, clearly? This question is difficult to answer. Part of the solution is that people often do not know their minds, do not know why they are saying what, do not know what they are feeling or thinking. Sometimes they are afraid to speak directly but can't help expressing what they are feeling. Metaphorical speech may then be a compromise between saying the feared words and hiding them. The careful listener may decipher true meaning. In the following example, had the therapist been listening for latent content, he might have intervened to prevent premature termination. At the end of the session, the patient declared that he would not return. He did not.

CASE 6.20. A 24-year-old man began his videotaped 16th session with a first year psychiatric resident by talking about a party at his house and how "I always manage to get myself in the center of attention." (He may have been referring to the camera and its potential audience.) He then said that he did not like being onstage and that he was going to stop seeing his woman companion (Linda). He ended the session by saying that he would not return to therapy. Therefore Linda appears to have been an analogue for the therapist. The therapist reported that he had been very directive with the patient, "He was one of my favorites, I was like his guru." Further evidence for the Linda–therapist analogue had come when the patient had stated his reasons for not seeing her. "It's a negative experience walking with her because she doesn't walk with you. . . . She'll just choose to cross the street at a point which I would not choose to cross the street. . . . She's very domineering in the way she walks. . . . One time it was like she was dragging me through the streets, you know, by the hair." (Both Linda and the therapist were highly directive.) A little later, the patient had stated that the only reason he went to her house that day was to get some marijuana. (He was also receiving medications from the therapist.) The patient had followed that possible parallel with a description of the relationship he hoped to have with Linda (and his therapist?): "When you establish a relationship with someone, I imagine that there is some work to be done and something to be accomplished, a mutual complement of one another's growth, especially in a relationship as intimate as the one I thought I may have had with Linda." Knowledge of this possible parallel, listening with a "third ear" for latent content, for indirect indications of termination, might have helped to prevent it or at least have helped the therapist to be less startled by the abrupt ending.

In the case above, how can one be certain that the patient was talking about the therapist? How does one know the proper interpretation of poetry? One looks at the context; one gathers corollary information to illuminate the symbols. In this case, multiple parallels between "Linda" and the therapist suggested that "Linda" was also a symbol for the therapist. One can, however, operate under a somewhat related assumption and come to the same conclusion. One may assume that the patient constructs his relationship with the therapist in the same ways that he constructs his relationship with others. Therefore, what he is doing with Linda may parallel what he is doing with the therapist.

RESISTANCE

Any failure to follow the ground rules of therapy or to subvert therapeutic progress may have its roots in a transference distortion. Talk of suicide often masks anger at the therapist; idle talk may mask sexual desires; silence may often blanket fears of the therapist's criticism and rejection.

"ACTING OUT"

The psychoanalytic term "acting out" literally means acting out a conflict instead of speaking or reflecting it.* Acting out of transference means enacting with another person the transference distortions toward the therapist. Thus, monitoring relationships outside the office may offer useful feedback about the nature of the therapeutic relationship. A patient in love with his therapist may have many affairs or enter a hasty marriage rather than discuss his feelings toward his therapist. A patient angry at her therapist may instead displace that anger onto her husband. On the other hand, positive developments in interpersonal relationships may reflect well on the psychotherapeutic relationship.

CASE 6.21. A 40-year-old woman with highly erotic fantasies about me early in therapy was deeply frightened about them because she feared that she would be unable to control them. She had been deeply hurt by her ex-husband and was terrified of intimacy with men. Gradually she became more relaxed in therapy by hiding behind a socially pleasant screen that broke down only through questions and severe work or social pressure. After 18 months of 30-minute once per week contacts, she described a platonic smooth relationship she had not mentioned before. Using the hypothesis that patients act out their relationships with their therapists, the patient was possibly stating indirectly that she was becoming more comfortable with me.

---

*The term "acting out" has come to be used more broadly to refer to any undesirable patient behavior.

PATTERN-SEARCH COUNTERTRANSFERENCE

Patients invariably attempt to induce therapists to respond to them, in ways that reflect their characteristic interpersonal distortions. Often these patterns are so subtle that they bypass the therapist's own conscious awareness and therefore emerge into the therapist's experience as an uncomfortable emotion, a set of inappropriate thoughts, or a series of inappropriate behaviors and techniques. Acknowledgment of this possibility can offer additional understanding of the ongoing intrapsychic and interpersonal patterns defining the patient's basic psychological difficulties.

In order to identify these influences accurately, therapists must be willing to accept their own vulnerability to patient influence. Furthermore, therapists are required to accept the possibility that their own psychological difficulties may play a part in generating their inappropriate reactions. Once the therapist's personal contributions to countertransference reactions are acknowledged, then the patient's influence may be more accurately defined.

One must be careful not to label all therapist responses as indications of countertransference because too great attention to everything the therapist does can lead to the conclusion that every response has a countertransference element. Therapeutic caring, empathic understanding, proper technique, previous clinical experiences, and theoretical knowledge can all contribute to non-countertransference-based responses. On the other hand, therapists must avoid the temptation to go to the extreme of blaming the patient for all their own odd and exaggerated responses to their patients. Each countertransference reaction probably contains some contribution from the therapist's own psyche; the degree or percentage of influence is critical (Beitman, 1983b).

Therapist-Induced Countertransference

Therapist-induced reactions have many sources. Classical countertransference has its source in the therapist's transference to the patient. The therapist reacts as if the patient represented someone from his or her past, as illustrated in the following example.

CASE 6.22. A 30-year-old woman therapist was treating a 60-year-old depressed man who had prostate cancer. She had difficulty with his statements about liking younger women and was confused by his mild but persistent sexual advances toward her. She was afraid to confront him on his sexual interest in her, fearing that he would terminate therapy.

On the other hand, she knew she needed to confront him in order to keep therapy moving. She remained paralyzed by these contradictory injunctions and, eventually, the patient slipped away from therapy, never to return. In discussing this case with a colleague, the therapist realized that although she knew that this man in some way resembled her deceased father, who was seductive toward her and had died of prostate cancer, she had not realized how much the similarity had paralyzed her. Among the possible interpretations were her wish for sexual contact and her fear of being reminded of his death. (Beitman, 1983b, p. 85)

There are many other sources of countertransference. Therapists may have "blind spots" about certain content and may fail to let certain ideas or emotions into their minds. Together patient and therapist may collude to avoid important areas of concern.

CASE 6.23. A financially troubled therapist had engaged a 28-year-old woman who was supported by investments made by her wealthy father. The therapist envied this woman's financial freedom and failed to address her complaints that therapy was too expensive, although the patient easily took spur-of-the-moment airplane trips to distant cities and purchased expensive clothing on a whim. When the therapist caught this blind spot, she uncovered the tremendous power the patient's father held over her with his threats of withdrawing support if she did not do as he requested. The subsequent discussion led to a much sharper understanding of this patient's underlying fear of displeasing her father and how her hatred of him was displaced onto other men.

Not only do the past and blind spots about such subjects as money, rage, homosexuality, and sexual attraction lead to countertransference reactions, but so do current professional and personal events. Training programs influence therapist reactions to patients through individual supervision, didactics, and program structure. Therapists who are angry at their work loads as trainees or who are fearful of criticism by supervisors may transfer their negative reactions to therapy patients.

Personal changes characterize not only patients but therapists as well. Therapists marry, divorce, become pregnant, are promoted, and experience grief when loved ones die. These life changes may affect therapeutic relationships indirectly or perhaps directly as suggested by the following case.

CASE 6.24. A therapist assumed that his psychotic patient needed information about his grieving for a loved one because of her shaky reality testing. He believed she must have noticed his changed demeanor. Therefore, he told her some details. The patient experienced the therapist's revelation as an overwhelming demand that she care for him, an experience that recapitulated her major childhood relationships. The revelation derailed therapy and led to a premature termination. The therapist later realized that he had needed to be cared for and had also wanted to deflect her rage at his emotional unavailability. (Givelber & Simon, 1981, p. 144)

Patient-Induced Countertransference

Once the therapist's contribution to a countertransference reaction is clearly identified, the patient's contribution may be examined. The therapist's distorted, personal response may then become a form of empathy.

CASE 6.25. A 34-year-old junior high English teacher was referred with the diagnosis of pedophilia made by a previous psychiatrist. He was unable to continue seeing that psychiatrist after four sessions because the patient's girlfriend was also in therapy with that psychiatrist for a long-standing character problem. The patient belonged to a fundamentalist religion which taught that sex before marriage was sinful. Although the patient had not engaged in intercourse with his girlfriend, he felt guilty for having experimented with naked sexual contact with her, his first such contact with any woman. His reason for entering therapy in the first place and continuing on with the second therapist was his fear of being caught caressing children. He found that they were often attracted to him and liked to play wrestling games with him. Sometimes he found himself getting an erection, which to him was wrong and frightening. Four years previously he had roomed with an 8-year-old boy during a church retreat and impulsively went over to the sleeping child and stroked his penis to erection. He did nothing more and the child was not awakened but he was greatly frightened by this lack of self-control. He was afraid that his reputation would be ruined if he were discovered. He was also disturbed by his failure to find a wife since getting married and having a family was his fondest dream.

During therapy he began dating a woman who showed interest in him. As the relationship evolved during therapy, his rules for "marriageable" women began to emerge. If someone liked him, he had to run from her. If she did not want him, he could chase her knowing that he could not have her. Was this new date a friend or was she more than a friend? When he went to her house with her he wondered what he was expected to do. Should he go in, should he touch her, should he kiss her?

He scanned her every movement, trying to interpret the meaning of her gestures, her tone, her words. In therapy while the patient was obsessively reviewing his attempts at interpersonal analysis, the therapist suddenly saw an image of a dentate vagina and was momentarily thrust back into his own frightening experiences with girls and women. His feelings during premature ejaculations washed over him. Now he could label those feelings! He was afraid! Coming out of his reverie he could see that these were also his patient's feelings now. He was frightened of women, frightened of what they could do to him.

In the preceding example, the therapist was quickly able to examine his own experience for the underlying trigger in the patient's description. In the following situation, I was not so quick in examining the patient's influence.

CASE 6.26. A 26-year-old woman was making the transition from severely disturbed borderline character to narcissistic–neurotic one. As she was making the transition, she took a position as a secretary in my psychiatry department in a different hospital, moved to an apartment near my home (the address of which she knew), and began a romantic relationship with a trainee I was about to befriend. As I reviewed these behaviors with her, I blurted out in a therapy hour, "I feel like a caged mouse being stalked by a lion." This metaphor did not seem to touch the patient, but I gave it considerable thought. In a previous intense relationship, my woman friend had declared her desire to cage and study me. I interpreted my remark as suggesting my own fear of giving in to her advances. The patient was very attractive to me and had fulfilled my therapeutic narcissism by making remarkable therapeutic advances. Much later in therapy, she was able to state how, indeed, she was looking for any clues I might give her that I might be vulnerable to her affection and be willing to step outside my therapeutic stance. Because I was caught up in my own difficulties, I was not able to perceive clearly how accurate my spontaneous remark had been in describing her intention toward me.

Complementary and Concordant
Patient-Induced Countertransference

Racker (1968), among others, attempted to delineate two subcategories of patient-induced countertransference reactions. Sometimes the therapist experiences the patient's internal state through exaggerated or inappropriate fantasies and feelings as suggested by the "dentate vagina" fantasy of Case 25 in this chapter. The term "concordant" encompasses this category by implying that the therapist is experiencing what the patient is experiencing but in a distorted way. Once cleared of its distortion, the concordant response becomes a form of empathy. Sometimes the patient attempts to induce the therapist to take roles that balance or complement the patient's preferred role. Some of the many forms of these fixed relationships include: patient grandiose and therapist depreciated, patient withdrawing and therapist rejecting, patient seductive and therapist stimulated, patient helpless and therapist rescuing, patient angry and therapist withdrawing, patient weak and therapist overly active or controlling.

Superficially, the distinction between complementary and concordant seems clear: The first is interpersonal and the second is intrapsychic. However, at least two sticky intellectual problems emerge upon closer examination. Deeply disturbed patients, by definition, have difficulty with self–other boundaries. If they cannot distinguish self from other very well, how can therapists make use of the distinction between complementary and concordant? Even when the distinction is viable, I doubt that any single countertransference reaction may be well delineated by one category. Many interpersonal manipulations reflect intrapsychic constellations and many intrapsychic experiences have interpersonal manifestations. In the "dentate vagina" case, the patient may well have been attempting to have the therapist confirm his fear of women. In the "caged mouse" example, the patient was driven to capture a vision of herself as having great power over others.

I suggest that the distinction between complementary and concordant are excellent places to start in dissecting patient-induced countertransference reactions. Therapists should keep in mind the possibility that they will overlap.

Transference–Countertransference Stalemates

Patients can induce therapists to behave in ways that confirm the patient's interpersonal expectations. One become the lock; the other the key. The mechanism then freezes.

CASE 6.27. A 28-year-old therapist was attempting to understand the personality pattern of her 24-year-old woman patient who was aspiring to become a psychotherapist as well. The patient repetitively badgered her therapist. "You are cold, you are unfeminine, no man could ever want you, you aren't helping me at all. I met someone just like you and I didn't like her." The therapist began to withdraw and had to reassure herself that men did like her and that she was trying to help and that she was trying to care. Nevertheless, their relationship took a fixed form in which the patient criticized and the therapist responded meekly. The therapist tried to break the deadlock by saying: "You seem to be trying to make me angry at you." The patient responded: "You don't have it together enough to become angry." During supervision, the therapist expressed her intense rage and helplessness. As she became more objective about her own reaction, she was able to see how frightened the patient was about revealing herself. Confrontation of this fear of developing a self-observer alliance broke the stalemate.

Other stalemates are illustrated in the section on transference in this chapter in Case 6.19 of the "epoxy borderline" and Case 6.11 of the jealousy-inducing manic-depressive.

Patients who deeply desire to fulfill the expectations of others may be particularly at risk to form stalemates, especially if the therapist requires certain responses to fulfill his or her own personal or professional needs. Ulman and Stolorow (1985) described a "transference–countertransference neurosis" formed by a patient's need to please and her analyst's need for her to fulfill his personal and professional needs.

CASE 6.28. An analyst needed an analytic "control" case to fulfill the requirements of his psychoanalytic training so, after 18 months, he asked a patient to increase the frequency of their sessions from two to three times per week and to lie on the couch. He needed her to excel as an analytic patient, and she felt this pressure from him. When she deteriorated after his vacation, she struggled to ease the pain of his distress over her dysfunction by complying with his suggestion for an increase in session frequency. As she improved, she indirectly expressed her fears that the therapist could not tolerate her separation from him. He acknowledged to his supervisor that termination would be humiliating and shameful for him. A critical point of therapy involved the therapist's ability to point out to the patient her compulsion to fulfill the therapist's needs because she feared that he would decay and then retaliate if she failed to do so.

While some giving to each other is essential to the psychotherapeutic relationship, the process of reciprocal mutual influence can stalemate a dyad if this possible resistance is overlooked.

THE INEVITABLE EMPATHIC FAILURE

Therapists are not perfect empathy machines constantly able to track the ongoing experience of their patients. Instead, we may miss understanding some key element of the patient's emotions or thoughts and thereby trigger anger, resentment, indirect criticism, or withdrawal. The more severely disturbed of our clients often have histories of not being received compassionately by significant people in their lives and are therefore more sensitive to these therapist failures. Countertransference often plays a part in these failures, yet with many patients they are inevitable. Most important is to reduce countertransference guilt and empathize with the pain for the client created by not being understood by one who is expected to understand. Resolution of the empathic failure through patient forgiveness is a very useful therapeutic exercise. But first the therapist must forgive him- or herself.

7.   *Process of Change*

Change in psychotherapy is relative to the context in which it is being measured. In psychotherapy there are many contexts. Change is relative to the viewer's perspective (Strupp & Hadley, 1977). For the prematurely terminating patient, change may be either entirely sufficient or completely impossible. To the patient's therapist, change may be promising but incomplete (otherwise the therapist would not label the relationship as prematurely terminated). To the patient's insurer, relief of symptoms sufficient to resume previous activities would represent adequate change, while to a spouse this level of change may be insufficient for the survival of the marriage. To the parents of a depressed adolescent, the appearance of rebellion against their standards of behavior may be too much change. For psychotherapy researchers, a satisfactory measure of change has yet to be found, although each has favorite instruments. How does one adequately balance the demands of therapist, patient, family, researcher, third-party payer, and society? Furthermore, how does one know when change has gained sufficient momentum to enable the patient to drop away from the therapist's influence without relapse?

Change is also relative to the basic personality and social skills of the patient. To the isolated heterosexual individual, simple discussion about the weather with a member of the opposite sex may be a major achievement. For a premature ejaculator, the achievement of adequate coital time marks a major advance. Acceptance of one's own limitations may also be a psychotherapeutic goal, although the economic limits of a corporation president and those of a single mother of two young children on welfare stand in stark contrast.

Causes of change are often judged by therapists to stem from specific psychotherapeutic interventions such as the mutative interpretation sequence of psychoanalysis, or the existential encounter of existential therapy, or the replacement of a "should" with an "it would be nice" in RET therapy. These views are ideological illusions that have their origin in the Newtonian notion of a single cause having a single effect. Instead, a single

170

event is likely to have multiple possible causes. Blinded by narrow perspectives induced by multiple competing views of change, therapists have tended to consciously ignore "common factors," "nonspecific factors," while placing excessive weight upon a specific theoretical concept linked to a prized technique. The following case illustrates the multiple possible influences outside of commonly held theories that could have contributed to the final positive outcome.

CASE 7.1. A 51-year-old, married woman whose metastatic breast cancer had miraculously gone into remission became depressed. For many months, she had trouble sleeping, had early morning awakening, had withdrawn from people, felt depressed and hopeless. She had gained 17 pounds. She readily discussed her thoughts during daily interactions and seemed to be an excellent candidate for cognitive-behavior therapy for depression.

This short, moderately obese, very talkative woman, very much resented being in a psychiatrist's office. Her oncologist, a friend of mine, had insisted that she come. She thought my fees were four times what they actually were and her insurance did not cover outpatient psychiatric treatment. Most notable in her history was the complete remission of her metastatic breast cancer, which she had been told would kill her. She had prepared for death and discussed it with her children (only the youngest was still at home but was preparing to leave) and her often-traveling husband. She had been married once before. After the divorce, she arrived home with another man. Her ex-husband suddenly appeared and killed him in a jealous rage. After hearing this story, all subsequent men stopped seeing her until she met her current husband of four years. The murderer, her ex-husband, was married to another woman while in jail. He was released after four years apparently "cured" of a psychiatric problem (I was astounded at this fact as well). Her greatest current anxiety was caused by the failure of her present husband to return home from out-of-town trips when he said he would. His work often delayed him. Before receiving the diagnosis of cancer she had traveled with him, often doing volunteer work in towns where he stayed for months finishing jobs. She knew she would have to "grin and bear it," to talk differently to herself; but she had not been able to do so.

By the end of the first session, she had come to realize that she felt she had only a little time left (although this was no longer true) and that she resented being robbed of the enjoyment of spending the remaining time with her husband. Because of her vegetative signs of depression and her belief that a medication would help her, I offered her a small dose of an antidepressant as an active placebo. I suggested a new perspective on her husband's absences. Perhaps his not returning on time reminded her of other untimely events: her ex-husband's murder of her friend and her failure to die of cancer. Both were unexpected reversals of expected events for which much recovery time was required.

When she returned the following week, we ended the session after 20 minutes because she was feeling fine. She reported feeling very well the day after taking the first pill and then stopped the medication after 3 more days. During the second interview, she was markedly more calm and more accepting of the fact of her husband's unpredictable extended absences. Two years later her oncologist reported that neither her cancer nor her depression had returned.[*]

How does one explain this rapid reversal of prolonged depressive symptoms? The single most important factor appears to have been the patient's own readiness to change. She was readily engaged in psychotherapy because I came highly recommended by her oncologist. Furthermore, she had identified a critical pattern in need of change: her attitude toward her husband's extended absences. In this way, she had quickly traversed the first and second stages of therapy. She was also deeply motivated to change. She did not want to see a psychiatrist, because she did not want to need professional help (she also believed my fee was four times higher than it was). In addition, the examination of "self-talk" characteristic of cognitive–behavior therapy fit neatly into her own personal psychological approach since she implicitly knew she would have to change the way she talked to herself. Perhaps my drawing a parallel between her husband's absences and the murder perpetrated by her ex-husband and her failure to die of cancer was somehow useful.

The rapidity of her change could have been influenced by the "miracle cure" background of her cancer treatment. Perhaps the antidepressant induced the parallel more convincingly because medications had apparently cured her cancer. She was certainly aided by the belief in her own self-mastery that she had obtained through work and volunteer experiences through which she had demonstrated skills at acquiring new and adaptive behavior. One could argue that the change occurred as part of the normal course of recovery or through the pharmacological effect of the antidepressant (again too rapid) or through some sudden environmental change: Her son chose not to leave or her husband changed jobs (although neither of these events took place). I believe the most critical factors were the patient's own readiness, desire, and ability to change.

---

[*]This case is discussed at length in Beitman (1986).

THE PROCESS OF CHANGE: GENERAL CONSIDERATIONS

The preceding case illustrates many of the variables influencing client change. It is truly difficult to assert that any one is necessary for every client. Experienced therapists have probably seen some patients who have changed without having been engaged, without apparent motivation, without knowing what they wanted to change, and within an environment apparently hostile to any change. On the other hand, there are patients who are apparently well engaged, well motivated, know what is to be changed, and are being encouraged to do so by friends and relatives, but may not change.

The process of change takes place in a number of contexts, each of which has some influence on whether or not it will go forward. The psychotherapeutic contexts include the strength of the therapeutic alliance and the specificity of the patterns identified for change. Without the support emanating from a firm engagement, patterns may not be clearly specified. Without the clear definition of maladaptive patterns, the required changes will not be obvious. Other major contexts within the possible control of the therapist and patient are the biological and the social. The social context includes work, school, family, and friends. With strong biological deficits (severe medical illness, mental retardation, untreated manic-depressive illness) psychotherapeutic change will be limited. With antagonistic spouses, employers, or friends, change is also likely to be impeded.

The process of change may be divided into three substages. First, the pattern(s) defined as in need of change must come to be viewed by the client as his or her responsibility — "Whether or not I have created this pattern, I am now maintaining it." This is the substage of responsibility awareness. It may be skipped over, disregarded, or passed through very quickly. (Some therapists are not interested in having patients know what the pattern is, and therefore do not insist that they become aware of their responsibility for it. Milton Erickson (*et al.*, 1976) was one such therapist.) Second, awareness of responsibility can lead to assuming responsibility. "Now that I recognize this pattern as my problem, I am the one who must do something about it." This is the substage of the initiation of change through beginning a new attitude or new behavior. The change is usually driven by some form of emotion (fear, hope, desire, guilt). A variety of techniques are useful in moving patients through each of these substages.

Third, after the initiation of change, the new way of acting, thinking, feeling must be practiced. The psychoanalytic term "working through" appears to be a kind of intrapsychic practice that often has behavioral elements outside the office. With a view of therapy as a cognitive change process, Raimy (1975) used the term "repeated cognitive review" to describe this substage.

During therapy and after termination, the new changes may be generalized to other circumstances. For example, the now assertive client stands up not only to her co-worker but also to men both at work and in social contacts. After termination, it is hoped that gains will be maintained. Therapists may need to predict environmental shifts that are likely to impede or to support the maintenance of change.

It is the therapist's responsibility to aid each patient's movement along the substages of change. All possible forces should be considered. Accidental occurrences may prove to be very helpful. The following case illustrates the use of multiple forces by which to build change-promoting contexts and by which to introduce a series of deviations from a current negatively experienced homeostasis.

CASE 7.2. A 30-year-old woman sought psychiatric help because she had a dissociative reaction. She had gone to the emergency room with chest pain, had mentioned she had been raped 3 months earlier, and then wandered off without any memory of what happened for the next subsequent 10 hours. During the first visit, she was extremely anxious and quite timid. Between the first and second visit, she completed a daily-activities schedule that revealed at least five major panic attacks and much incapacitating anxiety between them. She had experienced these attacks for 3 years beginning shortly after she separated from her husband. He had abused her verbally for the 4 years of their marriage, had had an ongoing affair, and finally threw her around the room and tied her to the bed. Her mother had resented her birth and repeatedly claimed that the patient's birth had almost killed her. Whenever the patient was sick, her mother insisted that she stay locked in her room until she was well past her illness. When, as an adolescent, the patient was involved in a very damaging auto accident, the mother was required to care for her. For many months, the patient could not move as she waited for her bones to heal. Her mother would rarely anticipate her needs and instead would require that the patient beg for a drink or some food.

My engagement of her included a confrontation of her tendency to want to look good to everyone, including me. This desire on her part was also useful because it encouraged her to do a thorough job on her diary. Her dissociative reaction and her reaction to my subtle probes of the rape indicated a need for me to avoid that subject until she was ready. Engagement as well as treatment included the prescription of alprazolam for her panic disorder. I also pointed out to her a recurrent pattern of victimization, first by her mother, then by her husband and others. One was an aggressive male coworker who intimidated her. In subsequent sessions, I repeated this theme and added confrontations of her meekness with me and her terrible fear of being wrongly accused by others. I suggested that much of this behavior had been adaptive in her relationship to her mother but that it was no longer useful.

Analysis of the weekly diary showed that her panics occurred most frequently at night before going to bed. I asked her to analyze her cognitions through the triple-column technique of Beck *et al.* (1979). She was then able to substitute rational thoughts for her terrible fear of going into the bed. The reduction of panics subsequent to her self-confrontations increased her sense of mastery. She stated during the seventh session that it helped her a great deal to have me in her life, she knew that someone cared. The following week, she spoke with a friend about problems with her aggressive male co-worker who frightened not just her but the other women as well. She suddenly became aware of the face of her rapist. It was her co-worker! During the next session, she was able to confront the horrible details of the event, all of which she had blocked out of her mind. She also decided to go to the police in hopes of remembering further details. She knew she did not want to run away from her current job. She recognized that she would have to stand up for herself. She was frightened to do so yet began to seek situations in which even minor problems of self-induced victimization could be altered. She could not control the rape or the choice of her mother, but she could control the selection of her husband. How else did she contribute to her own victim role?

Some of the crucial variables leading to the initiation of change in this case include:

1. The dissociative reaction defined herself to herself as a person in psychological difficulty. This perturbation of self-concept led her to seek help.
2. Engagement included a confrontation of her submissive character traits, avoidance of discussion of the rape, the clarification and pharmacological treatment of panic disorder, and the clarification of a recurrent pattern of victimization.
3. Through a diary, the patient defined those panic attacks escaping pharmacological management. As a result of gaining control of them through her own efforts, her self-opinion began to shift. Self-control was possible.
4. Her unconscious gave her conscious access to repressed memories during a conversation with a helpful friend. She permitted herself further access during psychotherapy and subsequently

began to take more aggressive steps against her assailants, both past and present, by going to the police.

Sometimes contexts must be developed in order to provide predisposition to change. The case of the raped panic disorder victim illustrates the necessity of therapeutic and possibly pharmacological contexts for behavior change. This patient needed to develop trust in me in order to permit herself to be influenced. She seemed to need pharmacological stabilization of her anxiety in order to work on elements of it. She also seemed to need to gain a sense of mastery over herself in order to confront her worst memories. Sometimes, a change provides a platform from which new changes may be initiated.

CHANGE AS ENGAGEMENT

Any deviation may provide patients relief from one level of dysphoria only to make them aware of other difficulties. Therefore a change may simply develop a new context, a new equilibrium from which future change may be addressed. This notion is illustrated in the case of the rape and panic disorder victim and is also shown in the following example.

CASE 7.3. A 29-year-old divorced mother of two young children worked on the assembly line of a small factory. She had been living with a man named Nick for 6 years. One year before seeking therapy she had decided to break up with him because he would not commit himself to marriage. She wanted to meet other men. Six months later, she decided she wanted him back, but he refused to return to her although they saw each other at work and occasionally for dates. During the 2 months before seeking help, she had been increasingly anxious each time she saw him. She became tremulous, her heart pounded and raced, "she felt as if she were going to pass out," and she felt unreal. Her history revealed that she had had an affair with another co-worker, John, but had lied to Nick about it. However, from her story it was clear that Nick had enough information to know that she had probably slept with John. The patient was extremely sensitive to lying because her mother had lied to her most of her life. She strongly valued "being up-front and honest." I suggested that she tell Nick the truth. What did she have to lose?

The patient's symptoms disappeared after the confession. Though this relief of symptoms was what she had sought, it was clear to both of us that the problems precipitating her anxiety were built upon attitudes and behaviors predisposing her to a recurrence. She decided to continue in therapy. Her relief of symptoms strengthened the therapeutic alliance, thereby providing another platform from which change could spring.

OUTSIDE INFLUENCES ON CHANGE

The individual psychotherapeutic relationship takes place within multi-layered contexts that influence the process of change. Biological age; genetic predisposition; current health; current family relationships; economic opportunities; prevailing racial, religious, sexist, and political climate are but a few of the backgrounds against which transitions must proceed. These influences may help or hinder the spiral of psychological change.

Of these factors, genetic predispositions and current family relationships are potentially within the reach of therapists through medications and family or couples therapy. Other factors may be extremely difficult to control. Following are brief vignettes of patients whose changes were influenced by factors beyond direct psychotherapeutic influence.

1. A 36-year-old divorced woman was determined to reduce her extreme perfectionism because her 8-year-old daughter had that irritating trait. She hoped that by changing herself, her daughter would follow her example.

2. A 26-year-old psychology graduate student was told by his therapist that he did not address the therapist as a person but rather responded to him according to the patient's own private image of him, which was that of a superior being. The client did not fully grasp the meaning of this comment, until during his course of work, he entered a role-playing situation in which an actress treated him as if he were the only person in the world who could help her. She extolled his personal virtues beyond his own opinion of them. Having been on the receiving end of such treatment, he now recognized more fully how by idealizing others he ignored their own experience of themselves.

3. As she completed 2 years of psychotherapy, a 36-year-old attractive divorced mother of two was ready to meet new men. As a result of her divorce settlement, she was able to live in a large house and had purchased an expensive sports car. Many men were drawn to her partly because of her economic well-being. Through this drawing power, she was able to practice dating whenever she decided to put out feelers of interest.

4. A 28-year-old chronic schizophrenic woman began to function more autonomously when her mother died.

5. A 26-year-old woman with multiple somatic complaints and several surgical failures for potentially correctable abdominal lesions was struggling to change during her second year of psychotherapy. She had no hope that she could accomplish her break from her mother and her long-sought-for independence. When another surgical attempt proved successful, rather than failing as usual, she seemed to gain courage that previously futile attempts at psychological change could possibly be effective. She was correct.

6. A 45-year-old married woman, depressed and in psychotherapy for many years, began to speak freely about being raped as an adolescent as television carried more stories about sexual abuse. The cultural recognition of the sexual abuse of children had lifted the guilt she had experienced during her adolescence when it was customary to blame the victim for the event.

In the following examples, outside influences dampened tendencies toward change.

1. A 24-year-old prostitute lived in a social environment in which people wanted only her sex, her money, or her drugs. She was therefore on guard continuously and at least slightly paranoid on many occasions. As she came to trust her therapist, she began to generalize this trust to others in her social sphere. She was immediately and repeatedly cheated.

2. A 63-year-old woman with breast cancer in remission was struggling in therapy with the failure of her 22-year-old daughter to leave home. When the patient finally began to let her daughter go, she developed a recurrence of cancer and faced the probability that she would survive only another 3 years. The recurrence reduced the energy she had available for the psychotherapeutic work on her daughter.

3. A 42-year-old woman was caught in a vicious spiral with her married lover who abused her verbally and sexually when she was in good spirits, left her alone when she became enervated by his assaults, and reentered her life to begin the cycle again after she had spent weeks and months recovering from his abuse. She believed she could not leave him because she depended upon his financial support to sustain her son and herself. He continued to insist that she could not survive without him, especially when she was beaten and depressed. Her lover enjoyed having a mistress and his wife passively accepted the fact. Psychotherapy was useful only to help her reestablish herself after he had fully abused her. Then the cycle would begin again.

The patient's presenting difficulty may hide difficulty in a family member or in the family dynamics. Family therapists seem to make this assumption for any presenting problem, while individual therapists must keep this possibility in mind whenever psychotherapy is apparently ineffective. Bisexual men, for example, may be covering the frigidity of their wives (Hatterer, 1974) and agoraphobics may be shielding the neuroses of their husbands. On the other hand, spouses and families dedicated to the personal growth of each other may accelerate personal change begun in psychotherapy. Furthermore, any relationship providing the opportunity for self-discovery will provide patients more rapid feedback loops through which to discover maladaptive patterns and try out potentially more effective ones.

Psychotherapy, itself, may have unforeseen consequences even when the desired goals are reached. "Successful" separation of an adolescent from the family unit has been followed by suicide or suicide–murder (Boszormenyi-Nagy, 1976). Following is a related example.

CASE 7.4. A 42-year-old devoutly Catholic executive, fired because of poor business decisions, entered therapy with a nun. He lived alone, was deeply attached to his family, had no friends, and had no heterosexual relationships. She successfully conveyed to him the value of a life of poverty and the acceptance of Christ. He began to destroy his house with an axe when he felt Christ was in direct communication with him and required brief hospitalization for an acute psychotic episode. Because of his isolation from work and social contact, his environment did not provide the buffer he needed to help put these ideas into perspective. He refused further treatment because he felt that he was following his religious convictions.

Careful reading of these illustrations will reveal that no specific environmental influence "caused" the described outcome, but, instead, each played a contributing role. Each of us has the capability to reconstrue our circumstances to find a "light at the end of the tunnel" or the "cloud with the silver lining." Otherwise, no poverty-stricken person could find happiness and no rich person could be suicidal; no paraplegic could be joyful and no healthy person could be disturbed. It is the way in which we construe our circumstances that seems to play the greatest part in the way we feel and act. On these constructions of reality, the therapist's influence is brought to bear.

THE STAGES OF CHANGE

The process of change itself has received minor emphasis among psychotherapy writers, who have preferred to emphasize techniques by which change can or should take place. This emphasis upon technique has obscured the relatively simple and basic sequence underlying therapists' efforts to promote change. Change in psychotherapy implies an enduring alteration of a major aspect of the patient's psychological functioning, a shift from a less desirable state to a more desirable one. The alteration may be one of mood (from depression to normal mood), of behavior (from drug abuse to abstinence), or of cognition (from a diffuse self-image to a more coherent one). More convoluted shifts may involve acceptance of normality where previously confusion and crisis were the ruling constants.

CASE 7.5. A 40-year-old executive had been raised by an alcoholic, abusive father and a deeply disturbed, picky, depressed mother. He had been divorced twice from narcissistic, drug-using, suicidal women, had a 16-year-old drug-abusing son who was in and out of jail, and had been unable to save money because of alimony and child support. During his entire life, external and self-generated turmoil had characterized his daily existence. Ten years of once-per-week psychotherapy between ages 25–35 had been useful but did not prevent his chronic moderate depression from returning. When he came again for evaluation of that depression, his life had become rather stable externally, yet he was continuing to cause crises. In a single session, he realized that he was not able to withstand a "bland" life because he was not used to it. Could he accept the quiet and stop creating unnecessary uproars?

Clients must go from one place to another, must give up something old for something new. Many simply wish to keep doing the same thing or substitute one pattern for a similar one (e.g., replace alcoholism with bulimia). True change requires a greater leap, a crossing of a larger barrier, a traversing of a dangerous, fearsome obstacle, the leaving behind of what is, and the traveling on to what can be. Consider the following parable:

A person lives in a small private territory of many known fears. He has periods of peace, but much of his life is devoted to fending off attacks by these fears. The methods of defense suffice when coupled with time, patience, perserverance, and occasional help from others. Occasionally, he wins a temporary victory by smashing one of his fears. However, he gradually tires of the constant struggles and runs away. He enters a new, unknown territory. He tries to conquer his fears of the new place with the same strategies but is unsuccessful. He yearns to return to the place where he at least knew how to fight. He meets a person on the road back who points him toward a cliff from which a narrow footbridge leads across a yawning abyss to another cliff. "Should you cross into that territory and should you keep in mind this way of thinking I tell you, then you should find a new day dawning in your life." He goes to the bridge and trembles at the sight of the deep emptiness staring back at him from below. He notes the constant wind ever shaking the narrow rope bridge. He looks back at the stranger and beckons to have him come along. The stranger shakes his head. "Can I trust this bridge, this person, this idea?"

The terms used by different writers to describe patients approaching and proceeding past this point are confusing. Some are based on the patient's perspective, others on the therapist's. Freud (1963) used "repeating and remembering" to describe the patient's expression of the maladaptive patterns. His followers used confrontation and clarification (e.g., Greenson, 1967) to describe the patterns back to their patients. Change then proceeded by the therapist's "interpretations" and the patient's "working through," terms that are but first approximations to complex concepts. From the research scientist–experimentalist perspective of cognitive–behavioral therapy, Mahoney and Arnkoff (1978) described the following steps: (1) identify causes or patterns; (2) examine options; (3) narrow options and experiment; (4) compare data; (5) extend, revise, and replace (p. 709). To describe change process, Hart (1983) used "need–choice–action–image" where the term "image" refers to a new personality image resulting from the need for choice and action (p. 189). Beutler (1983) chose the following terms: "magnify" (the patient's awareness of cognitions, behaviors, and/or emotions associated with the identified concern); "validify" (analyze the magnified patterns and test out resulting new insights or feelings through behavioral and interpersonal change); and "solidify" (develop social supports and reinforcements for changes) (pp. 147–149). To describe their view of the process, Prochaska and DiClemente (1984) used the terms "contemplation," "action," and "maintenance." They had originally postulated a decision substage between contemplation and action, but their questionnaire studies of outpatients in various stages of change did not discriminate decision as a separate stage. In order to confirm that a decision had been made, the clients had already to be in the action stage (p. 23).

Yalom (1980) and Schein (in Pentony, 1981) both paid a great deal of attention to the process of relinquishing the old pattern, of giving it up. Cashdan (1973) used the phrase "stripping the maladaptive strategy" to emphasize the therapist's contribution, which may sometimes be quite aggressive. Yalom placed great emphasis upon becoming aware of responsibility for the pattern and then taking or assuming responsibility for it by acting. Schein (and Kurt Lewin) used the more general term "unfreezing" to describe the process of loosening the pattern's attachment to the patient's ongoing experience. The subsequent stages they termed "transition" and "refreezing." As they emphasized, this sequence is not specific to psychotherapy but may also be found in brainwashing, religious conversion, indoctrination, and many other areas of socialization and resocialization including the raising of a child into the family belief system.

As described earlier in this chapter, my view of the process includes a strong emphasis on relinquishing the patterns. This process usually involves responsibility awareness and assumption, but need not. Responsibility assumption may be out of awareness and may not be necessary to the desired change (Haley, 1963). Nevertheless, therapists seem to believe that it is within the realm of each client's capability to alter his or her circumstances and to achieve a more favorable situation. Therefore, at least the therapist must become aware of the ways in which the client is maintaining current difficulties by not doing or thinking in patterns that would bring substantial relief. Many therapists like to help their clients discover their responsibility because this lesson may generalize to other circumstances.

SPECIFYING THE PATTERN(S) TO BE CHANGED

The search for patterns must culminate in the elucidation of something to be changed. The "something" should be as specific as possible. Whether or not the patient is aware of what is to be changed is a matter of debate. Erickson (*et al.*, 1976) was quite content to keep collaboration on specific pattern identification out of the therapeutic discussion. He spoke in metaphor, in limited behavioral injunction, but appeared to have in mind just what he wished to change. The majority of therapists, however, appear to strive to define collaboratively thoughts, feelings, and behaviors that, if changed, could lead to improvement in psychological well-being.

Beginning therapists often illustrate the tendency to avoid specificity in their remarks to patients.

CASE 7.6. After struggling with a 25-year-old man's inability to comprehend his instructions, a first-year resident in psychiatry stated, "I'm not your father." The resident was simply trying to tell the patient to respond differently to his directions, to forget about being rebellious and angry. However, he did not state these requests clearly. The patient looked at him once again as if he did not comprehend what he was saying.

The same problem arises during the identification of many different pattern contents. In dealing with depressed patients, it is insufficient to declare "you must like yourself better." Instead, the manner in which the client dislikes him or herself must be specified and challenged. When confronting patients with their interpersonal difficulties, it is insufficient to state that they tend to recreate similar relationships in a variety of different situations. The nature of the repetition must be clearly enunciated. In handling intrapsychic conflict, it is usually insufficient to state: "You have two sides warring within yourself." The nature of the war usually needs to be clearly defined. The following case illustrates the manner in which a pattern may be clearly specified.

CASE 7.7. A 33-year-old divorced lawyer was deeply enmeshed in the lives of his parents and relatives although he lived 2 hours from their small town. The parents had wanted him to take over their four flower shops, because his sister seemed to them incapable of the forward thinking, dedication, and intelligence required to run the successful business. The patient, however, decided to become a lawyer. When he left for college, his parents disowned him for failing to stay in the family fold. After a quick marriage and divorce, he gave his ex-wife a large cash settlement plus monthly payments without any court edict. He had always been generous, had always given money to friends and family, and was always quickly responsive to anyone's needs. His friends criticized him for doing so much for people in trouble that he had no life of his own. After he had become established as a lawyer, he often returned home to help in the flower shop, to give his parents money and presents, and to help them with medical problems. For 1 week he arranged for a series of physicians to biopsy a lump in his father's throat. After the procedure, the father went home and returned a few days later with flower arrangements for everyone involved in his care. The nurses, the secretaries, and the physicians all received bouquets. There must have been 20 in all. The patient laughed in amazement at his father's behavior — how could he do that? I asked, "What about all the arrangements you make for people?" In that quick question, he saw more clearly how he was still operating in the family business by making pretty arrangements to make people feel better just as his father did.

RESPONSIBILITY AWARENESS

As the maladaptive pattern(s) become more clearly defined, clients may come to appreciate their own contributions to the difficulty. The greater the specificity, the more likely it is that one will be able to identify that set of thoughts and/or behaviors that may be aiding the maladaptive cycle. It is the therapist's task to present the evidence (Raimy, 1975) indicating self-responsibility.

The question of self-responsibility remains an existential question interpretable in many ways. On the one extreme, is the belief that we are totally without free will, and, on the other, the conviction that all that ever happens to us is the result of decisions we have made. Most therapists seem to accept a middle ground, in which the person has some measure of freedom within biological, psychological, economic, and cultural constraints. Without some substantial attribution of responsibility to the patient for the problems he or she brings into the office, the therapist has no hope of change. Therefore a fundamental psychotherapeutic assumption is that each individual is in some critical measure responsible for maintaining his or her current level of psychological difficulty. Each therapist's task, then, is to discover what the client is doing to perpetuate the presenting difficulty.

Cause

The notion of cause is also an elusive problem. The manner in which a set of problems is being maintained is not necessarily the cause of the problem. That a certain set of thoughts and actions are maintaining the problem may be substantiated through altering them. Whether a certain series of events brought the problem into existence is another matter. Freud, who sought historical cases for current psychological difficulties, noted this dilemma:

> So long as we trace the development [of a mental process] backward, the connection appears continuous, and we feel we have gained an insight which is completely satisfactory or even exhaustive. But if we proceed the reverse way, if we start from the premises inferred from the analysis and try to follow these up to the final result, then we no longer get the impression of an inevitable sequence of events which could not be otherwise determined. We notice at once that there might have been another result, and that we might have been just as well able to understand and explain the latter." (Freud, 1950, p. 226)

All events are parts of causal chains and they are, in turn, chained historically to other events. Fixing upon one event as the cause of another event is a fiction, the main purpose of which is to provide alternatives by which change may be initiated and maintained (Strong, 1978). The following tale illustrates these points:

A 2½-year-old boy remains clinging to his 35-year-old father while avoiding attachment to his 30-year-old mother. The maternal grandmother finds this behavior intolerable because the boy is too old to cling, and if he clings, he should do so with his mother. The parents each feel guilty, wanting to please the grandmother and also believing that she may have a point. Where is the problem? In their marriage? in each parent's relationship to the child? in each parent's problem in being a parent? or in the child? Or, if the problem intensifies, should they seek a toddler psychotherapist, individual psychotherapy for one or both of them, couples therapy, or family therapy? Where should they look to find a "cause" that can lead to a desired change?

The couple could start with an attempt to persuade the grandmother that it was now more acceptable for men to "mother" their children. Or the husband could look at the number of times he picks up the child when he no longer needs to do so. Or the wife could examine her acquiescence to her husband's caretaking of the child when she could get up with her son in the morning and let him sleep. Or she could feed and bathe the boy and let her husband relax. The couple could also examine their own resentment toward each other. She continues to resent his absence during the childbirth. He perceives her as weak and unable to withstand the rigors of child rearing and resents her failure to live up to that natural role. He could look historically at his resentment toward his mother, who seemed chronically burdened by raising him and his sister. Was he trying to rescue his mother from himself? She could examine the way in which she was raised — as a princess of whom little was required. Was she permitting her husband to be the servant that her mother and maid were to her during childhood? Perhaps the toddler, himself, had been disturbed by these early resentments and now needs to act out in play therapy a revamped parental interaction pattern.

For the people caught in this psychological puzzle, effective insight requires the generation of causal options within the control of one or all individuals. In individual psychotherapy, the therapist may try to help the client develop causal attributions that can lead to the assumption of responsibility through the perception of potential control.

Free Will

Psychoanalytical and behavioral theories have developed from a belief that psychological behavior is determined by mechanisms beyond the individual's control. Although their practitioners implicitly recognize the need for responsibility assumption through the exercise of individual will, the notion of willing has been underplayed in these deterministic approaches. Existentialists and social psychologists have attempted to fill the vacuum. Nevertheless, the philosophical debate between believers in free will and believers in determinism continues. This point is well illustrated by material marshaled by Yalom (1980). In commenting on the radical behaviorist Skinner's contention that since we are determined by our environment, we can manipulate our environment to determine our behavior, Yalom argued that this argument is internally inconsistent. "Who is it after all, who is manipulating the environment? Not even the most fanatical determinist can contend that we are determined by our environment to alter the environment; such a position leads to an infinite regress. If we manipulate our environment, we are no longer environmentally determined; on the contrary the environment is determined" (p. 270). He also cited Binswanger's observation that Freud's own life contradicted his deterministic theories: "Those who, like Freud, have forged their fates with the hammer—the work of art he has created in the medium of language is sufficient evidence of this—can dispute this fact least of all" (p. 270). The point was further illustrated with a summary of an experiment described by Bandura that demonstrates the extra something that permits an individual to assert control over the environment.

> A researcher once studied schizophrenic and normal children in a setting containing an extraordinary variety of attractive devices, including television sets, phonographs, pinball machines, electric trains, picture viewers, and electric organs. To activate these playthings, children had simply to deposit available coins, but only when a light on the device was turned on; coins deposited when the light was off increased the period that the device would remain inoperative. Normal children rapidly learned how to take advantage of what the environment had offered and created unusually rewarding conditions for themselves. By contrast, schizophrenic children, who failed to master the simple controlling skill, experienced the same potentially rewarding environment as a depriving unpleasant one. (Yalom, 1980, p. 270)

People deny their responsibility in standard ways. Rather than perceiving themselves as the prime actors in their uncomfortable dramas, they try to find the "cause" someplace outside of their own realm of influence. Patients may blame their parents, their social class, their biology, their spouses, their therapists, their culture for their difficulties. They will inevitably be able to sustain their claims with well-founded and convincing evidence. Nevertheless, the causal chain has several links involving their own attitudes and behavior. The innocent victim may be playing a very important part in his or her spiral of dismay. The compulsively sexual person can make other decisions when confronted with loneliness and sexual urges. The therapist's task is to find ways to reconstrue the patient's misery in terms that suggest some personal control. In this way, the patient may begin to give up, relinquish, unfreeze the old pattern.

THE ABYSS

Many patients assume responsibility, decide upon a course of action, and take it. Some, however, proceed through the sequence in a more deliberate, more frightened manner. The assumption of responsibility and the relinquishing of old patterns leave holes in their attitude and behavioral repertoire. They do not know how to replace what is lost. They may need to mourn the loss of their old selves, dysfunctional but familiar. They become suspended between the past and the future. Some are filled with terrible anxiety and despair.

CASE 7.8. A 30-year-old woman had been living with a man for 4 years. They decided to marry, but shortly after they did, she became increasingly depressed. She sought help from a therapist who was little able to understand her plight. The patient's father had died 2 years previous to the marriage, and her mother had died when she was 15, after suffering for 3 years with metastatic breast cancer. She had felt terribly guilty about wishing for her mother's death, and when it finally came, threw herself into her father's life as the wife substitute. Ever since, she had remained her father's daughter and substitute wife, although she had left her home town. She had been very reluctant to be married, and now that she had finally done it, was confronted with giving up her image as a member of her father's family. She could not accept the loss of her old identity and accept her new one as part of her husband's family. As she began to mourn the loss of her old identity, she became terrified of trusting this new family member. For many months, she remained suspended between the two worlds, anxious, with recurrent panic attacks and with little help from her therapist. Finally she accepted her reality, and with the help of a new therapist proceeded to decide to create a child for her new family.

INITIATION OF CHANGE: RESPONSIBILITY ASSUMPTION

Therapists are largely responsible for engagement and for pattern development, but when the pair comes to change, only the patient can perform the necessary action. Those therapists who do not recognize patient responsibility in their theoretical conceptions may disagree with this contention. The behaviorist Goldstein (1973) and the multimodal Lazarus (Lazarus & Fay, 1982) each maintained that failures to change should be attributed to the therapist's inability to construct the proper treatment plan. When Wilhelm Reich (1945) found that he was not achieving the results he anticipated by following standard analytic procedures of the 1930s, he was told by his colleagues to "keep analyzing." Many analysts would agree that the fault is likely to lie in the analyst's own failure to manage the relationship and interpret correctly. Unfortunately, these bows to therapist omniscience ignore the hard reality of patient responsibility for self-initiated change.

During the middle phase of successful psychotherapy, therapist–patient pairs that fit well together experience periods of disequilibrium (Orlinsky & Howard, 1978). Perhaps the therapist is refusing to meet the patient's expectations for assuming responsibility for the progress of therapy. This backing off from doing it for the patient appears to be an essential step in the therapeutic progression.

In the schema presented here, the stage is now set for action. Awareness of responsibility through reconstruing of causes leads to new alternatives and the potential for relinquishing old patterns. And then . . .

Some patients decide. To decide means to commit oneself to an action and to carry it out. Without action (or the withholding of a designated action) no true decision has been made (Yalom, 1980). (One could say that without a change in behavior the patient has decided not to decide, a decision about deciding). Some patients say, "Yes, I know what is to be done now. Thank you for helping me see the alternatives more clearly. I want to straighten out this mess, quit hurting myself and other people. I'll do it." They say good-bye and, in follow-up, report that change has gone according to plan. Neat and clean.

More commonly, people decide in small increments, in gradual out-of-awareness steps. They don't know that they have decided. They keep it as a dark secret from themselves and others. The consequences of full realization are too frightening, and the secrecy permits retreat without self-recrimination. They cross the narrow footbridge of change in pieces, like an amoeba slowly bringing parts of itself into new territory, yet able to withdraw committed parts at a moment's notice.

CASE 7.9. A 52-year-old married mother of four was referred to me by a cardiologist because he could find no biomedical explanations for her faintness and palpitations. During our first interview, she pleaded with me to hug her as she described her tremendous need for physical affection. She hated me for not responding. She returned 1 month later, terrified of further discussions but driven by her physical–emotional discomfort. She was willing to describe the situation under which her symptoms worsened, and I quickly realized that she was unable to say no to any of her husband's many demands. I warned her that if she stayed in therapy, her relationship with him would likely change, while she reported that he was adamant that her behavior toward him not be any different. I suggested during our third session, 1 month later, that she decide whether or not she wished to continue. She decided that she would and returned, having accepted my role with her. She had much to tell me about herself that she had not told anyone else. She unburdened a life of repeated rejections: Her mother abandoned her at age 5; her father would not take her at age 9; the orphanage would not support her during a physical illness; and her foster father, an alcoholic, beat her. And yet, she had emerged as a competent administrator and successful mother of four children. We decided to meet once monthly for 1 hour. Over the next four sessions, her anger at her husband's contradictory demands arose. I supported her perspective and clarified it. She felt stronger at home and one day performed the following "daring" action, which she sheepishly reported: "I was always afraid that he would be angry at me if I changed the radio station in the car. I tried it and nothing happened." During the eighth session, she reported that she was ready to go back to work, but her husband had forced her into taking care of another one of his projects. She insisted upon going back to work and found herself becoming exhausted. Her physical symptoms recurred. He proposed another, more massive project. She simply stated that she would move out if he carried it out.

This woman had been terrified of displeasing her husband and had reached a point through therapy in which she was willing to give up the marriage to save it and also to save herself from her disabling symptoms. In retrospect, she had decided to change when, after three sessions, she committed herself to the therapeutic contract. It mattered little how frequent our meetings were or exactly what we talked about. Finally, she developed the courage to change the radio station, and then said no to one of his projects. She had started to change, but now she knew it.

Why is this choice so difficult? Why are decisions so hard to make? To decide and to change is often to journey into the unknown, to the chaotic, to the uncertain. At least when one is stuck in patterns, they are familiar, almost friendly. The lonely person is befriended by his habits. They are his companions, predictable and reliable. To change is to enter uncharted territory. Furthermore, the journey often requires traveling through frightening territory, whether one calls it a narrow footbridge over a wide and windy chasm or a walk through the valley of the shadow of death, the changing person is leaving the known and has not yet reached the other known. He or she is caught between two realities, leaving and not yet arriving. The woman-changing-the-station had begun her journey and was faced with the terror of losing her husband. Would she still have him when the process of change had been completed?

To choose is to lose what once was. To make a choice is to exclude other possibilities and to experience their loss. Choosing is another boundary experience that challenges the myth of personal specialness (Yalom, 1980). We cannot be all things. One cannot please one's husband in all ways and also maintain personal and physical integrity. Choice means limitation and loss.

PRACTICE

Once a change has been initiated, some clients are able to walk away from therapy without the need for further assistance. Perhaps the deviation has been so accurately placed that it was amplified through interaction between the self and the environment in a way that stabilized the change. Perhaps the client is able to continue to practice the new change through personal determination and the firm support of a caring relative or friend. However, most therapists are required to help their patients practice newly discovered changes. Like teachers, they must repeatedly review the new ideas; like coaches, they must encourage their players to try the new actions over and over again until they become part of their repertoire.

The clearest example of practice may be found in the behavioral treatment of phobias. Exposure is the key therapeutic mechanism (Marks, 1976, 1978). It may be prompted in many different ways. Whether *in vivo*, in imagination, slowly, or quickly the therapist encourages the patient to expose him- or herself to the feared object. Sometimes one session is sufficient; with proper instructions 15% of agoraphobics will accomplish their goals on their own (Mavissakalian, 1984). Others may take many months because they may be impeded by various intrapsychic and interpersonal barriers.

Patients must often redecide over and over (Yalom, 1980). Each practice session may require another decision to go ahead with it. Breaking up with a lover whom one sees daily at work takes persistence and support, especially if the lover resists the loss. Standing up to a parent who refuses to listen may require redecisions to separate from the parent–child relationship. The behavior itself may be less the issue than the decision to go ahead. Therapists must be willing to go over the same alternatives again and again.

The old and new attitudes may require repeated contrasting. For Raimy (1975), whose view of therapy concerns the alteration of misconceptions of the self, repeated cognitive review is a basic part of most therapies. "So widespread is the tendency of experienced therapists to help patients review their misconceptions repeatedly, on either a systematic or nonsystematic basis, that sufficient warrant exists to establish it as a general principle of psychotherapy" (p. 68). In Rational Emotive Therapy, clients are repeatedly confronted with their self-statements containing personal commands. The word "should" is repeatedly targeted as a word to be changed (Ellis, 1973b).

In classical psychoanalysis, the term "working through" represents intrapsychic practice. Freud (1963) wished to demonstrate to his patients the presence of their repressed instincts. Because many of his early followers had difficulty accepting their patients' failure to learn from one demonstration of these instincts, he counseled them in the following way:

> One must allow the patient time to get to know this resistance of which he is ignorant, to work through it, to overcome it, by continuing the work according to the analytic rule of defiance of it. Only when it has come to its height can one, with the patient's cooperation, discover the repressed instinctual trends which are feeding the resistance; only by living them through in this way will the patient be convinced of their existence and power. (p. 165)

Fenichel (1945) defined working through more generally: "A chronic process which shows the patient again and again the same conflicts and his usual way of reacting to them, but from new angles and in new connections" (p. 31). Fromm-Reichman (1961) emphasized the necessity to test insights time and again in new connections and experiences. Alexander and French (1946) placed a great emphasis upon the importance of working through in the here and now as have many other psychodynamic therapists.

Psychoanalysts have tended to avoid direct approaches to behavior change and instead to emphasize insight and, implicitly, awareness of responsibility. One of the major limitations to psychoanalytic clinical theory is the failure to emphasize behavior change and its practice. However, since therapeutic change often requires a period of practice, the repeated review of insights is likely to carry with it therapist lessons for what and how to change (Buckley, Karasu, Charles, & Stein, 1979). Many other change approaches are also imprecise and seem to be applied indiscriminately for each substage. The next chapter describes general and specific approaches to the change substages.

8. *Change Techniques and the Substages of Change*

Psychotherapists have devised a wide variety of approaches to psychological change. Some are very general and function as growth-promoting environments. Some are applied to each substage with minor variations. Others are applied to specific change substages. This chapter describes many of the common approaches to change as they are related to the substages of change.

GENERAL APPROACHES TO THE CHANGE SUBSTAGES

Some approaches to change provide general contexts within which positive growth is enhanced. The therapist provides an atmosphere conducive to the patient's finding a better alternative. The placebo response, the therapist's positive attribution, and the corrective emotional experience are three examples of therapist-devised growth-promoting contexts.

Placebo Response

The patient's faith in the healing process may be sufficient to bring movement from discomfort to relief without necessarily defining clear interpersonal, intrapsychic patterns requiring change. The therapist may indeed select a specific focus, but its relevance to the change process has far more to do with the patient's faith in the therapist and the healing ritual than its relevance to the patient's basic problem. The offer of medications for depression, for example, usually brings a 70% response rate, while the offer of placebos generally is correlated with a 30–40% response rate (Klein, Gittelman, Quitkin, & Rifkin, 1980). Medications are offered within medical healing settings by physicians who generally believe strongly in the efficacy of their treatment. The physician's belief and the healing setting serve to promote the patient's faith in the treatment. The patient does not know how to alter specific brain biochemicals or to alter specific cognitions. Nevertheless, faith seems to trigger movement along the sequence of change. An essential ingredient to the use of a placebo appears to be the development of a plausible, acceptable explanation for the problem and its solution. If the procedure somehow makes sense to the client, then the probability of the placebo response is increased (Pentony, 1981).

The Therapist's Positive Attribution

In addition to offering a healing ritual in which they believe, therapists usually peer into the dark corners of their clients' psyche to discover hidden potentials. Can the therapist assemble from the tattered pieces of each client's self-image, a vision of a future self that is more integrated, better functioning? Once the therapist constructs and conveys the outline of a more positive view of the client's future, the client is caught between two images of the self. If the therapist's view is impossible to realize, then the patient must discredit that view. If the therapist is holding an opinion that is within the client's grasp, then he or she must change in that direction in order to reduce the dissonance between them (Strong, 1978). The more cherished the therapist, the greater the likelihood is that clients will shift themselves in the desired direction in order to reduce the dissonance between them.

Corrective Emotional Experience

Franz Alexander (1980) coined the term "corrective emotional experience" to refer to the ameliorative aspect of the psychotherapeutic relationship centering around the fact that the therapist's actual responses to the patient's emotional expressions are quite different from the parents' original treatment of him or her. The fact of this difference forces the grown-up child to adjust his or her responses to current reality. Alexander carried the notion one step further by suggesting that therapists could increase the effectiveness of the corrective emotional experience by striving to create an interpersonal climate that highlights the discrepancy between the patient's transference attitude and the actual situation between patient and therapist. If the patient is a frightened son responding to a punitive father, the therapist should behave in a calculatedly permissive manner. If the father is all-forgiving, the therapist should then be more impersonal and reserved.

The term now has a more general meaning. It refers to any aspect of the therapeutic encounter by which the patient experiences an unexpected form of interaction that leads to change in self-concept and the relinquishing of old patterns. The warm, positive regard extended most patients is sometimes corrective in itself (no one has ever treated me this way) as may be the scientific collaborative style of cognitive–behavioral therapy. The present comes to be perceived as different from those of the patient's expectations that are based on past experiences. The patient must then change to meet this new reality.

SPECIFIC TECHNIQUES APPLICABLE TO EACH OF THE THREE SUBSTAGES

The placebo influence, the therapist's positive attribution, and the corrective emotional experience are terms for general influencing processes. They are less techniques and more positions or attitudes assumed by the therapists.

In addition to these more general approaches, some techniques may be applied to all of the substages. In this section are described single techniques that therapists use for all three substages, sometimes, perhaps, without knowing that the same technique is being used for different purposes.

Exhortation

"I think this guy needs a kick in the pants," said a frustrated therapist trying to move his patient along. Sometimes "a good swift kick" works. Usually a friend or relative has already tried it. If this approach would have been useful to the client, then therapy would not have been necessary.

The foot in the pants is very direct and nonverbal. It is also not generally accepted as a psychotherapeutic technique. In its slightly more subtle forms, the therapist states alternative forms of thinking and/or behavior that would appear to benefit the client. These positions are stated insistently with firm conviction.

RESPONSIBILITY AWARENESS

Exhortation to assume responsibility awareness takes the following general approach: "You are responsible for what happens to you in your life. Your behavior is, as you yourself know, doing you in. It is not in your best interests. This is not what you want for yourself . . . " (Yalom, 1980, p. 291). Therapists have developed a number of techniques by which to promote this message. If a patient excuses his or her behavior by saying, "It was not deliberate. I did it unconsciously," the therapist might counter with "Whose unconscious is it?" If someone irritates the patient, the therapist might ask the patient to say, "I let him irritate me." Any time the patient blames an external agency for a feeling or behavior, the therapist has an opportunity to say, "Own it. It is your feeling. It is your behavior" (Yalom, 1980, pp. 231–232).

Unfortunately, as suggested by Yalom, these simplistic techniques are often insufficient because they are little more than what has already been tried by others in the patient's social system. Furthermore, the authoritarian mode in which responsibility injunctions are delivered implicitly imbues the therapist with the responsibility for the patient's changing. In this way, a paradox is created between the content of the message and the form in which it is delivered. The content is responsibility awareness; the metacommunication is, "I know what is best. I am responsible for your responsibility awareness."

INITIATION OF CHANGE

Therapists may attempt to use their leverage as authorities, as knowers of what is best, as charismatic leaders, to urge their clients across the chasm of change. Through shouting, ridicule, guilt induction, therapists may try to push their clients along. Few therapists have been more vigorous in their exhortations than Albert Ellis (1973b/1984). The following dialogue illustrates his insistent, didactic approach to the initiation of change:

THERAPIST: All anxiety comes from *musts*.

CLIENT: Why do you create such an anxiety-ridden situation initially for someone?

THERAPIST: I don't think I do. I see hundreds of people and you're one of the few who *makes* this so anxiety provoking for yourself. The others may do it mildly; but you're making it very anxiety provoking. Which just shows that you carry *must* into *everything*, including this situation. Most people come in here very relieved. They finally got to talk to somebody who knows how to help them, and they're very happy that I stop the horseshit, and stop asking about their childhood, and don't talk about the weather, *et cetera*. And I get *right away* to what bothers them. I tell them in five minutes. I've just explained to you the secret of all emotional disturbance. If you really followed what I said, and used it, you'd never be disturbed about practically anything for the rest of your life!

CLIENT: Uh-huh.

THERAPIST: Because everytime you're disturbed, you're changing *it would be better* to a *must*. That's all the disturbance is! Very very simple. Now, why should I waste your time and not explain this — and talk about irrelevant things?

CLIENT: Because perhaps I would have followed your explanation a little better, if I hadn't been so threatened initially.

THERAPIST: But then, if I pat you on the head and hold back, *et cetera*, then you'll think for the rest of your life you have to be patted on the head! You're a bright woman!

CLIENT: All right —

THERAPIST: That's another *should*. "He *should* pat me on the head and take it slowly — *then* a shit like me can understand! But if he goes *fast*, and makes me think, oh my God, I'll make an error — and that is awful!" More horseshit! You don't have to believe that horseshit! You're perfectly able to follow what I say — if you stop worrying about "I *should* do perfectly well!" For that's what you're basically thinking, sitting there. Well, why *should* you do perfectly well? Suppose we had to go over it twenty times before you got it?

CLIENT: I don't *like* to appear stupid!

THERAPIST: No. See. Now you're lying to yourself. Because you again said a sane thing — and then you added an insane thing. The sane thing was "I don't like to appear stupid, because *it's better* to appear bright." But then you immediately jumped over to the insane thing, "And it's *awful* if I appear stupid — "

CLIENT: [Laughs appreciatively, almost joyously]

THERAPIST: " — I *should* appear bright!" You see?

CLIENT: [with conviction] Yes.

THERAPIST: The same crap! It's always the same crap. Now if you would look at the crap — instead of "Oh, how stupid I am! He hates me! I think I'll kill myself!" then you'd get better right away.

CLIENT: You've been listening! [laughs]

THERAPIST: Listening to what?

CLIENT: [laughs] Those wild statements in my mind, like that, that I make.

THERAPIST: That's right. Because I know that you have to make those statements — because I have a good *theory*. And according to my theory, people couldn't get upset *unless* they made those nutty statements to themselves. (pp. 218–219)*

Ellis ridiculed her way of thinking while acknowledging her intelligence. He grasped the pattern in the here-and-now, thereby making it more emotionally laden and obvious, while at the same time, he confidently proclaimed his superior theory. She felt empathically understood because he grasped her inner thoughts. He told her what is better and she accepted it, at least partly to avoid his punishing criticism. By shifting, she won him over.

PRACTICE

Exhortation may be a useful approach to practicing changes. Once clients have begun to try incursions into new territories, the therapist is less able to influence subsequent events. To encourage, cajole, and cheerlead persistence can be of great use to some patients. It can require, however, relatively great expenditure of therapist energy.

Interpretation

In classical psychoanalysis, interpretation is the ultimate and decisive instrument of therapeutic change (Greenson, 1967). To interpret is to assign meaning and/or causality to symptoms, behaviors, emotions, and thoughts. In psychoanalysis, meaning and causality are assigned from analytic theory, of which there are many competing divisions. These theories are maps of unconscious functioning thought to influence daily behavior and to lead to the formation of symptoms. Identification of cause and elucidation of meaning are believed to bring about basic (structural) change in mental organization that leads to relief of symptoms and more adaptive functioning. While younger therapists might hold out a belief in the one dramatic interpretation that will change a patient's life, the reality of analytic work indicates the slow, piecemeal, laborious nature of the interpretative process. The psychoanalytically oriented therapist

---

*From "Rational–Emotive Therapy" by A. Ellis in *Current Psychotherapies* edited by R. J. Corsini, 1984. Reproduced by permission of the publisher, F. E. Peacock Publishers, Inc. Itaska, Illinois.

generally begins this process with a specific symptom, behavior, thought, or emotion that the patient can agree is worthy of further examination. This step requires a firm agreement between the patient's self-observer and that of the therapist. The identified focus may then be examined for its reality triggers and the reality reasons for the patient's response. This step resembles the S→O→R sequence of cognitive therapy. It is probably common to most therapies, as suggested by Hart (1983). Then, drawing from psychoanalytic theory, past knowledge of the patient's life, empathic understanding, and intuition the psychoanalytically oriented therapist offers a possible cause, motivation, or meaning to the behavior, emotion, thought, or fantasy under examination. If the interpretation is correct, the patient will confirm it by adding additional relevant information to flesh out its understanding or by symptom relief. Usually patients come up with new resistances, new ways of thwarting the investigation of unconscious phenomena, and/or new symptomatic fantasies, behavior, or thoughts. The interpretative process must then be begun again. A brief vignette will illustrate some of these elements.

CASE 8.1. Mrs. E. W. was a married woman with hysterical symptoms who was well into her therapy when the bar mitzvahs of a number of her friends' children led to the exploration of her disappointment and rage that her husband had never given her a son. In this context, in the session to be described, the patient spoke in detail of her longing for a son and of some of the surface real and fantasied reasons for this intense wish: A son would take care of her; he could please her father who was also sonless; and he would give a sense of completeness to her family structure. She then described a fantasy of meeting her therapist at a party and of feeling embarrassed by it. It was toward the end of the session and the therapist made this interpretation: Mrs. E. W. wanted to meet him socially because she imagined that he could give her a son. She responded that she had not mentioned it, but she had experienced a good deal of anxiety on her way to her session, and had been thinking of the couch in the therapist's office and what it might be used for. She went on to describe a discussion with her dentist in which she had gone out of her way to find out if he had a son, and learned that he had two. (Langs, 1973, p. 452)

Langs explained this session in the following way:

The intervention made here was a transference interpretation of unconscious fantasy related to the therapist, with probable genetic ties (not alluded to in the intervention) to the patient's father. The session began with expressions of the patient's conscious but frustrated wish for a son.

In this context, the sequence, in which the next set of thoughts related to
meeting her therapist socially, provided the clue to the patient's currently
central unconscious fantasy and intrapsychic conflict: Mrs. E. W.'s wish
for the therapist to impregnate her and give her a son, and the anxiety this
evoked. This fantasy, of which the patient was not directly aware, was interpreted to her and confirmed through recall of the previously repressed
thoughts of the therapist's couch, and of her displaced interests in her dentist's sons." (pp. 452–453)

Although he did not discuss this specific case any further, Langs
would argue that this interpretation did not take place as an isolated intervention but, instead, deals with a section of unconscious fantasy life
that the therapist is attempting to elucidate. It is the rare interpretation
that uncovers the entire core conflict; instead, each one elucidates a facet
of the multifaceted psychoanalytic objective. No doubt the patient's incestuous wishes toward her father and her own self-recrimination for not
having been a boy herself are part of the therapist's interpretative objectives.

But how do such forays into hypothetical constructs of unconscious
activity lead to change? How can all the analytic schools be correct in
their concepts of the unconscious? Some emphasize the id impulses (mur-
derous rage, incestuous wishes, homosexual yearnings, sexual perversions,
sadomasochism). Some emphasize self–other boundary distortions. Some
see all maladaption in terms of oedipal conflicts or preverbal experiences.
What is a correct interpretation?

To the theoretical researcher, correct interpretations are those that
match and extend the therapist's theory of the unconscious. If, for example, the therapist in the case just presented is looking for a nuclear unconscious fantasy that is composed of oedipal, self-destructive, and lesbian (with her daughters and mother) yearnings, then the successful
presentation of these elements in terms compatible with the patient's current fantasies and behavior would be termed a correct interpretative sequence. On the other hand, if the patient does not change, then the
pragmatic therapist would argue the interpretative process is not correct.
For the pragmatic therapist, correct means effective. Among many psychoanalysts, correct (according to theory) interpretations may have become idealized to the point at which they are no longer effective (Applebaum, 1975).

The wide variety of meanings and the question of correctness distort
the precision with which the interpretative process may be aligned with
the substages of change. Therefore, therapists who interpret may not
think in terms of substages but, instead, may apply interpretations with-

out awareness of the specific effect they are intended to have in regard to movement along the substages.

RESPONSIBILITY AWARENESS

Before interpretations are offered, psychoanalytically oriented therapists usually confront patients with their resistances to insight. Confrontation is the verbal holding of a mirror in front of patients to show them what they are doing now. It is an attempt to point to symptomatic behavior and thinking — a way of delineating a maladaptive coping strategy, interpersonal style, or security operation. Repeated over time, a series of confrontations may become a clarification. The pattern is delineated. Because the patient is involved with the same pattern at different times, the therapist directly or indirectly encourages the patient to consider himself or herself as the originator of the pattern. Since many psychoanalysts prefer indirection, the likelihood is that the clarifying statement will be repeated until the patient "discovers" his or her own responsibility for the pattern. As will be suggested in the section on specific techniques for specific substages, demonstration of repeated patterns is one of the effective methods of raising responsibility awareness.

INITIATION OF CHANGE

Although suggestion may be an inevitable part of psychoanalytic practice, major psychological change is thought to take place through interpretations that remove the effects of suggestion (Stewart, 1975). Interpretations are intended to undo repression, alter superego functioning, and help the patient to function autonomously from the therapist. Can these and the many other goals of psychoanalysis be understood in less theoretical terms?

Psychoanalytic interpretations are based upon the analyst's guesses about unconscious motivation. The analyst learns to decipher patient metaphors, to discern latent content, in order to understand unconscious functioning. As patients watch their analysts performing this deciphering, they are likely to identify with this analyzing functioning. Indeed, the acquisition of self-analytic functioning is one of the common outcomes of psychoanalysis (Schlessinger & Robbins, 1983). However, analysts do not seem to consider the possibility that their analysands are also learning to decipher what the analyst is saying and that perhaps there are lessons latent in that material. The following example, taken from a case of fantasied psychoanalytically oriented psychotherapy, demonstrates the indirect manner by which psychodynamic therapists convey one of the primary lessons of psychoanalytic therapy.

CASE 8.2. The therapist has had to discontinue therapy because of an attack of jaundice. She returns 3 weeks later and is greeted by a very constrained patient, who speaks about trivialities. She suggests that he is avoiding feeling because he cannot face the pain of his loss of her. He responds by becoming more animated and says that during the past 2 weeks, he has been preoccupied by the loss of his previous two girlfriends. She suggests that these thoughts may have been set off in him by the loss of her. He says, "Yes, it's funny, but the thought did cross my mind, 'what if she never comes back?'" Noting the similarity between the patient's current feelings and his reaction to his mother's death, the therapist states that if she had not returned it would have been exactly the same as had happened to his mother. He sobs heavily and recounts details of the day in which she had unexpectedly died, details he had not recalled in years. (Malan, 1979, p. 84)

The lesson indirectly offered is a common psychoanalytic message: The past is not the present; now is not then; you must decipher the present more carefully to avoid confusing it with what happened to you. The message is delivered in a highly personal context, tailored to the individual's experiences of then and now, within the highly charged therapeutic relationship. As suggested by clinical and research experience, for some patients this is an excellent medium for change and for some it is not.

PRACTICE

In order to be effective, interpretations usually are repeated again and again in different contexts with different symptoms until a basic lesson is transmitted. Further interpretations may then be necessary for subsequent problems. The process is veiled in theory and metaphor. One analogy goes as follows: Working through is like the ocean waves bringing precious shells on shore and then sweeping them back. The patient watches this repeated showing of shells until he or she is ready to grasp them and take them permanently on shore (Green, personal communication, 1985).

The analogy implies processes working outside the patient's responsibility. The ocean is the unconscious moving at its own pace. The shells are plucked from the waves by the hidden force of the analyst. Suddenly the patient decides to take responsibility for the shells. How this step takes place is not clearly defined.

Working through sometimes resembles behavior therapy for phobia.

The patient is exposed through a variety of means to wishes, fears, fantasies, memories that are terribly frightening. Through repeated interpretations, the analyst is trying to show the patient that his or her fears are now unfounded. They may have had a basis in the past, but the past is now passed. Anger can be confronted and controlled. Destructive fantasies do not have to be acted upon. Working through then becomes an intrapsychic practice. Once the internal fears can be confronted, their analogues in the external world may also be faced.

Working through may also refer to the process of resolving intrapsychic conflicts the poles of which have already been defined. One intrapsychic personality or agency is confronted with the demands of another. The confrontation is most dramatically illustrated in Gestalt chair-doubling exercises but may be carried out in simply verbal ways.

The many definitions of the term reflect its ambiguity as well as the fact that working through was the first term used to describe this substage.

Therapist Self-disclosure

As a cornerstone of existential psychotherapy (Havens, 1974) and as an anathema in classical psychoanalytically oriented therapy (Langs, 1976), therapist disclosure is controversial. In Haven's view of existential psychotherapy, the therapist strives to be with the patient in the here and now, to comprehend and experience the ongoing state of the other. Often this objective requires attempts to shift, to go with, to keep looking for the ever-changing experience of the other. Sometimes the therapist may require the patient to stay with them. In order to do this, therapists may be required to express their own feelings. In this way, the process is somewhat reversed; the patient must meet the therapist. This coming together in the here and now may create an existential moment or existential encounter through which the isolated individual called patient comes to experience the existence of another. According to Havens, this reduction of emotional distance can be curative.

The idealization of the existential moment resembles the idealization of the mutative interpretation. In one sweeping maneuver, the patient is transformed. While such occurrences do take place, the more common reality is likely to be the repeated going over of similar territory. Persons do not learn of the existence of another at one moment as often as they discover the other in little experiences over time.

If the therapist is to self-disclose, what is to be revealed: past history, dreams and fantasies, current traumas, specific reactions to patients? What should therapists not tell their patients?

Weiner (1983) has attempted to systematize some of the answers to these questions. Fundamentally, the question is not how much of what should the therapist disclose or not disclose, but rather, what specifically is to be disclosed, in what manner, and in what context (p. 58). As in any other therapeutic intervention, the therapist must keep in mind his or her objectives in disclosing. What effect is the self-disclosure intended to have?

During engagement, some patients very much want to know personal demographic data about the therapist. How much information is needed in order to promote engagement? When does further information unnecessarily distort the therapeutic process? While the therapist's professional experience and technical orientation may be standard information, should the patient also be informed of the years of marriage, place of worship, and major recreational activity? What are the patient's reasons for asking for this information?

On the other hand, what are the therapist's reasons for talking about the troubles he has during his divorce proceedings, or discussing his financial or professional problems? What is the therapist asking for when she invites a patient to listen to the pain of her mourning for a recently deceased loved one? Why is a therapist telling his lovely young patient that he finds her sexually attractive? In each of these instances of self-disclosure, the therapist may be responding to personal needs rather than to the needs of the patient.

Therapists must often judge their patient's need to know. Sometimes therapists are forced into long absences from their work due to illness or other catastrophe. If reality, however we define it, is the touchstone of psychotherapeutic work, then therapists must consider letting their patients know what is going on to the limits of their desire to know. When discussing the implications of life-threatening illness like metastatic cancer or relapsing leukemia, physicians must also follow the guidelines implicitly set up by each patient. In the following case the therapist judged correctly the patient's need to know.

Case 8.3. A patient in her 20s who had been sheltered as a child from the facts of her father's psychiatric hospitalization was gratified by her therapist's simple acknowledgment that their many canceled hours had been due to the therapist's mother's illness and death. The facts the therapist provided did not inhibit the flow or analysis of fantasy. The young woman felt she had been treated like an adult and experienced a heightening of self-esteem. (Based on Givelber and Simon, in Weiner, 1983, p. 107)

On the other hand, therapists may misread their patient's desire to know, as illustrated in Case 6.24. In that relationship, the therapist incorrectly judged the patient's needs.

Therapist fantasies may be useful in promoting therapeutic change in many ways. In the following example, a slow-moving patient was stimulated to further self-exploration by self-revelation.

CASE 8.4. As the patient rambled, his therapist was greeted by a visual image of a Galapagos Island turtle lumbering along a sandy shore. Discussion of this simple image drove home to both participants the patient's extreme reluctance to confront a very embarrassing situation. (adapted from Singer & Pope, 1978, p. 18)

RESPONSIBILITY AWARENESS

Therapist self-disclosure may be very useful in promoting patients' awareness of their effects on other people. As a representative of all the persons with whom the patient has extensive contact, the therapist may describe how he or she feels in response to the other. Because the therapist is minimally involved in the outcome, and because the therapist is being paid to render psychological information, these descriptions are often readily accepted when the pair has a strong self-observer alliance.

CASE 8.5. A 19-year-old college freshman was struggling with her studies. If she did not pass, her father was not going to continue to support her in school. Her future looked bleak. She was moderately depressed and had begun to experience a number of panic attacks. In therapy, she revealed her frustration with studying. "I've never studied so much in my life. I keep trying and trying but my grades don't get any better. You understand what I'm saying?" She peppered her monologues with this latter question. Each time she asked it, I felt uncomfortable and then decided to wait for an opportunity to comment on it. She described how she was able to manipulate her father into giving her money and repeated a dialogue with her mother in which she had sharply put her down. Nevertheless, she felt helpless in her current circumstances and did not know what people meant when they called her manipulative. I called her attention to the question "You understand what I'm saying?"

PATIENT: Yeah, my girlfriend Helen used to say that to me all the time and so I picked it up from her. I say it because I'm afraid people aren't understanding what I'm saying.

THERAPIST: I'd like to tell you how it effects me. Is that OK with you?

PATIENT: Yeah.

THERAPIST: I know you are saying it because you are afraid that I am not understanding you. But the way it effects me is that I feel criticized by you. You or your parents are paying money for me to listen and understand and here you are accusing me, indirectly, of not listening.

PATIENT: No, I'm just afraid that you won't understand me because of the way I'm saying it.

THERAPIST: I understand that. But I'm just trying to tell you how it might effect other people since it affects me this way.

PATIENT: So, maybe I do manipulate other people. But I really don't see that because they can make their own decisions if they want to.

This was the beginning of her seeing the possible effects she has on others.

INITIATION OF CHANGE

Therapists may reveal their fantasies, dreams, feelings, and desires toward their patients without knowing just what effect they are likely to have. Some skillful patients are likely to maneuver some forms of self-revelation into psychotherapy for the therapist. While therapists also acquire much information about themselves from the caring responses of their patients, limits on these ministrations must be ethically drawn.

Rogers (1961) used the term "congruence" to indicate the therapist's ability to be without facade, while expressing his or her current feelings and attitudes. Rogers (Meador & Rogers, 1973, p. 139) insisted that intuition be the guide for therapist decisions to thrust "his own organismic responses into the situation." He believed that the therapist's willingness to be "real in the relationship provides the client a reality base he can trust and takes away some of the risk of sharing himself with another."

The following case illustrates how self-revelation about the patient's effect on the therapist helped to initiate change. Again a strong self-observer alliance is required through which the patient joins the therapist to understand the therapist's experience.

CASE 8.6. A 33-year-old therapist was trying to help her 45-year-old patient to understand how he subtly encouraged young women to quit working for him. He had been divorced for 3 years and had a series of unsuccessful relationships. He preferred young aggressive women who were moving to the top of their chosen fields. They seemed to find him attractive, but after a few months of knowing him found some excuse to leave him. The therapist too had found him attractive at first, but after a few months of once per week therapy found herself becoming frustrated with him. He seemed to dimly appreciate the manner in which he was condescending toward women, how he attempted to control them through making them into little daughters. The patient, however, did not grasp what she meant. After 4 months of once weekly therapy, the therapist made a billing error. The bill went directly to the patient, rather than to his insurance company. In a very condescending way, full of veiled criticism, he said, "I'm very disappointed in you." She felt as if her father were talking to her. With this thought in mind, she rummaged through her memories to check whether or not she had also felt this way with her father. While her father had triggered responses something like this one, there was also a qualitative difference. Coming from her patient, the feeling was more negative, more foolish and embarrassing. Yes, it did appear to her that she was experiencing what the other women must have been experiencing. She asked if he would allow her to discuss her reaction to his statement of disappointment. Even as she asked, he seemed to stir. As they discussed it, he recognized very clearly the manner in which he had spoken to his employees and lovers. This began the discussion of how to change that set of responses.

PRACTICE

The use of therapist self-revelation is limited during practice. The objective of any technique during practice is to help the patient persevere. To make a statement like "I'm disappointed in your progress" would likely be as counterproductive as it was for the previously described patient in Case 8.6. Perhaps the way to use self-revelation is for the therapist to state that he or she too has struggled with such difficulties and, through perseverance, has mastered them. For example, during a certain period of my own life, I was excessively paranoid. I have found myself telling my excessively paranoid patients about this difficulty whenever they had begun confronting their own. I have usually reaffirmed the necessity to test out hypotheses about reality by asking other people for their opinions of the situation in question. I had to repeat this project over and over again for myself until some outline of a more plausible reality emerged. I suggest that they need to do the same.

Self-revelation of this type is a request that the patient copy, imitate, or identify temporarily with the therapist. It may not work, especially if the issue is crucial and self-revelation has not been part of the therapist's style up to that point, as suggested by the following example.

CASE 8.7. When I was 30 years old, I was in therapy with a 45-year-old psychoanalyst in twice weekly, psychoanalytically oriented psychotherapy. I filled the hours with detailed descriptions of my past history, while the therapist passively listened. I knew somehow that I was avoiding getting into more important information. My therapist, however, said very little. After 6 months, my insurance was running out and I saw little reason to continue. I told him I was going to quit in 2 weeks. During the next session, as we discussed termination, he told me something of himself. "I, too, wanted to quit my therapy after a few months, but I stayed with it. And I'm glad that I did." I found his testimonial weak motivation, particularly in light of his remarkable passivity up to that point. I quit.

SPECIFIC APPROACHES TO RELINQUISHING OLD PATTERNS

Bandura (1976) and Kopp (1977) are among many writers who believe that much maladaptive thinking and behavior is the product of past learning once appropriately applied but now carried forth unnecessarily into the present. A child may adapt to an inconsistently punishing mother by steady compliance and intense willingness to please. Although these behaviors may have had little impact on the mother, the child gains some hope that she or he has somehow moderated the mother's influence. The child, however, carries these excesses into adult life, failing to learn that these extremes are no longer necessary. People are often terribly afraid to give up their once-adaptive patterns, fearing the catastrophe they were designed to prevent. Phobias represent the simplest form of such adaptive behaviors. The child once frightened by a relatively large dog stays away from any dog during adult life. As in the treatment of phobias, thoughts and behaviors that are maintained by irrational fears must be changed through some kind of exposure that disconfirms them. The patient must somehow come to believe that as long as he or she maintains the current attitudes and engages in current behaviors, the satisfactions sought will be beyond reach.

Many clients are demoralized when they enter therapy because their repeated efforts at adaptation have been fruitless. They are aware that something has not been working. It is the therapist's task to add specificity to this sense of demoralization in order to provide a way out. The client must come to a clear notion of the causal chain in which his or her pain is embedded. Then he or she must determine a point at which a change under his or her control is likely to lead to a deviation in current homeostasis toward a more agreeable one.

Unfortunately, such a rational analysis is not usually sufficient. Some emotional shift appears to be required. "Emotion is the very life of us," said Fritz Perls (1973). It drives us to move. Knowledge, understanding, vision are by themselves only ideas. Energy is required to propel a reluctant person out of a deeply engrained pattern in search of another. Techniques aimed toward helping patients relinquish old patterns require elements aimed toward generating the necessary emotion for the change process. Three such techniques are: (1) the clear elucidation of recurrent patterns, (2) delineation of consequences of maladaptive patterns, and (3) description of major discrepancies or contradictions.

Elucidation of Recurrent Patterns

If a person finds himself or herself in the same situation time and time again, attributing the cause to external forces becomes increasingly more difficult with each recurrence. However, human beings are quite capable of construing differences for situations with similar features and/or conveniently ignoring salient facts that would show the striking similarity between the past sequence and a current one. For some people, the public discovery of similarities is embarrassing enough to drive them toward relinquishing the pattern.

CASE 8.8. A 29-year-old mother of two entered therapy in a desperate attempt to regain Bill, her most recent love. She had insisted he leave her home because he was cruel to her children and made no financial contribution to the household. He had been increasingly cold to her as well, yet she couldn't bear to be single again and to be without him. When she had met him 4 years earlier he was out of work, without a car or place to live. She invited him to stay with her, got him a job, and tried to make him part of a family with her two children. Her ex-husband, Jim, had come from a poorer family than hers, had a reputation as a lazy, fun-loving boy, and was looked down upon by her family and friends. She became pregnant by him. The day before they were married, he told her of a sexual encounter with another woman; his affairs continued during their 5-year marriage. She supported him and their two children. When I clarified her pattern of picking men who were less capable than she of earning a living or giving emotionally, she could only remark that she wanted to feel superior to men, not inferior. She was embarrassed to realize that this desire implied that she was not good enough for men who might treat her well. She was forced to look at her own negative self-opinion.

Public embarrassment in the privacy of the therapist's office may be sufficient to motivate people to change. The recognition of responsibility through pattern definition has played an important part in psychodynamic psychotherapy, although psychodynamic writers do not formulate the effects of their interpretations in this way. Menninger (1958) and Malan (1979) attribute more theoretical objectives for identifying recurrent patterns as part of the process of change. The analysis of transference in order to make the unconscious conscious is the common explanatory purpose. More realistically, the psychodynamic therapist who points out a recurrent pattern between a parent, a lover, and the therapist is placing the patient at causal center for the recurrence. The indirect message is: "You are responsible for maintaining this pattern. Implied in these details are the means to stop it."

The simple intellectual demonstration of recurrent patterns is often insufficient to generate the emotion of change. Further leverage may be required. The continued emphasis in classical psychoanalysis upon the oedipal conflict may in part be explained by its potential for inducing shame. Although not generally discussed in this way, the shame-inducing power of the oedipal interpretation may explain its endurance. A young woman or man involved in destructive relationships is told that he or she is unconsciously seeking sex with a parent. The incest taboo is implicitly evoked, shame induced in a susceptible person, and emotion generated to relinquish the old pattern.

CASE 8.9. A 26-year-old woman entered short-term dynamic therapy because she had found herself wandering into the prostitute-filled section of her city but could not explain her action. She attempted to resist the urge to go but was only temporarily able to control it. Her relationships with men repeatedly centered around sex. When affection and commitment appeared on the horizon, she tended to start another sexual relationship. However, she was most disturbed by her inability to control the urge to go to the red light district. In discussing her father, the patient offhandedly mentioned that he often visited prostitutes in this very section of town. After further discussion of his behavior and the outwardly cool reactions of her long-suffering mother, the therapist made the following interpretation: "You are looking for your father. You are hoping to be a prostitute for him." (Sifneos, 1976)

The presentation of evidence for ongoing incestuous feelings serves to shame the patient into change.

Delineation of Consequences

A related approach is to emphasize the consequences of patterns and choices. Inevitably the patterns are demonstrated each time their consequences are outlined. The delineation of consequences adds an important emotional element. By showing the effects of a pattern upon marital discord, upon children, upon financial well-being, upon social contacts, and/or upon job performance, therapists indirectly imply that their clients are foolish to continue to hurt themselves and their loved ones in this way. Since the message is usually delivered within an evenhanded, noncritical presentation of the evidence, the shame is not directly acknowledged and may be preserved for the motion of change.

Inducing Discrepancy

The human desire for self-consistency has been studied under conditions in which subjects are placed in psychologically inconsistent situations. The "cognitive dissonance" resulting from these experiences generates discomfort, driving the people to reconstrue the situation in a manner consistent with their self-opinions. Therapists may point out inconsistencies between clients' avowed intentions and their consequences. They may point out aspects clients have distorted, denied, or deleted. Therapists may also offer different standards for evaluating perceived events and different relationships among the event elements (Strong, 1978).

The term "reframing" has been used to describe the introduction of a new theory that resolves contradictions. "If a person comes to 'know' a theory about his behavior, he is no longer bound by it but becomes free to disobey it" (Howard, quoted in Watzlawick, Weakland, & Fisch, 1974, p. 100). Through reframing, confusion may evolve toward explanation. A weak understanding may be replaced by a more effective one. The person confronted with newly discovered alternatives generated by the new theory becomes ready to change in order to reduce the discomfort caused by the now obvious discrepancies.

For example, when therapists notice patterns by which patients are reacting against models offered by a disliked parent, the stage is set for a discrepancy induction. Inevitably going to the opposite extreme means that the parent is still determining the patient's behavior since the opposite sets the inverse standards. Usually the oppositional position is not complete because the patient has also incorporated some of the hated characteristics without being aware of it. Therapists can evoke the energy of change by organizing evidence to show that the patient is still being controlled by the disliked model through out-of-awareness identification and through allowing the model to set the inverse standards.

In the following example, the patient was confronted with evidence clearly defining inconsistency between his behavior and his beliefs.

CASE 8.10. A 36-year-old bisexual married man came to therapy because he was languishing. He worked part-time in his parent's business, took drugs and alcohol regularly each day, and, when he felt the urge, cruised for homosexual liaisons among his three regular friends. He did not want to stop his drug use; he did not want to stop his homosexual activities. However, though he felt being gay was natural for him, he felt guilty about his continued sexual encounters with men because he had promised his wife that they would stop. He felt guilty about taking money from his parents for his major expenses, and he felt angry at his wife for resenting his not bringing in sufficient money.

At first he blamed his wife for his difficulties. "Why should she want to stay married to a man like me? Is she a lesbian trying to deny her homosexual feelings by converting me to a straight?" Then he thought that perhaps his best approach would be to divorce her and leave town. Further analysis revealed that he had not told any member of his family that he was gay. He felt he was protecting them, but then he heard himself say that they did not need protection. He had insisted that being gay was natural for him; he believed that his family would accept him under most circumstances, and yet he had not told them. He realized that his favorite fantasy centered around bringing his male lover home for Christmas. Why had he not lived up to his beliefs about himself? Why was this man who insisted upon honesty and living up to one's personal values not being the person he knew himself to be with those people who loved him the most? This set of discrepancies led him to see his responsibility for his current languishing state.

In helping patients to relinquish old patterns, the therapist must strike a careful balance between providing psychological safety and disconfirming of old patterns (Pentony, 1981, chap. 2). The strength of the therapeutic alliance may be tested by the shame, guilt, or dysphoria sometimes accompanying attempts to encourage giving up of the old patterns. Some therapists prefer to emphasize the power strategy of straightforward declaration that the current pattern is unacceptable. Cashdan (1973), for example, called this substage "stripping." His approach involved aggressive confrontation to yank the pattern away. Others prefer the use of gestures of goodwill designed to bring about a cooperative working out of the problem. Most seem to alternate direct and indirect forms of stripping with gestures of support and concern.

SPECIFIC APPROACHES TO THE INITIATION OF CHANGE

As the old pattern is sliding away, clients confront an empty space where once a familiar strategy for handling self and others had been. They search for a replacement, since the psyche, too, seems to abhor a vacuum. Milton Erickson recognized the vulnerability to influence persons feel when caught in a situation without clear alternatives and therefore sought to create this experience in any way he could. The following incident led him to develop an unusual method of hypnotic induction called the Confusion Technique:

> One windy day . . . a man came rushing around the corner of a building and bumped hard against me as I stood bracing myself against the wind. Before he could recover his poise to speak to me, I glanced elaborately at my watch and courteously, as if he had enquired the time of day, I stated 'It's exactly ten minutes of two,' though it was actually closer to 4:00 P.M. and walked on. About half a block away, I turned and saw him still looking at me, undoubtedly still puzzled and bewildered by my remark. (Watzlawick *et al.*, 1974, pp. 100–101)

Erickson had failed to respond in the socially expectable way but instead had offered another response that was factually incorrect. The result was confusion, unalleviated by any further pieces of the puzzle. Subjects caught in this dilemma are eager to grasp any piece of information that will help them organize the situation. They are thus open to influence. At this point in therapy therapists may: (1) describe alternatives, (2) offer themselves or others as models for new behaviors, or (3) describe specific behaviors or thoughts for the client to try.

The Description of Alternatives

What can the client do? Given the data of the current situation, the therapist can describe the available alternatives. Many therapists believe that they are offering evenhanded options and that they are not invested in the outcome. Nevertheless, alternatives are usually value laden and it is therefore likely that the therapist will in some way or another encourage the choosing of one alternative over another. A cognitive–behavioral colleague quoted himself talking to a client: "You are like a hungry person confronted with a table of food. You can choose to go hungry or come to the table and eat." Until I reflected back to him what he had said, he did not know that he was attempting to leverage his patient toward his own belief system. Many therapists are probably just as unaware of how they attempt to interject their beliefs.

Modeling

Human observation of others provides much information about alternatives. Children watch their parents and imitate them. Adolescents model their successful peers and avoid behaving like their unsuccessful ones. Television sports provide many examples to which young athletes may aspire. Mothers and fathers observe the interactions between other parent–child pairs to gather information for their own alternatives. Therapists are usually closely observed by their clients, especially those who wish to become therapists themselves. Trainees learn a great deal from watching their teachers perform psychotherapy as well as from hearing them talk about it.

The mechanisms involved are complex. Bandura (1969, 1976, 1977) has played a major role in using and describing modeling during psychotherapy. Most of his efforts have been spent on externally definable behavioral problems (e.g., snake phobics, assertiveness training). In psychoanalysis, identification with the therapist is recognized as a crucial part of treatment. In discussing change for the relatively more disturbed patients, Chessick (1977) suggested that interpretations were often relatively unimportant. Of greater importance was the therapist's nonanxious, observing attitude and his or her compassionate, studious, and sincere approach with which patients identify and that they incorporate as part of their own self-opinion. The warm, empathic regard promoted by Rogers and integrated into the approaches of many other therapists also provides a compassionate model with which to alter one's own self-opinion (if my therapist thinks of me this way, perhaps I can think of myself in this way also). The cognitive–behavioral therapists Mahoney and Arnkoff (1978) were quite explicit about encouraging client identification: "The therapist is sharing years of professional training by making the client an apprentice in therapy" (p. 709). Through actions and attitude, the therapist models alternatives. These alternatives are most persuasive when the patient is seeking a new way.

Direct Instructions to Act Differently

Homework assignments are a common therapeutic strategy. Therapists request a new behavior (diary, assertiveness, special requests, regular meeting with spouse) and the patient is to carry it out. Stories about Milton Erickson's selection of behavioral instructions are tantalizing reminders of what can be done in this mode (one of his cases reported in Haley, 1973, pp. 225–226, illustrates this well). Erickson seemed to grasp how to select the "right" small behavior that would create a deviation-amplifying feedback loop leading to a more desirable homeostasis:

CASE 8.11. This husband and wife had been running a restaurant business together for many years and they were in a constant quarrel about the management of it. The wife insisted that the husband should manage it, and he protested that she never let him do it. As he put it, "Yes, she keeps telling me I should run the restaurant. All the time she's running it, she tells me I should do it. I'm the bus boy, I'm the janitor, I scrub the floors. She nags at me about the buying, she nags at me about the bookkeeping, she nags at me because the floor needs scrubbing. I really should hire someone to scrub the floor, but my wife can't wait until somebody comes in and applies for the job. So I wind up doing it myself, and then there's no need to hire some one to do it."

The wife took the reasonable position that she wanted her husband to take care of the restaurant because she would rather be at home. She had sewing she wished to do. And she would like to serve her husband at least one home-cooked meal a day with special foods he liked. Her husband replied, "That's what she says. You can hear it, I can hear it. But she'll be in the restaurant tomorrow morning!"

I [Erickson] learned that they locked up the restaurant in the evening at about ten o'clock, and they opened at seven in the morning. I began to deal with the problem by asking the wife who should carry the keys to the restaurant. She said, "We both carry the keys. I always get there first and open up while he's parking the car."

I pointed out to her that she ought to see to it that her husband got there half an hour before she did. They had only one car, but the restaurant was just a few blocks from their home. She could walk there a half-hour later. When she agreed to this arrangement, it solved the conflict.

[Erickson explained the solution in the following way:]

"When the husband arrived a half-hour before his wife, he carried the keys. He opened the door. He unlocked everything. He set up the restaurant for the rest of the day. When his wife arrived, she was completely out of step and way behind. So many things had been set in motion by him, and he was managing them.

Of course, when she remained behind at home that half-hour in the morning, it left her with the breakfast dishes and her housework to do before she left. And if she could be a half-hour late, she could be thirty-five minutes late. In fact, what she hadn't recognized when she agreed to the arrangement, was that she could be forty-five minutes or even a hour late. In this way, she discovered that her husband could get along at the restaurant without her. Her husband, in turn, was discovering that he could manage the restaurant."*

Erickson seemed to understand not only what instructions to give but also how to give them in order to maximize the likelihood that his clients would comply with them. According to Haley's account, he asked the woman who liked to manage if she would see to it that her husband arrived a half-hour before she did. She was put in charge of the assignment and, therefore, was willing to accept it.

Watzlawick *et al.* (1974) also placed great emphasis upon the manner in which an instruction was to be given, insisting that it be placed in the client's frame of reference:

> To the engineer or computer man we may . . . explain the reason for this behavior prescription in terms of change from negative to positive feedback mechanisms. . . . With somebody who seems a poor prospect for any form of cooperation, we shall have to preface the prescription itself with the remark that there exists a simple, but somewhat odd way out of his problem, but we are almost certain that he is not the kind of person who can utilize this solution. And to types like ourselves, we may even lecture in terms of Group Theory, the Theory of Logical Types, first-order change and second-order change. (p. 126)

The offer of behavioral suggestion must also take into account the patient's reactance (Beutler, 1983). How willing is this person to follow directions from others? How much does this person fight authority and need to do the opposite? The latter group of people will require indirect instructions. The masked directives of psychodynamic interpretations serve this purpose well for many patients.

---

*Reprinted from *Uncommon Therapy, The Psychiatric Techniques of Milton H. Erickson, M.D.*, by Jay Haley, by permission of W.W. Norton & Company, Inc. Copyright © 1973 by Jay Haley.

SPECIFIC APPROACHES TO PRACTICE

Among the most alluring qualities of Milton Erickson's work is the very short term contact required with him. He needed very little therapeutic time for practice. As illustrated in the case of the restaurant couple, he was able to conceptualize their interlocking system with sufficient precision to allow him to introduce a small shift that snowballed in the desired direction. His prescriptions were often more efficient than effective medications because his clients were required to follow them but a few times. Subsequently, the power of the deviation carried them into a new, more desirable homeostasis. Practice was therefore built into the successful intervention.

Many therapists offer behavioral advice without Erickson's magnificent intuitive grasp of the context within which the difficulty is being maintained. These more ordinary prescriptions require practice to permit them to be integrated into the patient's repertoire and accepted by the patient's significant others. Shelton and Levy (1981, pp. 37–77) have presented a systematic outline of the variety of ways in which behavioral suggestions may be practiced.

1. The therapist should be sure that assignments carry specific detail regarding response and stimulus elements relevant to the desired behavior. For example, many socially isolated clients receive the instruction "take a volunteer job." This instruction is too general for most patients needing to consider it. Take a job where? Whom to call? What to say? How to say it? These are but a few of the questions requiring specific answers. Each may require discussion, role-playing, and several real-world practices before the goal is achieved.

2. The therapist should give skill training where necessary. Erickson's restaurant couple did not need skill training in order to have the wife come a few minutes later than her husband. However, many clients require practice in behavioral skills in the office before they attempt to try them outside. Complex behaviors should be practiced in order to reduce the probability that they will be punished by persons in the environment. After assessing the client's skill level, the therapist proceeds to give verbal and perhaps written instructions, as well as reasons that the target behavior is important. After the therapist models the skill, he or she then coaches, prompts, and reinforces the client toward successive approximations of the desired goal.

3. Practice for desired behavior should be reinforced. Reinforcement comes from three major sources: the therapist, the client, and significant others. (a) Therapists reinforce by direct compliments, in the office or by telephone. Therapists may decide to schedule the next appointment

contingent upon the client's successful accomplishment of the next step in the practice sequence. Or they may reduce the length of sessions, while charging the same fee, if assignments are not completed. Behavioral contracts should be clearly specified and usually written out and signed. (b) Self-reinforcement can be vital to maintaining practice schedules. Target behaviors can be supported by self-praise or by external rewards. For example, upon completion of a successful behavior, clients can reward themselves with positive self-statements ("I'm doing a good job; I know it will work out.") Or they can take themselves to a movie or buy something nice to eat or drink. (c) Reinforcement by significant others is the most desired form. Fish (Pentony, 1981, pp. 61–62) elaborated on this concept. He drew attention to the often overlooked fact that when a person begins to behave in a noticeably different manner, people who know him or her well are uncertain how to respond. Efforts should be made to ensure that they do respond positively. One possibility is to provide them with an explanation to account for such change. The explanation should be couched in terms that indicate the change is real and not superficial. There is no need to attribute the change to therapy if the person who is to understand does not believe in psychotherapy. The explanation should be couched in explanatory terms that can be accepted by the listener.

4. The therapist should begin with small homework requests and gradually increase assignments. If the client is an active participant in determining the therapeutic activities rather than a respondent to heavy demands from the therapist, the chances for compliance are increased.

5. The therapist should use cuing, prompting or reminding clients to carry out assignments through any available means. These include phone calls by the therapist, cuing from significant others, timed buzzers, calendars, and dated pill dispensers.

6. The therapist should elicit a public commitment to comply. One of the best predictors of client behavior is the response to the question whether or not the person is going to carry out the suggestion. Written contracts seem to increase the likelihood of following the suggestion.

Shelton and Levy (1981) described three other approaches that might possibly enhance the practice phase: cognitive rehearsal, attempts to reduce the negative effects of compliance, and the close monitoring of the target behavior from as many sources as are possible.

CHANGE PROCESSES IN A CASE OF AGORAPHOBIA

The written word cuts planes through the complex process of psychological change. Description of the general and specific approaches described in the previous sections captures the separate perspectives. A case report can convey the blending of these elements as they affect a single person.

Agoraphobics usually have had panic attacks that usually decrease in frequency if the patient stays home. The patient's spouse often plays a part in the difficulty, especially once it has begun. Therefore, treatment may be composed of three or four prongs: (1) management of the panic attacks themselves, usually with medications (Grant, Katon, & Beitman, 1983); (2) exposure treatment for the agoraphobia; (3) analysis and alteration of the spouse's contribution; and (4) possibly in-depth examination of the patient's psychological predisposition to panic (Shear, 1985).

CASE 8.12. A 42-year-old woman was referred by her gynecologist for treatment of episodes of intense anxiety. The patient had been married for 22 years and had three children ages 21, 17, and 12. Her husband had become a minister after working in a factory for most of their marriage. He had felt the calling, quit work, and went to school to become a minister. The patient enjoyed the life at the university since there were many other women like her here. She resented, however, having to leave her newly bought home, with the new fence and the friendly neighbors. Her husband received an appointment at a small church in a small town in Missouri. As they drove through St. Louis during rush hour, she was overcome with anxiety, sweating, faintness, palpitations, and chest pain. She pulled over and her husband, following in a pickup truck, pulled over behind her. That was her first panic attack. She had many more. Once in the new town, she found herself unable to go to the large shopping malls 40 miles from town. She was frightened to go more than a block from her home, because she feared that she would have an attack. Her life became increasingly restricted. She would go nowhere without her husband. During her premenstrual period, she was extremely irritable, cried easily, and slept as much as she could. She was becoming despondent because she did not know what to do.

The first step in therapy was to define her primary difficulty as panic disorder with subsequent phobic avoidance. I suggested that medication was likely to be helpful. Because of her history of responsiveness to low doses of medication, I started her on a low dose of imipramine. I also explained that slow steady exposure to greater and greater distances from home would be the only treatment for her fears. I invited her husband in for the first interview and asked him to understand and help her in her efforts. She returned 2 weeks later, having started to increase her distance from home. She feared the panics less because she believed that the medications would help to stop them. She asked that her husband not be present during the second meeting and described in further detail how angry she was with him for bringing her to this small town where being the minister's wife meant nobody truly accepted her as an equal. She despised her husband's sermons because he spoke an uneducated English. She hated him for teasing and tickling her when she did not want it from him. She wanted him to get a secular job and move closer to her family in Illinois. She decided to discuss these issues with him.

During the third session 2 weeks later, she had traveled 20 miles with a friend, not her husband. She had become tired but pushed herself anyway and then had a panic attack. However, she noticed that she was far less irritable during her period and wondered if the medication had helped that. Because she was experiencing episodes of dizziness, she thought she might have to reduce the medication. I agreed. She reported that her husband was willing to quit his job and find secular work in another town. She also found that she could accept his poor use of English if he would listen to her when she did not want to be teased or tickled. She had been able to walk 1 mile from home and back without trouble.

The fourth session, 1 month later, marked a great increase in her self-confidence. She had changed her hair and driven the entire 2 hours to the medical center by herself with her husband beside her. She was able to drive around this large town without fear. In fact, she enjoyed seeing all the cars and people. She felt she could live in a bigger city now. She was not sure her husband would be able to find good secular work but she was less bothered by this possibility. Her last period had been preceded by moderate discomfort. She wondered if she should raise the medication to the previous dose the 10 days before her period was to start and lower it after it began. I agreed. Her follow-up appointment was set for 2 months later.

She called 2 weeks before that appointment wanting to see me sooner. She came in at week 7 instead of 8, feeling depressed and anxious. Her husband could not get a job near her relatives and they had just bought a new house in their small town. Her traveling had become somewhat restricted but she felt she could overcome that. She wanted to restart the now stopped medication but the Beck Depression Inventory was 10 (within the normal range). She simply felt frustrated with having to stay there. Would they ever accept her? I asked her to consider whether she would accept them. These people were rural, farm people like her husband. Could she accept herself as the wife of a minister to farmers?

In this case, change had been initiated through three different and interlacing mechanisms: (1) The medication served to bolster her confidence in the possibility that she would not become panicked. Whether this would be best called a pharmacological effect or a placebo effect is difficult to determine in this case because the patient's tendency to panic may also have been dramatically reduced. The frequency of panic attacks seems to shift throughout a person's life. (2) Exposure in a slow and steady manner to the feared situation by putting greater and greater distance between her and her home offered the central approach to her initial complaint. Her ability to carry it out quickly bolstered her confidence to speak with her husband and get a positive response from him. (3) Marital therapy was initiated during the first interview by making the husband part of the solution and thereby implying that he also might be part of the problem. When she asked that he not attend the second session, she wished to use the session to make further inroads in changing their relationship.

A fourth mechanism became obvious during the end of the second to last session described in this report. The patient kiddingly described how women patients often fall in love with their psychiatrists and expressed her deep gratitude for the help she had received from me. She seemed to want to please me as well.

Unfortunately, for the science of psychotherapy, patient states at the end of psychotherapy do not necessarily continue. Sometimes patients improve on these end states and this is our fondest hope for them — that they take from us ideas and information that will help them to continue their psychological development. However, forces in the environment often work against these fond hopes by pushing patients back toward undesired states. She had wanted to escape that small town, to live closer to her relatives, to live closer to her daughter. Now she had to adjust to life in this place. I suspected that I would see her again. The problem of the maintenance of change is discussed in Chapter 11.

9. Change: Therapist Lessons

In the previous chapter, change techniques were linked to substages of change, but they were not linked to specific content of the pattern search. Should not therapists be able to identify certain patterns and derive a set of techniques to help to change these patterns? Unfortunately, this apparently logical linkage does not take into consideration the fact that therapists seem to use change technique as a way to teach their own values and coping strategies. The techniques of change provide ways for therapists to attract their patients' attention to new ideas. When therapists are able to induce their patients to enter into that often frightening transition point between relinquishing old patterns and not yet having begun any new ones, patients are particularly vulnerable to therapist influence. The identification of patterns to be changed provides a language through which the therapist lessons can be specified in a mutually understood language.

Among the common self-deceptions perpetuated by psychotherapists is the value-free nature of the therapist's influence. Techniques are smoke screens by which therapists can pretend to "remove blocks to individuation" or "make the unconscious conscious" or "increase self-efficacy" while actually directing clients' thinking according to therapists' own beliefs. Research evidence has strongly confirmed the value-laden aspects of psychotherapy. In a survey of 81 psychodynamic psychotherapists, most of whom had been in psychoanalysis, Buckley *et al.* (1979) found that most of the 81 respondents generally agreed the therapist should not impose his value system on the patient. Nevertheless, half the group believed that an important aspect of therapy was encouraging the enrichment of the patient's social, educational, or vocational pursuits. Successful psychotherapy seems to be characterized by changes in patient values and beliefs toward those of the therapist, even though therapists vary widely in belief and value postures (Beutler, 1983; Strong, 1978). If these findings are to be accepted, therapists must begin the difficult process of clarifying their values, beliefs, and coping styles. Whether aware of it or not, therapists are teaching their patients to be like them or to assume roles of which they approve. After reviewing some teaching mechanisms, this chapter describes many of the common values and coping styles taught by psychotherapists.

TEACHING MECHANISMS

The methods by which therapists teach their patients require more precise delineation. Most of the techniques therapists call change inducing, as well as many pattern-search methods, would probably be included. For example, the apparently innocuous empathic reflection can be used to reinforce certain speech content and presumably certain attitude and value changes as well. Exhortation is perhaps the most obvious and direct form of teaching.

One of the remarkable curiosities of modern psychotherapy is the lack of awareness of many therapists about how and what they are conveying to their clients. How often have therapist and patient mused together toward the end of a successful therapy about who is responsible for the change? The patient often prefers to give most credit to the therapist while the therapist may take a variety of overt and covert positions. Those who believe that change is the client's business and that the therapist is simply a facilitator will be hard-pressed to allow themselves to accept responsibility either silently or to the patient. Those who believe themselves to be behavioral technologists may prefer to take full responsibility for the change. However, such therapists may also believe that clients should leave therapy with an increase in their own sense of mastery and, therefore, may describe the gain as a team effort or largely the client's doing. A more precise answer to the question may lie in the degree to which the therapist persuades the patient to assume a set of attitudes, values, and coping styles.

The curious tendency among some therapists not to assume responsibility for their own influence over patients implies some value to this perspective. How has it been useful for therapists to believe that they are simply "facilitating change" rather than also influencing clients in well-defined directions?

Freud, Rogers, and many existential–humanistic therapists have led in the development of therapist self-concept as a passive facilitator of psychological change. To use a biological analogy: Therapists act like enzymes to promote transformation without lending anything of themselves to the transformation. The patient–client is a potential force striving to be liberated from its encrusted blocks; the therapist simply helps to remove the blocks. There is something pristine, immaculate, and reassuring about playing the role of the uninvolved yet necessary element for psychological growth. Yet enzymes wear out and need to be replaced. How can one touch without touching, participate without participating?

The passive therapist's self-identity has very definite practical advantages. Many patients learn better from their therapists if they are taught indirectly. The carefully placed reinforcers of accurate empathic statements, of certain nods or voice changes can produce responses without clear patient objection and rejection. If the therapist is unaware of the direct intent of these techniques, he or she does not have to feel guilty for "manipulating" the patient and can feel comfortable in attributing the change to the patient's efforts. Consider the following example:

CASE 9.1. A 32-year-old, unmarried accountant, very withholding of emotional expression, became angry at the idea that his past relationships with his parents might be influences on his current behavior. He did not understand why people described him as condescending and why he procrastinated at small household tasks, especially when he knew that accomplishing them would make him feel better. He was tormented by conflicted emotions in relationships with women and wanted relief from these pains. He readily admitted being very angry at his parents: his mother for overprotecting him and his father for rarely spending time with him when he was growing up. He feared that expressing this anger would "destroy" his father.

The therapist tried to show him that the past was alive in the present by suggesting: You remain afraid to express your anger at your father and you inhibit your expression of feeling to others now because you are still afraid that your emotion might hurt them. He seemed to grasp the idea and after careful thought said, "I should not be afraid to express my feelings to others."

This self-statement was the indirect lesson of the past–present interpretation that implied that he might as well get angry now; he wasn't going to hurt anyone. The therapist made a standard psychodynamic statement. Embedded in it was a directive. The patient had to work to understand it and make it his own.

One of the powers of indirectness is that it leads the persons to draw the conclusion themselves without having been directly told to do so or think so. Any time the therapist comments on the patient's behavior, the therapist is implying something is wrong and needs to be changed. However indirect the comment, the patient will often attempt to perceive the embedded lesson if the alliance is strong. If not, the comment is more likely to be perceived as a criticism.

Those therapists who emphasize the interpretation of latent content serve as models for their patients, who, in turn, tend to interpret the latent content of their therapist's utterances. Therefore, patients gradually learn to understand the latent messages in their therapists' responses. Perhaps one of the reasons psychoanalysis takes so long is because the therapist speaks so infrequently and in such theoretical terms that the patient takes many years to piece together his underlying value system.

The political and economic consequences of many therapists' failure to acknowledge their own influence over patients may be far-reaching. If therapists are not really doing anything (having an effect), why should they be paid? If therapists do not accept that they are actually influencing their clients, how can they argue for their effectiveness? How can therapists be "working" without "effecting"? This paralytic paradox must be broken in order to clarify therapists' self-identity and to more clearly make the case for society's support for psychotherapists. Breaking this paradox will help to better define the qualities of excellent therapists who are by definition effective communicators of adaptive values and coping skills.

WHAT DO THERAPISTS TEACH?

Realization of therapist influence leads to an even more complicated question. What lessons are most effective for which patients seen by which therapists?

People become clients because they have difficulty adjusting to the stresses and strains of their existence. They have problems in living, immature defense mechanisms, ineffective coping strategies, blocks to individuation, poor control over the contingencies governing their behavior, and/or misconceptions of themselves in relationship to others. These terms converge on a common theme: The person is having difficulty regulating the self and/or the self in relationship to the environment. The regulating mechanisms currently being employed are ineffective and need to be readjusted. Therapists attempt to aid their clients in making this readjustment. The manner in which alternatives are selected for specific patients is, unfortunately, not systematic.

Therapists tend to cherish certain beliefs about the world, certain ways of regulating internal states, certain ways of relating to other people, and certain attitudes toward the self. These ideas are nurtured by culture, educational training contexts, self-selected schools of psychotherapy, critical personal life events, and the challenges of the therapist's current life cycle stage.

Western cultural values are greatly concerned with the preeminence of the self, while Eastern values emphasize the self as part of a greater

social context. Western therapists tend to emphasize individual responsibility, power, and influence, while Eastern teachers tend to subordinate
the individual to the greater good of the group. One of the preeminent
tasks of earth culture is to reach a compromise between these two extremes, to create a culture in which both the identity of the individual
and the well-being of the group are nurtured and preserved.

Geographical location, early schooling, college, and graduate education also influence attitudes toward the world and ideal ways of living.
Small-town cultures may tend to encourage the helping of one's neighbor,
while larger cities may teach people the dangers of trusting others living
on the same block. Liberal-arts colleges may promote a love for the history
of ideas, while large state universities may emphasize technology and implicitly foster the insignificance of the individual. Medical school may
train therapists to treat patients as physiological mechanisms; social work
school to treat them as members of social networks; and psychology
graduate school to treat them as information processing units. Choices
of therapeutic orientation may be influenced by a number of factors
(student personality, visibility of a theory, peer pressure, opportunity)
(Cornsweet, 1983). This decision then increases the likelihood that certain
ideas and values will receive greater emphasis and others will be ignored.

Finally, the therapist's current age presents him or her with specific
bicultural challenges that serve to highlight certain problems and their
potential solutions. Beginning therapists are often in their 20s and are,
therefore, struggling with their professional autonomy and their ability
to form lasting relationships with peers and lovers. Beginning therapists
may therefore teach lessons related to professional autonomy and romantic love. For the 40-year-old therapist, reapproachment with family of
origin may take on great significance, while the tragedy of a patient's
divorce may not seem so terrible as it did during the perhaps more romantic earlier years in the profession. Therapists in their later years may
be less invested in any outcome and more able to accept inevitable events.
This passivity, strongly influenced by physical decline and the loss of
acquaintances through death, will have differential usefulness to patients.

These many influences upon the being and perception of therapists
determine in part the types of messages therapists send to their clients.
Ideally, therapists will formulate concepts and behaviors that will suit
the needs of each individual while also keeping in mind Rollo May's (1975)
hope that authentic values should best emerge from the patient's own
development. This paradox of influence without influence may be resolved by noting the continuous readjustment therapists must make to the
emerging needs of their clients.

What are some of the common teachings emerging from the psychotherapeutic encounter? Please keep in mind that what follows is a selection of ideas biased by my own beliefs, values, and experiences. Like the content of the pattern search, the specific lessons of psychotherapy need greater specification, clarification, and discussion.

The Problem of Meaning

Human beings appear to be meaning-seeking creatures trying to comprehend the world around them. However, there appears to be no absolutely correct world view unless one chooses to believe that a specific perspective is the only correct one. The only true absolute may be that there are no absolutes (Yalom, 1980, p. 423). Viktor Frankl (1955, 1959) for example, believed that his role as therapist required him to help his patients find a meaning by which their lives could take value. During his concentration camp experience during the Nazi holocaust he had noted that individuals without a sense of meaning were less likely to survive. Human beings appear to function better when imbued with a sense of purpose that gives significance to their daily existence. For Frankl, a great many people enter therapy because they are without that vision. Consider the following Frankl example.

CASE 9.2. A colleague, an aged general practitioner, turned to me because he could not come to terms with the loss of his wife, who had died 2 years before. His marriage had been very happy, and he was now extremely depressed. I asked him quite simply: "Tell me what would have happened if you had died first and your wife had survived you?" "That would have been terrible," he said. "How my wife would have suffered!" "Well, you see," I answered, "your wife has been spared that, and it was you who spared her, though of course, you must now pay by surviving and mourning her." In that very moment his mourning had been given meaning—the meaning of sacrifice. (1955, p. xiv)

Belief in a Supreme Being has provided millions of people with an enduring sense of mission, purpose, and significance, thereby preventing the suffering that often accompanies meaninglessness. Although I find much reprehensible behavior among those who firmly believe in their own religious righteousness, I am also impressed with the security and self-confidence that many of these individuals possess. Furthermore, those who have in some way grasped the connection to a higher source often radiate a beatific glow most enviable and alluring. Can humankind evolve toward religious belief that does not posit the superiority of one diety over another or encourage the decimation of one religious group because they believe differently? Should the concept of a Supreme Being be eliminated entirely or better clarified? Pastoral counselors are by definition therapists who are seeking to help their clients discover or rediscover their connection to a Higher Power. Wapnick (1984), for example, stated explicitly his belief that all guilt rests ultimately with the sense of having separated from the Supreme Being. The belief in this separation is, according to him, the sickness bringing people to therapy. The function of therapy is then to reestablish the link, thereby bringing about psychological and spiritual healing.

Alcoholics Anonymous and other religiously based self-help groups also rely heavily upon developing or recapturing flagging religious beliefs by which their members can regain a sense of coherence and mission. These organizations also provide membership within a social group, the opportunity to advance up a social hierarchy, and a mission to help similarly suffering people. Individual psychotherapy is generally unable to supply so readily these meaningful social bulwarks against the chaos of purposelessness.

CASE 9.3. A 35-year-old, married man with one child was a recovering alcoholic who had reached the highest rung of his work in Alcoholics Anonymous. He had also been in psychotherapy for 5 years in another town, and it was as a result of this treatment that he had been able to join the organization and get married. He found himself deeply agitated, believed he had hypoglycemia, thought he was depressed, and kept up sexual affairs with two other women. He was sought out by AA members because he was well respected, had a good job, and was self-confident. He could not find someone within AA in whom to confide his troubles. His major difficulty appeared to be an overarching self-criticism coupled with an impossible list of expectations. Through our encounters he was able to reduce some of these self-demands, to relinquish his affairs, and to devote more time to his wife and child. He seemed to accept his limitations. He repeatedly complained about the energy drain of his AA connection. He wanted to go less frequently; he wanted to quit the organization. When I confronted him about this possibility, he became anxious. Further discussion only heightened his anxiety. He realized that he was afraid to leave despite his discomfort with its demands. I invited him to return to therapy when he wished to leave AA. After 6 years, he had not stopped going to AA. Apparently he accepted the need for that social role and the meaning it gave to his life.

For those many therapists who embrace secular personal meaning rather than cosmic religious ones, there are many alternatives. The emergence of science as a tool for comprehending reality has created a new, often antithetical, perspective: *scientism*. Scientism refers to a belief only in what is provable by the scientific method of controlled experimental trials analyzed by accepted statistical methods (Hine, Merman, & Simpson, 1982). Believers in scientism tend also to accept only those who share like beliefs, thereby forming rational clubs of like-minded individuals who are less predisposed to criticize each other. Thus another social organization can be formed providing social meaning and purpose.

There are a number of other secular meanings that can provide believers with a coherent, supraordinate pattern to life and a role into which to fit (Yalom, 1980).

Through *altruism* many people find important roles and useful purpose. Dying cancer patients sometimes wish to convey to others their discoveries while living without a personal future. The here-and-now becomes so much more vital, human contact so much more beautiful, that they wish to share their experience, perhaps in part with the hope of living on through having influenced another. *Selfish altruism* is that form of helping that also serves the helper. Psychotherapists and other helping professionals are rewarded in many ways by their interactions with patients. Parents caring for their children experience many joys and the sense of living on through them, as well as the worry and pain inevitable to the nurturing process. Unselfish denial of one's own needs may prove to be an excellent strategy for maintaining long-term relationships (Cashdan, 1973). Two partners who unselfishly meet the needs of the other provide each other with enduring and committed interaction.

Through *dedication to a cause*, individuals take themselves outside their own personal pursuits and place themselves in a higher context through which their efforts can take on greater meaning. Causes, whether the family, the state, secular religions like communism or facism, a scientific project, a sports team, or religion, often have altruistic underpinnings. Through *creativity* individuals produce something new and unique. No matter what the area, art, science, cooking, administration, or romance, the creation of something unique and the sense of being able to create more, provides a light against the darkness of meaninglessness.

For many, the answer is the *hedonistic solution*, not uncommon in the more affluent sections of modern America. Money and power become ends in themselves. Drugs, food, clothing, or social position become the guiding principles. In the broader sense, any activity that brings pleasure, including altruism, could be called hedonistic, but here I mean a selfish indulgence of one's own whims while shunning the needs and values of others.

How can therapists dedicated to the accumulation of wealth fail to instill this value in some of their clients? How can therapists who strongly believe in Christ as the Savior avoid influencing some of their clients in this direction? Short-term contacts may be less likely to provide the opportunity for value transfer, but longer relationships seem to provide ample opportunity.

Values

Values are special forms of beliefs and attitudes that have to do with modes of conduct and end states of existence. To say that a therapist has a value is to suggest that he or she "has an enduring belief that a specific mode of conduct or end-state of existence is personally and socially preferable to alternative modes of conduct or end-states of existence." The difference between preferable modes of conduct and preferable end states of existence is the distinction between means and ends, between instrumental and terminal values. Statements about instrumental values take the form: "I believe that this mode of conduct (honesty, courage, sharing, sexual fidelity) is personally and socially preferable in all situations." Statements about terminal values take a similar form: "I believe that this end state of existence (world peace, emotional awareness, loving relationships, great wealth) is personally and socially worth striving for" (Rokeach, 1972, p. 160).

Once a value is internalized through parental, social, or therapeutic persuasion, it becomes a standard by which to guide actions, to justify one's own actions and the actions and attitudes of others, to morally judge the self, and to compare the self with others. Take, for example, the common psychotherapeutic value that therapists should not have sex with their patients. Patient advocate groups and many state legislators have condemned this form of sexual contact. Nevertheless, as in cases of rape and child abuse, only the most flagrant violators are punished and, therefore, restraint is primarily a matter of personal ethic. How does a male therapist who strongly believes in sexual fidelity but who is caught in a difficult marriage in which sex is minimal manage to hold back from the lovely invitation of a passionate patient who declares that simply holding hands will bring ecstasy? How do such therapists manage to look into those pleading eyes while sensing the other's intense sexual arousal and refuse the warm invitation to physical union? Furthermore, what is the message in such refusals?

In addition to learning that sex cannot always be used to alter power imbalances, therapists also teach, by their restraint, that sex plays a part in a limited number of relationships. In this way, the therapist models commitment to one partner and implies that there are benefits to such commitments. Restraint helps to indicate that the therapist is interested in maintaining the therapeutic relationship that otherwise would be destroyed by sexual contact, and to suggest that sexual contact is not necessary for all caring heterosexual relationships.

Psychotherapy Values

Perhaps the most pervasive, though often-unstated, value taught by psychotherapists is self-responsibility. Therapists differ widely in their beliefs about degrees of self-responsibility, ranging from those who believe that the self is totally responsible for everything that happens (Ajaya, 1984; Ellis, 1962) to those who believe in a narrow range of freedom within many environmental restraints. Part of the reason for this wide range of opinion lies in each therapist's different perspectives and life experiences. Some can and prefer to see their own power as the controlling influence on their directions in life, although they too are limited by biological and environmental constraints (e.g., aging and social and financial limitations). Others prefer to place great attention on their limitations, although they too are free to emphasize what is within their control. Despite this wide range of variance, therapists appear to ask much the same questions:

1. What is the domain of reality over which this person has control?
2. What are this person's resources within these limitations?
3. What is this person doing that thrusts him or her repeatedly into the same undesirable end point?
4. What is preventing this person from acknowledging what he or she has influence over while accepting what is relatively beyond influence?

Answers to these questions lead patients to define themselves within their social and environmental contexts, thereby defining self-responsibility and its limitations.

By their very emphasis upon the individual's experience, psychotherapists reflect a basic Western regard for the primacy of the self. The existence of more than 200,000 professionals with a major interest in psychotherapy (Beitman, 1983c) testifies to how strongly American culture supports the individual's attempt to stand out from the group. Although therapists vary in the ways they express it, they all share a desire to help people differentiate themselves, to define more clearly who they are, to understand more fully what they can be, to remove impediments to realizing their potentials. Psychotherapists have been criticized for this emphasis (Wallach & Wallach, 1983) because it urges a selfish "me-centered" philosophy that ignores the social context. Psychotherapists have also been criticized for training their patients to accept the status quo without recognizing the political and economic constraints that are contributing to their difficulties (Agel, 1971). During the Vietnam War, for example, some psychoanalysts interpreted the motivation for the protest movement as a mask for personal inadequacy for which psychotherapy was the cure (A. Freud, 1968). In fact, aside from moral questions, these people were facing an increase in the possibility of premature death for themselves and their friends. Some therapists, male and female alike, may be still encouraging depressed women to accept their roles as wards of their husbands. Among the less controversial cultural values that most psychotherapists emphasize are encouragement toward better education; mature heterosexual intimacy; financial self-support through work; good care of the body, including moderation of drug and alcohol intake; honesty; politeness; and respect for law. Therapists are representatives of the culture, often licensed by the state and trained by its institutions. They are likely to promulgate the widely accepted values of the cultures through which they pass.

This dialectic between individual and cultural values illustrates a critical question for psychotherapy values clarification. When and for whom should a therapist emphasize individual concerns and when should cultural values be emphasized? How can they be brought to merge?

The clarification of one's own values and the values of others can be a very tricky problem. Consider the question of religion. During the 1980s, fundamentalist religion began to play an increasingly important role in American politics and, as a result, psychotherapists began to examine more carefully the meaning of religion to them and to their patients. To be religious does not define one's value orientation because there appears to be an important continuum of religiosity upon which believers distribute themselves. Allport called one pole *extrinsic*, attributing utilitarian, self-centered, and opportunistic characteristics to the people located there. At the other end of the continuum he found the *intrinsic* person, characterized by basic trust and a compassionate understanding of others, so that "dogma is tempered with humility" (Allport, cited in Rokeach, 1972, p. 194). In a study of religiously minded students, all enrolled at one denominational college, two distinct groups emerged. One was open-minded and tolerant and the other was closed-minded and highly prejudiced. While they expressed similar values in college, 6 years later, their values had diverged. Both groups still rated religious values highest but there they parted company. The open-minded group put social values next and theoretical values third. The closed-minded group put political values second in importance and economic values third. Thus it is obvious that to say a patient or therapist is religious does not sufficiently define his or her crucial values (p. 195).

Values are essential to human adaptation because they provide guides to action. When one has values, each decision point in life does not require a complete analysis but instead can be judged according to these superordinate standards. In addition, values add predictability to social life (Kluckholn, quoted by Yalom, 1980, p. 464) since those who belong to a particular group are defined by their beliefs about what behaviors and ideals are best. If a fundamentalist Christian psychotherapist who supports conservative politics meets a client with a similar self-description, they both know that they share a great many attitudes. If a liberal Jewish therapist from a large city meets a liberal Jewish patient from a large city, they will also recognize many beliefs and attitudes in common. If either of these clients is considering marriage, should the therapist encourage marriage to someone of the same religious background? One could argue very persuasively that such marriages are likely to produce less conflict in critical areas and, therefore, may be more adaptive. On the other hand, one could criticize the therapist for imposing his or her religious views.

Psychotherapy World Views

The schools of psychotherapy share with religions high-level constructs about the nature of the world and the best ways of dealing with it. If prayer is the answer for certain deeply religious people, then dream analysis may provide comfort and direction for Jungians. If ritual brings solace for an anxious religious person, relaxation exercises may work for a student of stress management. If studying the Holy Book brings answers for the confused religious person, then examination of ones own cognitions may provide a reorientation for a student of cognitive therapy.

These and other psychotherapeutic coping techniques are embedded in philosophical attitudes about human existence that are implicitly conveyed to patients in psychotherapy. These school-bound philosophical positions are blended with each therapist's own value system. Freud (1933) saw human beings as buffeted about by forces beyond their individual control. On the one hand, civilization was making increasing demands for organized, conforming behavior and, on the other hand, the primeval forces within each psyche were relentlessly demanding expression. Rogers (1951) struck a more optimistic note with his Midwestern belief in the goodness of each person and his or her ability to find the best for the self and for others. Speaking for most cognitive therapists and many existentialists, Kelly (1955) insisted that the world can be construed in many different ways. Therefore, a limited number of highly flexible principles that could be molded over the data of observation would best serve the individual. Radical behavioral therapists have tended to see the world as beyond individual control; all responses are conditioned or determined by environmental events. Milton Erickson seemed to delight in an awareness of the systematic interrelationship of multiple events that could be altered by simple well-placed interventions. (Watzlawick *et al.*, 1974).

Coping

Although values and world views are important for human adaptation and are often taught by therapists, patients usually need to discover better ways of coping. Lazarus and Launier (quoted in Coyne & Lazarus, 1980, p. 154–155) define coping as "efforts, both action oriented and intrapsychic, to manage (that is, to master, tolerate, reduce, minimize) environmental and internal demands and conflicts which task or exceed a person's resources." This definition distinguishes adaptation from coping by emphasizing that coping covers only stressful situations, that is, times when the person's resources and limitations are exceeded. It is under conditions of excessive taxation that patients often come to therapy implicitly requesting a broadening of their resources. Therapists generally try to improve intrapsychic mechanisms (e.g., defense mechanisms) or provide better problem-solving methods or some combination of the two. Schools of psychotherapy survive probably because they are able to provide followers with coping strategies that work for clients or their practitioners.

Many therapists share a strong belief in helping their clients to "face their fears." By doing so, the unknown becomes more comprehensible and, therefore, alternative responses become more evident. This strategy has been most systematically developed in the treatment of phobias by exposing the sufferer to the feared object. Apparently, the specific form of exposure matters little, whether it be in imagination or *in vivo*, rapid or gradual (Marks, 1976). Similar approaches have been adopted for unconscious phenomena; in these cases, therapists may expose their patients to deeply rooted conflicts, either rapidly, through penetrating interpretations (Greenson, 1967; Klein, 1932), or slowly, through uncovering by confrontation, clarification, and just-below-the-surface interpretations (Greenson, 1967).

Underlying many approaches is a firm conviction that clear acknowledgement of reality through the search for truth is essential (Ellis, 1962). Unfortunately, one truth of human existence is that reality is encased in many covers, any of which may be labeled the true reality (Bandler & Grinder, 1979; Kelly, 1955).

Therapists may select from a wide variety of coping responses. Coping has two general functions, either to change the situation for the better or to manage one's own subjective or somatic responses in order to avoid damaging morale or social functioning. The situation may be changed for the better either by altering one's own behavior or by changing the damaging or threatening environment. One's own subjective responses may be changed by altering the environment, for example, by avoiding it or by denying its potential harm, or by altering the self (by avoiding negative thoughts or taking drugs) (Lazarus, 1981). The choices therapists make about what clients should learn seem to depend in great part upon their own personal experiences with what works as well as what society dictates to be within the normal range of coping responses.

Many therapists fully believe that medications can play an extremely useful role in the treatment of some patients. Psychiatrists, who are therapists licensed to prescribe psychoactive medications, report having more than 35 % of their psychotherapy patients on medications (Beitman & Maxim, 1984). Psychologists (and other nonmedical psychotherapists) also regularly refer psychotherapy clients to physicians for psychoactive medications while continuing to see them in psychotherapy (Beitman *et al.*, 1984). On the other hand, many therapists, including some psychiatrists and many nonmedical therapists, are strongly opposed to the use of this coping strategy. Some are ideologically opposed to any kind of drug "dependence" while others simply cannot prescribe it and do not wish to have someone else interfering with their treatment. Psychiatric medications can also be viewed as providers of an extremely useful coping strategy that each potentially responsive patient may learn to use (Ward, 1984).

Relaxation techniques of all kinds, further elaborated by self-hypnotic instructions (Spiegel & Spiegel, 1978) represent nonpharmacological methods that clients may learn to use to self-regulate under stressful situations. These exercises may be prescribed for specific frequencies during the day, much as a medication would be prescribed. The effects are measurable physiologically as well. Others may advocate learning to speak to oneself in more adaptable ways through soothing, complimentary words, or self-encouragement, or a reduction in self-criticism (Ellis, 1962; Meichenbaum, 1977).

Some prefer to speak of emotional self-regulation in terms of defense mechanisms and may ascribe a hierarchy of defenses from the narcissistic through immature to mature (Meissner, Mack, & Semrad, 1975). Therapists may wish to move their patients upward along the continuum, for example, from projection and somatization to rationalization and reaction formation to sublimation and humor.

More effective alteration of the environment may derive from improved self-regulation. Relaxation may improve performance, reduction in the frequency of depression may improve a marriage, and more constructive self-talk may improve confidence at work. Many therapists also insist upon encouraging direct action toward others through assertiveness training, political action, career changes, and flight from dangerous circumstances. Reduction in frequency of destructive behaviors like bingeing–vomiting, narcotic ingestion, and wife-battering exemplify goals of behavioral inhibition.

Ultimately, therapists hope to instill in their clients coping strategies that will serve them after therapy has been completed. More likely than not, they will attempt to transmit strategies that have worked and continue to work for themselves. Mahoney among others (Mahoney & Arnkoff, 1978, p. 709) embraced the "problem solving" approach using the acronym SCIENCE.

S   Specify general problem
C   Collect information
I   Identify causes or patterns
E   Examine options
N   Narrow options and experiment
C   Compare data
E   Extend, revise, or replace

Some strongly believe in using synchronicity to guide their decision making. Synchronicity is an acausal principle by which personal meaning is given to coincidences (Bolen, 1979; Jung, 1973; Koestler, 1972). Others pay great attention to dreams as guides to living (Bonime, 1962; Freud, 1938; Jung, 1954, 1964). Emotional awareness seems to play a vital role in guiding the lives of many therapists (Perls, 1969; Reich, 1961) and, therefore, of their patients. For still others, the principles of operant conditioning allow them to understand the controlling variables of their own lives and those of others. Systems theories describing the interrelationship of the parts to the whole provide maps for many therapists and patients alike. The concept of deviation amplifying feedback is a crucial lesson for psychotherapists and their patients. How are undesirable spirals initiated and maintained? How can they be interrupted? How can desirable spirals be initiated and maintained? Perhaps the single most important value espoused by me through this book is the encouragement in both therapists and patients of the development of a flexible, moldable, adaptable aspect to their theories of themselves and the world. This flexibility is characterized by the ability to revise our existing concepts — to provide metaprograms for our human biocomputers (Lilly, 1972). There are many options by which to perceive reality and many guidelines by which to organize our responses. The ability to revise smoothly when confronted with new information appears to be a useful coping mechanism that is value laden. Some people choose to hold tenaciously to old ways of thinking that are impervious to new information.

Therapists differ in their values, their world views, and their preferred coping strategies. Each therapist needs to clarify these preferences in order to better understand what he or she is likely to try in order to help clients to learn. Like it or not, many clients are expecting to be taught something, as suggested by this note from a patient to a psychodynamically oriented therapist:

CASE 9.4. Dr. T: Is this basically what you were saying about dealing with people? (By the way, I don't care what other people say, I really like you, and I think you help me a lot!)

I need to adapt — not please.

First, I need to size up a person, which I actually do quite well (quite accurately).

Then I need to do something with this information, which I do quite poorly, and can correct (both for my good and the individual's). What *I* do with the information is as follows:

I ignore it — and hope things really aren't the way they are. I live in a dream world — if only I give enough, try to please enough, am nice enough, am perfect enough —

Then, THEN maybe my impossible dream will come true — that person will be what I want, a true-blue wonderful friend. Not the cold, hostile person he or she may be.

Instead — realistically —

1. I need to see the person for what he or she is, and accept it.
2. I need to adapt my actions to them, so that I remain feeling good and the other remains unirritated (as much as possible) without trying to please them.

3. I must believe it's OK not to be best friends with everyone I meet, particularly not people or persons in authority.
4. I must learn to feel content even when things aren't exactly the way I wish they were

See you Tuesday. Have a nice week, W.

The process by which this patient came to these conclusions was long and arduous. She had four previous therapists, two of whose spouses she threatened to kill. Another one she verbally abused through rage and intimidation while accepting the lithium treatment that seemed to help calm her roller-coaster emotions. By the time she reached the therapist to whom she had written the note, she had become fully acclimated to the therapeutic relationship, realized some of her basic self and other distortions, and was ready to listen.

These lessons are often difficult to deliver. Some of the ways in which patients and therapists get in the way of their delivery and how these blocks may be utilized in the service of change are described in the next chapter.

10. *Resistance to Change*

From the beginning of therapy, patients tend to avoid having to change themselves. Despite presenting themselves for help, they often wish just to lose their symptoms or to have others change. Therefore, resistance to change may be identified at many different places along the psychotherapeutic journey. This chapter will focus on the common impediments present during the process of change itself. The first third is concerned with general resistances, the second with transference distortions, and the third with the identification and use of countertransference reactions.

GENERAL RESISTANCE TO CHANGE

As patients stare into the abyss that yawns between their current and future selves, they often find themselves frozen. The difficulty may be ascribed to many sources, including (1) the patient's fundamental inadequacies, (2) the patient's intrapsychic conflicts, (3) a patient–therapist impasse, or (4) the technical limitations of the therapist or therapy.

CASE 10.1. A 17-year-old woman returned to inpatient treatment having a clear psychotic episode. She felt as if she were in a different dimension, that she was out of sync with everyone around her, that no one could understand her. She was deeply perplexed by the meaning of this state of mind. She had been hospitalized just 1 month earlier, after a suicide attempt, but had had no evidence of psychotic thinking. When she was much younger, her father had sexually abused her, and her mother had failed to acknowledge her complaints about it. Subsequently, her brother had also forced her to have sex with him and his friends. Her mother now believed her father's abuse, but still did not believe that her son had done the same thing. The patient had been furious with her mother for many years. She was in psychotherapy for the past 3 years. Prior to this second hospitalization, she was confronted in therapy with what it meant to change. To her, it meant acceptance of the adult view of reality and the consequent loss of desire to punish her mother for not understanding and acting. "What if you know everything was wrong and yet everyone else thought everything was fine? What would you do?" Rather than make the leap into the world view offered by her therapist, she became psychotic.

This series of events could be construed in a number of different ways:

1. *Patient deficits, limited resources.* The patient has a genetic disorder now manifesting itself. This is likely the beginning of chronic schizophrenia. The patient is biologically predisposed to react this way under sufficient stress.

2. *Intrapsychic conflicts.* The patient is so angry at her mother that she cannot tolerate forgiving her. To forgive her would mean to lose her only connection to her, which, however painful, is still a connection. Her psychosis is the result of a powerful ambivalence about her mother.

3. *Ideological conflict, patient–therapist impasse.* The therapist pushed the patient too hard. She was not ready to accept his insistence upon forgiveness, upon seeing that the worst was over. They had an ideological conflict about the best way to perceive her reality.

4. *Therapist inadequacies.* The therapist had missed the signs of incipient psychosis and should have referred her for evaluation of neuroleptic medications. Furthermore, the patient was so enmeshed in her family that family therapy offered the only possibility of change. Since the father refused to come, as did the brother, change was practically impossible.

The most optimistic perspective is to ascribe the difficulty to the patient's own conflict about separating from mother, to consider the episode to be a brief psychotic reaction that more clearly delineated the conflict and to proceed with individual psychotherapy in combination with neuroleptics.

The following section expands upon the four sources of general resistance introduced above.

Limited Resources

The initiation of change frequently requires the giving up of old behaviors and the beginning of new ones. Sometimes clients can be poised on the brink of change but cannot take the next step, although they want to take it. They may not have the necessary information about when to do it, or they may lack the ability to carry out the necessary behavior. They may be unduly anxious before carrying it out, they may be hampered by feared consequences, or they may have moral and ethical reservations (Goldfried & Davison, 1976, pp. 238–240). Assertive behavior serves as a useful example of these variations since many therapists hope to instigate in their clients positive self-expression in the face of a threatening environment.

CASE 10.2. A 30-year-old man who worked as an assistant prosecuting attorney reported that he could not put up with his wife's demands and abuse each time she became drunk. She continually ignored his feelings; he became more withdrawn. Her own work had become draining, the child by her previous marriage was having trouble with his new family, and her parents were continually intruding on her life. He began a passionate affair with a married woman, but soon broke it off when he realized that she would not leave her husband because of financial ties. His behavior with his own wife was characterized by repeated deception about even the smallest things. He lied about the cost of new suits and about time spent away from home. He justified the deceptions by believing that he was protecting his wife from exploding at him. She became furious whenever he overspent or wasted time. During therapy, he realized how silly but ingrained many of these deceptive behaviors were. Furthermore, when he wrote his father about this behavior, his father replied that he must have learned it from him since he had always "protected" his mother by these little white lies. Yet, he could not stop himself. He did not know what else to do. He was startled when I asked him whether or not his wife wanted him to lie. He thought "yes" and "no" were both absolutely correct. She wanted to know what he did, but she did not want to be angry at him. He remained paralyzed. He realized that if he did not take the opportunity to express his wants, beliefs, and needs to her, then he would suffer in silence and yearn for another affair. He wanted children. His therapist pointed out to him that he needed to be able to negotiate with his wife. "But that's what I do everyday in my job. I should be able to do that at home!"

In this case, the patient's resistance to change was due in part to his failure to realize that he had developed at work some of the requisite skills. When he realized that, he became more able to apply them in the anxiety-provoking arena of his marital relationship.

Intrapsychic Conflict

Change is a boundary experience (Yalom, 1980), an event that defines ones own limitations by clearly defining losses as well as gains. To change is to lose one identity for another one, to risk the unknown, and to become transformed. The threat of change triggers intrapsychic conflict about the past and the future, about the tried and untried ways of being. No matter what the details of the proposed transformation, trembling on the brink is very common. For the assistant prosecuting attorney, change meant commitment to his wife, relinquishing his role as his father's son, and grasping the chance to become a father and husband. For the 17-year-old psychotic, change meant giving up her angry attachment to her mother. For all patients, change means giving up the need for their therapists. Some obviously relish this possibility while others find it discouraging and threatening.

Patient-Therapist Impasse

Therapist and patient may find themselves locked in reciprocal roles that prevent change. One not uncommon form is ideological conflict over the nature of change.

CASE 10.3. A 64-year-old professor had far exceeded most of the women her age in her professional achievements. Nevertheless, she was deeply distraught over the state of her marriage, but firmly believed that nothing could be done to save it. She had presented to me with chronic variable somatization that was relieved by focusing upon the pains of her family life. However, she insisted that there was nothing to be done. I persisted in repeated examination of her place in her family. She seemed to tolerate these incursions, occasionally became enthusiastic about them, but usually told me that other psychiatrists had tried the same thing without success. The best I could do was to encourage her to take a sabbatical, during which she blossomed, away from the stresses of her family life. Until her death of recurrent cancer, I plodded away at her family relationship, but only when death was certain did she and her husband have the reconciliation she had so longed for. I persisted in believing that something more could have been done, but she did not agree. She may simply have wanted a pleasant companion in her lonely life. I had tried to break the impasse by pointing out how she was reacting with me, mirroring the obstinate, noncompliant relationship she had with her mother and that her daughter had with her. But insight could not overcome this conflict with me.

Other impasse forms will be discussed in the transference and countertransference sections.

Limitations of Therapy and the Therapist

Although therapists often hope to have their patients leave therapy armed with sufficient information to prevent any return to treatment, they often have to accept far less. Some patients appear to need to keep coming in order to maintain reasonable functioning. Others commit suicide. Still others fail to change for discernible reasons, among the most common of which is the fear of the effect of such change on a spouse.

CASE 10.4. A 45-year-old woman had been treated with insight-oriented psychotherapy and with antidepressant medications, but she remained intermittently depressed. I saw her after her third psychiatrist had tried to treat her in individual psychotherapy. She rapidly idealized me, thought my understanding of her was exquisitely accurate, and showed evidence of tremendous ability to produce insights about herself. She was clearly a "good insight patient," but she had failed to change. I asked her to invite her husband to the next session. She was startled, and replied, "I want to keep him out of this." Indeed, her efforts at being a good patient, at idealizing her therapists, at developing multiple psychiatric complaints, appeared to be ways to avoid her difficult marital problems. Her husband was at first reluctant to consider himself part of the problem and instead saw himself as a consultant to me. He soon accepted the possibility that both of them were contributing to the difficulty, but he continued to behave as if he were trying as best as he could while she was the one with the problems, despite evidence to the contrary. When this conflict resolved, they were more able to confront the mutual difficulties to which they were both contributing.

This limitation to individual therapy takes many forms. Sometimes parents are afraid to become more assertive with their children because the children threaten to commit suicide or take drugs or run away. Wives are afraid to develop professionally, fearing that they might better their husbands. Children are afraid to leave home or assert themselves because parents might withdraw their love. People on disability may be afraid to change because they would lose their disability payments. In a yet more convoluted example of the influence of external factors, a 19-year-old boy was reluctant to improve his academic performance or social life because these difficulties were being reinforced by the upset they caused his father whom he detested (Goldfried, 1982, p. 111). One might also expect this pattern to be transferred to the therapist working with him.

RESPONSES TO CHANGE RESISTANCES

Therapists' responses to resistance depends upon the manner in which they construe the cause. The most common cultural response to the psychological problems of a dear one is to encourage and exhort, "C'mon. You can do it. Just keep going and everything will be OK." The effectiveness of this form of folk treatment is difficult to measure because those who are aided by it do not present themselves for psychotherapy. Therapists sometimes incorporate this perspective into their own work, yet training as psychotherapist requires that many more options be available. Resistance is to be expected because the very nature of the patient's need for outside help implies that some forces are operating to prevent the desired transformation. On the other hand, therapists inadvertently step into roles that perpetuate the problem either because of their own difficulties or because the patient has masterfully encouraged them. How much is the patient's problem, how much the therapist's, and how much is the limitations of therapy?

Reevaluate Patient Resources

If the patient cannot perform the desired activity, perhaps the fault lies in an improperly designed therapy strategy in which the therapist does not take into consideration the patient's limitations. To use the assertiveness example: If the patient cannot act because he or she lacks information about what can be said or done differently, then direct didactic instruction coupled with selected readings may be useful. If the patient is not able to carry out the behaviors, then modeling, rehearsal, and periodic feedback would be useful. If the client is burdened with anticipatory anxiety though he or she knows what to do and how to do it, then systematic desensitization with relaxation exercises would be helpful. If the problem is unrealistic fears about how others will react, then these fears of rejection and loss of respect can be addressed. If such people can see that by being unassertive they are generating the kinds of consequences they are trying to avoid, then perhaps they can be won over. Many people are afraid of losing the respect of others by becoming assertive, when they are actually losing respect by being unassertive. On the other hand, some employers and spouses and parents simply do not like to see increases in assertiveness and will make every effort to nip the change in the bud. These environmental limitations must also be addressed (adapted from Goldfried & Davison, 1976, pp. 238–240).

The process of change is extremely frightening to some deeply disturbed patients and, as a result, can lead to major psychiatric difficulties, including major depression and psychosis. Although it may be possible to predict these reactions, they may be very difficult to prevent. Antidepressant and/or an antipsychotic medication and possibly hospitalization may be necessary to help them past their immobility.

Therapists may find themselves emphasizing insight about maladaptive patterns when the patient in fact needs to push on to behavior change. Therapists who idealize insight to the exclusion of behavioral transformation may find their therapies longer and more arduous. Insight lacking in practical application outside the office may be offered as gratification for the psychotherapist's analyzing ability, as a way to deaden feelings, and as a resistance to behavioral change (Applebaum, 1975).

Interpretation of Intrapsychic Conflict

Beginning with the belief in a conflict between the "devil" and "angel" in each of us, two internal warring elements have played key roles in Western understanding of intrapsychic events. Superego versus id, parent versus child, top dog versus underdog, depreciated versus grandiose self are but a few of the labels for these combatants. While each term is embedded in different models of human psychological functioning, they share in common a dualism between superior and inferior elements, each of which gains control over the ship of the mind at different times. At the point of change in psychotherapy, the conflict often becomes severe, the switches in control oscillate more frequently, and anxiety tends to increase. Oscillating patients may be approached in a number of different ways.

The warring elements can each be carefully delineated in terms that make sense to both participants. The words and symbols often employed by the patient are most useful. They may be reconstructed as images of parent and child relationships from the past. They may be construed as being reenacted in the present therapeutic relationship. Each may be given names of separate elements of the self trying to reach a compromise. Fundamentally, each patient seems to be struggling with the fears of going beyond the dualist conflict to greater internal harmony. The problem for therapists is to formulate the fear of individuation, of greater maturity, of loss of the dualistic struggle in terms that permit the patient to take control over these elements through increasing their mutuality.

Breaking Stalemates

Consultation and supervision are often the only ways out of situations in which both participants are feeding the resistance to change. The highly perfectionistic therapist with the highly dependent patient, the controlling therapist with the dependent patient, the nurturing therapist with the needy patient, the sadistic therapist with the masochistic patient, the inexhaustibly helpful therapist with the help-rejecting complainer, each represent common stalemates.

Paradox

While paradoxical injunctions span a wide range of poorly categorized responses, they are intriguing because they go against therapeutic common sense. Paradox often simply extends the patient's reality into the future. As Watzlawick and his colleagues (1974) repeatedly declared: "The solution is the problem." And the solution may be undone by extending it into the future.

CASE 10.5. A 52-year-old engineer was receiving disability insurance from his company because of depression and his unwillingness to face the unhappiness of his marriage. He suddenly left his wife to live in an apartment with no furniture except for a few pillows and a mattress on the floor. He felt lonely, isolated, and bored and wanted me to help him. At first I suggested small behavioral excursions. No help. I tried to interpret his anger at his wife and at himself for staying with her so long. He did not budge. Finally, I saw that his life-style resembled that of an Eastern mystic searching for enlightenment through isolation and meditation. I set about trying to help him become the "Best Sitter" in the city since he said that was all he did — sit. I described meditation, placed him with the Indian cave meditators, described how he had completed his life as a family man, and, like them, was sitting in a cave waiting to escape the Wheel of Reincarnation. I was serious. He became serious. And then he sabotaged my scheme by getting odd jobs and eventually returning to work.

Paradox is an alluring approach to resistance, but tricky to use (Greenberg & Pies, 1983). The psychoanalytic approach to resistance closely resembles the more flamboyant paradoxical techniques. Psychoanalysts suggest that therapists accept the resistance, label it as a defense that illustrates an intrapsychic conflict (Greenson, 1967), and go with it through understanding it. Freud did just that with his transference resistances; instead of trying to sweep them out of the way, he invited them to grow and thereby established a fundamental tenet of psychoanalytic technique. Gestalt therapy also emphasizes the need to accept resistances, to go with them, to see where they lead (Fagan & Shepherd, 1970; Polster & Polster, 1973). This ability of therapists to take what is given to them as a threat to therapeutic change and to turn it to therapeutic advantage marks one of the great differences between ordinary human interchange and psychotherapy.

TRANSFERENCE REACTIONS TO CHANGE

The confidence built up through a good engagement and the extended intimacy of the pattern search leads many clients to view change as a threat from which the therapist can rescue them. The manner in which they attempt to evoke protection varies with the interpersonal maneuvers learned earlier in life, particularly from parents, and the subsequent modifications incorporated as a result of other significant relationships. In addition, change is the true beginning of separation, of termination. Therapists often come to represent safe interpersonal havens in the rocky, windswept seascape of human relationships. To change is to begin to leave and to venture out on one's own.

The major resistance to change for many patients may also represent an excellent way to promote it. The manner in which they cling, plead, demand, or seduce therapists into avoiding transformation can be utilized to overcome the resistance.

There is relatively little debate among classical psychoanalysts about the utility of transference interpretations. In psychoanalysis, they are the ultimate instrument for therapeutic change (Greenson, 1967). Among the short-term dynamic therapists, there is also little controversy. Malan (1963, 1976b), Davanloo (1978), Mann (1973), and Sifneos (1972) each strongly stated that direct attention to transference reactions through interpretation may be exceedingly useful in short-term psychotherapy. Malan (1976a) has marshaled evidence to support the possibility that transference interpretations are associated with better outcome. While according to Frances & Perry (1983), there are many shortcomings to Malan's research design, a great weight of therapeutic experience supports this notion.

However, there is no need to insist that transference interpretations be held out as the only effective therapeutic technique. Nor need they be totally ignored. Instead, therapists must recognize the individual variation among their patients. Some will tend to form very fixed, easy to recognize transference distortions. Some will form them, but be unable to step back and speak about them. Transference may not be relevant to the therapeutic task, or there may not be enough time left in therapy to work on the distortion (Frances & Perry, 1983).

Occasionally, the transference reactions are so intense that therapy will be disrupted if attention is not paid to them.

CASE 10.6. A 25-year-old mother of three children, married for 9 years, decided to divorce her husband. She had made numerous false starts, but finally was beginning the long difficult road to independence. She had met and married him immediately after graduating from high school, had never dated other men, and was simply trying to find someone who would take care of her so she could get out of her parents' house. She never thought the marriage would last. However, it did. Finally, she had taken steps, with my aid, to break away. During most of the sessions, I had felt some sexual tingle in her presence, but during this session, I felt none.

CLIENT: Almost every time I leave the office, I feel funny. I can't help it, but when I'm riding home in the car I think of being in bed with you. I feel a tremendous urge to do that with you. I don't know, perhaps it is to reward you for helping me, like I reward my husband with sex when he is good to me. This is hard for me to talk about, I just don't know. Maybe because I haven't slept with anyone in such a long time.

THERAPIST: You feel like you'd like to be in bed with me and somehow it has something to do with rewarding me, like you did with your husband.

CLIENT: Yes, it's something like paying you off, giving you something from me. It is the only thing I have to give, I guess. [She was shaking as she talked.] My stomach feels all tied up in knots. My body feels so tight.

THERAPIST: What would happen if we had sex together?

CLIENT: I don't know, but I feel it would change our relationship entirely. Just wouldn't be the same and that would be no good.

THERAPIST: How do you mean that?

CLIENT: I'm thinking of Mike, who I kept trying to get in bed and trying and trying. He said we shouldn't do it because it would change our relationship completely, and he wanted to keep it as it was. Maybe because I was still married and he thought that if I slept with him while I was still married, I might also sleep with someone else if I was married to him. Anyway, I finally got him to bed with me and our relationship changed. We didn't see much of each other after that.

THERAPIST: What would happen if we had sex?

CLIENT: I don't know. Thinking of Mike, I think it would change. This is really hard for me talk about. I'm surprised I even brought it up.

THERAPIST: Why were you able to do it?

CLIENT: If I didn't, I wouldn't be able to come back. It bothers me too much.

There ensued a period of time which I do not recall directly, but during which the emotions between us were rising. She knew her feelings were inappropriate, yet she was being consumed by them. She shook, she looked at me longingly and was also a little frightened. I was deeply impressed by an image of her being afloat on a stormy sea of feeling, trying to keep her self-observer intact while it was being washed over by waves of emotion. I thought of using the psychoanalytic procedure of withholding my reactions and letting the feelings develop so that we could explore the fantasies behind her feelings. But I had a good idea about the origin of her sexual bartering. I opted for a reality statement that would give her something solid to grasp and that I also hoped would aid us in the progression toward understanding and change.

THERAPIST: You will not be having sex with me.

CLIENT: [She stiffened] That felt like an icy chill through my body. It feels like you don't like me.

THERAPIST: [Defensively] Does that mean you aren't coming back?

CLIENT: No, no. [She said laughingly and assuringly] I was just reporting to you what I was feeling. [I had misunderstood her report as coming from her experiencing self when it was her observing self reporting what she had felt. I was too caught up in my own concerns to read her accurately, but she corrected me.]

THERAPIST: [Recovering] So my refusal means I don't like you.

CLIENT: Yes, that is what I feel.

THERAPIST: What do you think of that feeling?

CLIENT: I try to use sex to get someone to show that he cares and then I end up feeling used. It is a vicious cycle of my own making.

We further discussed the value of her describing her reactions toward me, spoke about a few other matters, and adjourned. This woman had an excellent self-observer. It allowed her to stand back and observe her own reaction to me with interest and curiosity.

Malan has described the standard form of transference interpretation as the pair of triangles described in Chapter 4 (see Figure 6). The transference–parent link is most prized. The triangle is completed by including someone in the patient's current life. Integrated into this ideal form is a second triangle describing the intrapsychic conflict being enacted in these relationships. In the case just described, the links were made between the therapist and current and past relationships. The patient grasped the significance of the pattern without also discussing her father's and brothers' sexual abuse of her. The conflict was clear: Am I a worthy person without having to give sex to a man? She subsequently was able to stand up to her father's demands in ways she was not able to before.

A major function of transference interpretations is to correct distortions one has about oneself in relationship to parent figures. The child is asked to grow up, to see his or her parent as another person with faults and potentials like the self rather than as some omnipotent, self-worth-determining dictator. Though parents did once have control over their children's lives, that influence has decreased significantly and yet the person continues to search out relationships in which the parent–child role can once again be reenacted. This behavior may be understood as fixation in the past, or in an image of self as immature and unlovable. Another view is that when grown-up children enter intimate relationships, they fall back on behavior patterns that characterized their interactions with previous intimates because these are the only patterns they know. When they start living with others, they are reminded of those previous relationships with family because family members represented their first experience in living together. Marriage and children further define the spouse as parent. The previous person called mother or father was the person's mother or father.

CASE 10.7. The 30-year-old son of a physician could not maintain living-together relationships with women. He was an attractive, verbal, and intelligent man, but something happened each time he moved in with a woman. He was dashing and romantic in the courtship stage, filling her needs for love, adoration, and sex. But when they paid rent together, he became picky, arrogant, and intolerant of minor flaws in her character. They broke up and he moved on to search for the next woman to conquer. By the time he came to me, he had been in therapy for many years with three different therapists. He liked being a patient. It seemed to provide him an excuse to avoid commitment because that problem seemed to underlie much of his behavior with women. Had I been a woman, he would likely have reenacted some of his idealization–depreciation with a more sexualized tone. Instead, I became the respected adviser who was to guide him through the torment of sexual frustration and loneliness. I was to replace his aloof but loving father, who died of a heart attack a few years after he had left home for college. He felt responsible for that death because he believed that his father wanted to keep him around because he kept his father feeling young. More likely, the patient liked feeling young, liked staying home. He described those times in very idealized tones. He also did not want to leave therapy. To leave therapy would be once again to leave his father. Would I die somehow or would he die? Weren't his failures to commit based on a desire to remain in the limbo between his past family and the future feared one in which he replaces his father and his son(s) replaces him? Wasn't he reenacting that sticky transition with me? Our relationship ended without a satisfactory resolution of these questions.

For those children who have lost a parent through death or other forms of disappearance, working out distortions in real life seems to become so much more difficult.

Eroticized Transference

Sometimes patients become fixed in a love for the therapist that prevents any discussion of its meaning. The patient finds in the therapist a potential lover who seems to promise all that is needed to sustain that person's emotional life. Any discussion of these feelings becomes an admission of its impossibility. The patient insists that their love must be consummated outside the therapeutic arena. The patient extends invitation after invitation to join the therapist in erotic trysts or requests that they live together or promises endless affection. He or she wants to embrace the therapist and may see each therapeutic encounter as another seduction opportunity. Each session also comes to represent devastating rejections that engender increasing amounts of anger, but the patient fears that if the anger is expressed, the potential for union is decreased. In such cases, patients may suddenly terminate, act out their anger by precipitous marriage, or make suicide attempts. Freud (1963) recommended that therapists withdraw from such circumstances. Consultation with a colleague is clearly indicated because the therapist's contribution to the stalemate is likely a factor in the stalemate.

CASE 10.8.* In order for me to experience patients like the ones my trainees were seeing, I "picked up" a 25-year-old prostitute in the emergency room as a patient. She had previously attempted suicide numerous times using large doses of meprobamate and codeine that were being prescribed for her by a primary care physician. She came to each of our videotaped sessions (which I was preparing for the trainees) high on these drugs. Eventually I was able to help her stop taking them. Because I thought she had a minimal brain dysfunction, I prescribed Dexedrine and desipramine. She was able to go to beauty school and to concentrate reasonably well. She spent one year relatively happy, getting along with her new roommate, and finding herself able to "enjoy the flowers" again without drugs. (Subsequently, I could call this a transference cure by which is meant that most of her conflicts were now contained in her relationship to me.) However, she soon found herself in difficulty at school and was confronted with a choice to try something else more suitable to her abilities. She decided to go back to beauty school and failed. She sent

*See Vignette 4 in Beitman, 1981.

me a card revealing her positive affection for me and then asked me to go to bed with her. I was surprised and shocked that I had not been looking for evidence of her erotic attraction to me.* She refused to discuss it and instead quit therapy in a rage, had sex with many different men, and became psychotic on an overdose of Dexedrine. She was hospitalized, saw me once, then went home and took an overdose of desipramine and was found dead 2 days later. In the middle of the night that she took that overdose, she called me to tell me that she was in a "different world."

My blindness to the obvious likelihood that a prostitute was likely to try to control me through sexual interest has been a source of repeated guilt. Had I seen it earlier, perhaps I might have been able to develop the necessary self-observer alliance to subvert this disaster.

Transference as Practice

The enactment of transference distortions generally falls upon a person who does not respond to them in the expected ways. Simply accepting them in a nonattached but understanding way seems to demonstrate to many patients that the fears of rejection and criticism do not always have a basis in reality. Discussion of the sources of the distortions probably helps to pinpoint them. The experience of expecting the negative result and not getting it may be very useful and resembles the systematic exposure of phobic patients to feared objects. Intimacy is greatly feared by many people and the gradual, safe exposure of tender feelings increases one's sense of mastery over them and increases the likelihood that others may also respond with less condemnation.

COUNTERTRANSFERENCE TO CHANGE

Among beginning therapists who are deeply invested in positive outcomes for their first few long-term patients the prospect of change is often elusive. Not only because their patients are not changing, but because they

---

*Among the contributions to this blindness was the experience of presenting the first six sessions of this psychotherapy to a well-known psychoanalyst in front of 200 psychiatrists at the Washington State Psychiatric Association meeting in Seattle in 1977. He was brutally critical and I was psychologically battered. I believe that this experience imbued in my mind a great fear of the patient's ability to harm me, since she was directly associated with his attack. I also became more wary of seeking consultation with colleagues. This trauma and its consequences, coupled with ongoing personal difficulties, made therapy quite difficult.

are so invested in maintaining the relationship, so afraid that the patient will leave, so accustomed to viewing the patient as malfunctioning, and so doubtful of their own abilities, that change sometimes happens without their noticing it. Supervision must then help them to ease up on their involvement, to let the patient go. The situation resembles that repeated challenge to parents at each stage of development that requires a further letting go, an increasing realization of the child's ability to function yet more autonomously. Much as the late adolescent break from home is the last in a long series of lettings go, termination is but the final separation in a series of separations between therapist and patient.

CASE 10.9. A 32-year-old psychiatric resident had an infant son who, like many children, had learned to cry with sufficient precision at bedtime that she had great trouble not returning to him. She had learned to nurture as a way to cope in her early family life; her son appeared to be able to manipulate this tendency of hers. For 2 years, she had been seeing a 34-year-old lesbian who had a long psychiatric history that included multiple suicide attempts, many hospitalizations, and who was currently taking high doses of psychoactive medications. However, the patient had made great progress. She had not been hospitalized in more than 2 years, had made no suicide attempts, was much more able to manage the minor stresses of her life, and in therapy was hinting that the therapist need not be so concerned about her. Nevertheless, the therapist persisted in behaving as if the patient needed much direction and much support. Rather than allow the patient to generate alternatives for a specific problem, the therapist leaped in with a few and asked the patient to select. Rather than ask the patient how she felt about a certain success, the therapist complimented her. In supervision, I was able to point out the discrepancy between the therapist's behavior and the patient's improvement while touching briefly upon the therapist's own transference to the patient. She was able to back away slowly and allow the patient more room to grow.

On the other hand, therapists may react quite negatively to the patient's process of change. They may notice improvement and back away too quickly. Or they may find themselves frustrated with the often fits-and-starts movement, particularly of borderline patients.

CASE 10.10. A gentle, kind, and eager-to-help 3rd-year psychiatric resident was treating a 26-year-old woman who became psychotic intermittently and needed neuroleptic medications. She did not want to take neuroleptics because they seemed to prevent her from getting high on street drugs. He combined his medication management with a reality-oriented psychotherapy during which he pushed her to examine alternatives that she had ignored. After a year of once per week half-hour sessions, sprinkled with additional meetings at times of stress, she received word that her divorce was being finalized. This was a rejection of catastrophic proportions to her; she began to decompensate. She spoke more often of suicide and had to be hospitalized twice. She continued to deteriorate and asked for antidepressant medications in addition to her neuroleptics. At first, the therapist, fearing an overdose, gave them to her for only short periods of time, a few days, perhaps a week. But he became frustrated with her lack of progress and did not know what to do. Unfortunately, he did not share his concern with his immediate supervisor but rather continued on by himself with her. One day he gave her a month's supply of antidepressants and only briefly wondered why. A few weeks later, after some missed appointments, the patient returned and spoke indirectly of her not being around anymore after a few weeks. Again, the therapist sensed suicide in the air. She talked about the therapy with him as being the only success in her life, the only refuge. Work had been the other success in her life, but now she believed that the people there were trying to poison her. Because of the association in time between her talking about him and then work and the fact that she was angry about having to take pills from him, he suggested that perhaps she was afraid that he might poison her. She agreed and talked about her anger at him for having to take pills. He then related her anger at him to her anger at her father. The therapist had succeeded in making an ideal transference interpretation. He had related the past to the near present to the transference in one sweep. Three days later the patient killed herself with an overdose of antidepressants given her by the therapist.

In our postmortem discussion of the case, the resident discovered his frustration in not having been able to help her, and, in fact, watching her decompensate. In his frustration with this deterioration, the therapist felt compelled to produce: he delivered for the first time in their therapy a transference-based triangle interpretation. He had discussed this case in an ongoing psychoanalytic seminar during which such maneuvers were presented as ideal. Ignored was the idea that in order for an interpretation to be well accepted by a patient, the patient must have a well-developed self-observer that had some distance from the experiencing self. This woman was decompensating and becoming paranoid. It is likely that she took the statement "you think I am trying to poison you" as confirmation of her fears rather than as disputation of them, since she had little self-observer. His frustration was aided by his own need to cure the patient and his anger at the patient for not living up to his expectations.

There is no way to know with certainty the therapist's contribution to the patient's suicide, whether a different set of responses might have kept her alive. Rather than make his triangle interpretation, the therapist might have explored the reality base of her ideation to determine the degree of her psychotic thinking. Then he might have attempted to increase her neuroleptics or considered rehospitalization. These maneuvers would have been in keeping with the reality-based, supportive psychotherapy he had been doing. In addition, he should have examined more carefully his motivation for giving her a month's supply of medication. Only in retrospect was he able to identify his intense anger at her.

One of the great paradoxes of psychotherapy is the therapist's need to care about the patient's well-being without insisting that the outcome be positive. The balance between insisting upon a convergence between their values and upon letting go without insistence upon how the patient should be is a repeated therapeutic challenge.

USING COUNTERTRANSFERENCE IN CHANGE

By accepting the possibility that patients evoke distorted responses from them, psychotherapists enter an exciting new area of personal and professional discovery. Not only does countertransference awareness impel therapists to examine the personal influences of past and present that are contributing to the distortions but it also encourages them to understand the nature and manner of the patient's interpersonal influence. By attempting to tease out the strands of interpersonal causes from personal ones, each therapist is performing a necessary exercise in individuation — the differentiation of self from other. Since therapist personality is so much a part of the psychotherapeutic instrument, these intrapsychic and interpersonal refinements offer the possibility of increasing therapist effectiveness as well as aiding personal growth.

If therapists accept that patients are often aware of countertransference reactions, then they may allow themselves to acknowledge their patient's accurate perception. Such acknowledgement does not necessarily require elaboration of the origins. Rather, acknowledgement may validate the patient's ability to perceive reality and, like any crucial event in therapy, may then become the subject for discussion: How does this therapist response affect the patient? Without acknowledgement of countertransference, therapists may suggest that the patient is perceiving the therapist according to a transference distortion, thereby continuing a process of disconfirming the patient's ability to comprehend others accurately.

When the therapist's personal contribution to a countertransference reaction is reasonably well separated from the patient's contribution, the remaining information is simply another form of knowledge about the patient. Like data collected from direct patient description, latent content implications, family members, or homework assignments, patient-induced countertransference information must be confirmed by other data and then formulated into interventions. Therefore, the manner in which patient-induced countertransference information is to be used depends upon each therapist's preferred psychotherapeutic techniques.

CASE 10.11. A 23-year-old homosexual man with multiple, shifting physical pains that had no discernible organic etiology was referred to a male psychiatrist but was to be followed concurrently by his primary care physician. The patient appeared erratically at their weekly sessions, usually promising to appear the following week, often skipping for months. Confrontations about his failure to keep appointments were ineffective. After 12 months, during a crisis in which he may have inadvertently given a friend herpes through an unplanned sexual encounter, he hysterically called the psychiatrist. The therapist helped to ease the patient through the emergency and that night had a dream in which his 14-month-old son turned into a rat who scurried around the house. He awoke with a start and immediately associated to the patient whose attendance at meetings was inadvertently harmful in a way vaguely reminiscent of the manner in which he had exposed his friend to herpes. The therapist decided to bring the issue of regular appointments to the next meeting. The patient began that meeting talking about how he needed to lay down some rules for another friend who was taking advantage of him. The therapist silently interpreted this latent content as confirming the need for an intervention about regular appointments. The patient was at first defensive about the confrontation. But, as a result of it, discovered how difficult it was for him to say directly that he needed the therapist's help. Apparently, he feared that he would be abused once again in another in a long series of such incidents that began with his being physically beaten many times by two separate foster fathers.

Perhaps the most controversial use of patient-induced countertransference knowledge within psychoanalysis is to express the information directly to the patient. Tauber (1954), for example, suggested telling patients dreams, feelings, and thoughts in which they appeared, while Weigert (1954) suggested that such responses be expressed only during termination. Langs, on the other hand, stated that "such maneuvers are implicitly something of a hoax, a seduction and a conflicted imposition of the analyst's problems onto the patient" (1976, vol. 2, p. 288).

Outside of psychoanalysis, Meador and Rogers (1973) advocated genuineness in addition to warm, empathic regard and nonjudgmental acceptance. By "genuineness," he meant direct expression to the client about how the therapist was reacting to him or her. Such reactions can provide useful feedback about how others may also respond to the client. This behavior may also serve as a model for the patient's own self-expression. Among the chief advocates of direct self-expression are existential therapists who tend to believe that direct emotional encounters between patient and therapist are healing (Havens, 1975). Yalom (1980, pp. 402–403) provided a series of anecdotes demonstrating that therapists believed their patients changed because the therapists were willing to encounter them in a real and human way. Weiner (1983) has compiled a number of different circumstances under which therapists may safely and effectively disclose their responses to patients.*

In the following case direct expressions of my feelings seemed quite useful.

CASE 10.12. A narcissistic student learned the distinction between self and not self through didactic instruction and experiments in which he tested out whether others could indeed read his mind and whether he could read the minds of others. In addition, when confusion occurred in his environment, he was instructed to determine rationally whether he was the cause and whether he was responsible for settling things down (he had felt he was the cause and cure of many family difficulties and his parents had made him into their peacemaker). As he learned what was not him, he noticed one day that his grumpy supervisor was possibly not angry at him, but may have had his own problems. This man became his first "three-dimensional person," as others had all seemed part of him before. He discovered a few more of these people. During this time, he thought of me as sitting on his shoulder telling him how better to think about the world. He was certain I was thinking about him when we were not together. During a trip with his parents, he first fused with them and then began to see them as separate from him. His mother's needs were no longer commands for him to follow. Despite his apparent progress, I felt empty and unrecognized during most of our sessions. My stomach often growled and I thought about food. He rarely seemed to acknowledge my existence. My energy was going toward him, but little was coming toward me; I was experiencing a state of "narcissistic depletion"

*Material in the preceding section has been taken from "Categories of Countertransference" by B. D. Beitman, 1983, *Journal of Operational Psychology*, p. 89. Reprinted by permission.

(Altschul, 1977). When he returned, I told him how frustrated I felt sitting with him and asked him to discuss the source with me. He had thought of me as a saint (much as he thought of himself), listening, but asking little. He discovered in my reaction a repetition of feelings he had sensed from others that seemed to originate in his withholding of emotion from them, keeping a stone face. The next week, he looked and felt separate from me. He recognized that he was trying to make me into the father he had wanted. He preferred to make his life on his own, although he was not quite ready to leave therapy. He expressed his emotions much more smoothly and seemed to recognize my existence as well. The countertransference confrontation of my frustration with him had seemed to define to him my boundary as something against which he could build his own.

These cases and the controversy about therapist disclosure seem to indicate that therapist self-revelation may function as yet another psychotherapeutic technique, the use of which must be judged in relation to the therapist's personality, the patient's needs, and the stage of psychotherapy.

THE PATIENT'S POSITIVE INFLUENCE ON THE THERAPIST

Not only does analysis of one's own reactions to patients accelerate one's self-understanding, but patients also attempt to increase the therapist's emotional growth.

Like any other technique, the expression of a therapist's personal feelings and thoughts can lead to difficulty, as in Case 6.24 in which the therapist told a psychotic patient about his grieving for a loved one. This revelation recapitulated the patient's major childhood relationships in which she was overwhelmed by demands to care for others. Therapy terminated prematurely.

Searles (1975) attributed what he had observed to each person's innate striving toward helping others mature and to the patient's genuine concern that the therapist thrive as a result of his or her caring.

Kaiser (1962) took this perspective to a logical extreme in his play *Emergency*, in which a psychiatrist's wife sought help for her husband from another psychiatrist under unusual conditions. The designated patient refused to admit that he needed any help, and, therefore, would not seek treatment. Would the psychiatric consultant please become a patient of her husband's and thereby treat him? The body of the play describes the manner in which the "patient" successfully treated the psychiatrist.

I also recognize I have benefited from the ministrations of my patients. In the following example, my patient's observations helped to reinforce a difficult lesson in my conduct with my wife.

CASE 10.13. A few months after she told me that she did not want to talk about our relationship, my patient showed increasing signs through latent and overt references that she now wanted to talk about her reactions to me. I had known her for 4 years and had been seeing her once weekly for 30 minutes. Our objective was to help improve her relationships with men to the point that she could tolerate being intimately involved with one. As the pressure built to talk about her here-and-now reactions to me, I asked her whether indeed she wanted to do that. She had said she wanted me to act as a consultant to her problems. After numerous challenges to her desire to reopen transference discussion, she agreed. She admitted that she did not want to talk about her feelings toward me and her observations of my reactions to her because *I blamed her for my feelings just as her ex-husband had.* I would not admit my contribution to these reactions. I told her that my wife had recently said just about the same thing. She remarked that it was courageous of me to admit that. She helped me to change my relationship to my wife, because, subsequently, whenever I tried to blame her for my feelings, I questioned myself. I also kept this observation in mind with future patients.

The Jungian belief in meaningful coincidences (synchronicity) has led many to evaluate the relationship of each patient's problem to the struggles of the therapist. "As an analyst, it seems to me that my patients come through my office door bringing with them the opportunity and necessity for encountering aspects of myself" (Bolen, 1979, p. 54). This perspective makes each chance meeting personally meaningful and reflects a concept of self-in-the-world that places each person in a matrix of personally meaningful events. These events can be read like dreams for understanding of the current self and possible future directions. Like all filters on the data of experience, therapists must decide when to use the idea of synchronicity and when to pass or ignore it.

The following case demonstrates the potential resemblance between synchronous events and dreams. It also demonstrates a patient's attempt to treat the therapist and the use of therapist's self-revelations.

CASE 10.14. I had known her for more than 9 years and we were once again attempting to separate. She read my caring about her, my sexual attraction to her, my desire to help her as indications that I wanted to leave the therapist's role and enter into a sexual and possibly long-term relationship with her. She was passionately committed to her image of me but was gradually coming to realize that this commitment to me prevented her from making any real-life commitments, and that I was not going to stop being her therapist. She had become a psychotherapy addict, while I, in many ways, was becoming frustrated with her. She had stuck her claws into the image she held of me and would not let go. My frustration came out in my attempts to show her that she did not know who I was, that she was responding to an image of a potential father and lover who was not me but her characterization of me. Why wouldn't she take "no!" for an answer. As my frustration began to build and her marriage became yet more rocky, she was attempting to cross a street on the bicycle trail near her home, when a car sped by almost hitting her. As she looked up to curse the driver, she was taken aback. I was the driver. To her I looked happy and content, with my wife sitting next to me and my child playing in the back seat. During subsequent sessions, she referred to this event in the following way: "You almost ran me over. That tells me you have much anger against me. I see it in the way you talk to me, when you get frustrated. You want to kill me." I felt she was trying to rub my nose in the event, that she was indeed angry at me, which she easily admitted. But I also tried to answer her interpretation. "Yes, I am mad at you. You do not accept me for what I am. And I cannot find a way to have you not do that." She said, "Your emotional expression means that you still do care about me and that perhaps you will change your mind." I then could see that she was taking true observations (my anger, my interest, my sexual attraction to her) and exaggerating their significance. When I described this back to her (for not the first time), she could grasp the meaning more effectively. We agreed to continue to look for these exaggerations in the future, not just with me, but also with her husband and her father with whom there was evidence she did just the same thing. As for her interpretation of that synchronous event between us, perhaps she had exaggerated its meaning as well. Although I came close to hitting her, I did not. Instead, I suggested that the event meant less that I wanted to kill her and more that I wanted to get her attention — to have her look at me as I am, rather than the image she carries of me.

As suggested by Loewald (1970, p. 66), "To discover truth about the patient is always discovering it with him and for him as well as for ourselves and about ourselves. And it is discovering truth between each other, as the truth of human beings is revealed in their interrelatedness."

11. *Termination*

Occasionally patients will discover a critical pattern, declare an effusive thank-you, and walk out, never to return. Follow-up information may indicate that some of these patients continued the work of therapy on their own: they practiced new behaviors and new ways of thinking and succeeded in integrating these changes into their personal lives. Many other patients are unable to perform this integration on their own and, therefore, require further assistance. In 1914, Freud (1963, p. 165) was compelled to counsel his followers in this matter because often they felt that the mere naming of a pattern was sufficient for change. Patients, however, behaved otherwise. "One must allow the patient time to get to know this resistance of which he is ignorant, to work through it, to overcome it, by continuing the work according to the analytic rule of defiance of it. Only when it has come to its height can one, with the patient's cooperation, discover the repressed instinctual trends which are feeding the resistance; only by living them through in this way will the patient be convinced of their existence and power." Some psychoanalysts linked working through to the compulsion to repeat — the tendency for the sexual and aggressive drives to be discharged in the same recurrent pattern. "The process requires demonstrating to patients the same thing again and again at different times or in various connections . . ." (Fenichel quoted in Sandler, Dare, & Holder, 1970c, p. 618). Fenichel also emphasized the mourning aspect of working through since each patient is forced to lose, through change, a familiar although troublesome aspect of her- or himself.

Kraus (personal communication, 1980) suggested the following metaphor for working through: "Imagine a bar of soap underneath a dripping faucet. Working through resembles the slow persistent erosion of the soap by the dripping water." The bar of soap represents a nuclear unconscious conflict. Each drop is an interpretation that carries away a bit of the irritant. Working through may also refer to transformation of the grandiose versus depreciated self into a more realistic and cohesive self-concept or to any other thoroughgoing acceptance of an in-

261

trapsychic concept of psychopathology (Horowitz, 1974). These foci of change illustrate the psychoanalytic valuing of intrapsychic change perhaps to the detriment of behavioral change. In a retrospective study of the psychotherapy of borderline patients, Waldinger and Gunderson (1984) found that those who had had psychoanalysis showed greatest improvement in measures of object-relatedness and sense of self, but when compared to those who had shorter forms of psychotherapy showed least improvement on measures of behavior and ego functioning.

For others, "working through" refers to the application of self-understanding in new and different circumstances (Mendel, 1975; Sandler *et al.*, 1970(c). New knowledge about the self is applied to the world outside the office and becomes part of the patient's history and life-style.

The term "practice" captures more succinctly the basic thrust of the third substage of change. The pattern is defined, the objectives clarified, and the client pushes forward through resistance, ignorance, and fear to leave the old ways behind. Homework assignments may play an important part in the practice substage by encouraging patients to perform specific behaviors outside the office. The use of family members to support and encourage specific alterations may be quite useful. In the treatment of agoraphobics, for example, the use of a spouse to help the patient continue exposure in a gradual manner to feared excursions seems to improve the rate and durability of change (Barlow & Beck, 1984). The many other possible strategies for reducing homework noncompliance (e.g., Shelton & Levy, 1981) may also be extended into the practice phase and later. Therapist reinforcement, definition of cues to elicit desired behaviors, and diaries are but a few of the means by which new behaviors may be maintained.

Ultimately, therapists hope to encourage patients to believe in their own abilities. The term "self-mastery" describes the ideal of control over one's own drives, emotions, thoughts, and self-opinion (Frank, 1976). Bandura (1977) used the term "self-efficacy" to describe the belief in one's own competence to perform expected behaviors. Perhaps the term "self-regulation" may represent the best compromise since it has been used by spokespersons of different theoretical orientations (Goldberg, 1975; Grotstein, unpublished; Karoly, 1980). Therapists can help to develop the patient's self-observer to elucidate clear patterns of difficulty and to encourage the utilization of effective means of change. Using these methods, patients can come to master their inner lives through understanding and tolerance and to develop confidence in their abilities while also accepting their limitations.

And then they are supposed to leave.

But when is "then"? How do therapists, how do patients, how do therapist–patient pairs come to define the end point of therapy? How does the termination stage relate to the objectives of therapy?

THE GOALS OF TERMINATION

A child is attempting to ride a bicycle without training wheels. An adult is balancing the bike from behind, running along with his hand on the rear fender. The child feels confident because the adult is there to balance the bike in case he loses control. He rides up the street, moving ever more quickly, enjoying the houses passing by. He wonders how the adult could keep up and looks back. The adult is shrinking in the distance; he is riding all by himself.

It is to be hoped that the child will not be startled by the loss of his balance insurance and, instead, will recognize and accept his own competence. Therapists also hope not to shock their clients with their loss; they too want to avoid causing a relapse to former levels of ineffective self-regulation. For many therapists, this is a real fear: "Failure to adequately explore and work out feelings during the ending period may result in weakening and undoing the completed therapeutic work" (Levinson, 1977, p. 481). Although there are probably times when the inadequate resolution of the meaning of termination results in permanent loss of therapeutic gains, I doubt that the frequency of this relapse is very high. A research project aimed at answering this question would be a useful addition to the psychotherapeutic literature: What problems, with types of patients in what kinds of therapy require attention to termination issues in order to maintain the gains of therapy and/or to lead to further improvement? In their study of short-term dynamic therapy with grieving patients, Horowitz *et al.* (1984) found that patients with low motivation for therapy and poorly integrated sense of self showed improvement with attention to termination issues while those with high motivation and well-integrated sense of self responded negatively to the exploration of termination reactions. While this conclusion was only mildly supported by the data, it is consistent with the positions of Sifneos (1969) and Davanloo (1978). They emphasize the need to address reactions to termination in patients more disturbed by loss and recommend against elaborate interpretive work in separation with better functioning patients.

Aside from the question of enhancing or reducing the results of the previous work of therapy, termination triggers universal human dilemmas regarding the passing of time, loss, and death. Humans are repeatedly confronted with separation and its impact upon the individuation process. The link between time and reality is insoluble (Mann, 1973, p. 3).

We live in a three-dimensional space in which time is the fourth, but uncontrollable, variable. We can modify our subjective experiences of time, but it moves inexorably forward. We cannot go backward; we cannot get off this incessantly ticking line. Through future space flight, a few of us may skip far ahead. Nevertheless, our bodies are limited to their own time, to their own number of heartbeats and respirations. Saying good-bye marks a boundary and defines our limitations. Whether addressed thoroughly or not, termination strikes a chord that reverberates to the souls of the participants.

Since separation evokes universal conflicts about time, death, and commitment, therapists may take the opportunity to study the manner in which specific patients react to this often-difficult experience. Most of us have had singularly painful separation experiences that linger on in our minds. To these have been added a series of other painful losses. The termination stage offers the opportunity to reexperience these traumatic events in a more objective and supportive context, thereby providing the opportunity to master the experience.

METHODS OF TERMINATION

Termination alternatives parallel the several patterns by which two human beings may say good-bye to each other: They both can agree that the time has come; one can insist while the other disagrees; external events can force the separation against the direct wishes of either or both.

Mutually Agreed Termination

In those settings in which therapy may proceed indefinitely, ideal termination is marked by the separate intuition of both participants that the time has come for parting. One implies that a great deal of work has been done. The other makes the implication overt by stating that termination should be considered. Although more work could be done together, both participants generally feel satisfied.

Rather than rely simply upon the intuitions of either or both participants, the achievement of initially agreed upon goals would appear to be the ideal signal for termination discussion. However, goals are often difficult to elucidate and may shift as therapy progresses. In the case of simple phobias, goals are quite easily defined (increasing ease when confronted with the feared circumstance), but in the more complex personality disturbances, the achievement of one goal may serve as a vantage point for the discovery of yet other important ones. For example, a paranoid patient may challenge his irrational fears only to discover intense loneliness. He may overcome his intense loneliness, only to discover a greater fear of failure at work. A snake phobic may achieve sufficient trust in a helpful behavior therapist to unburden physical abuse in her marriage. There are always more psychological battles to win. How does one determine when enough victories are sufficient?

One response to this dilemma has been to agree upon a maximum number of therapy hours at the outset. This number may be firmly set, as did Mann (1973), when he set a maximum of 12 hours. Some may have general upper limits to which the therapist asks the patient to conform. Malan (1979) suggested 20–40 and Beck *et al.* (1979) used 20 as the upper limit. If the patient requires further treatment, some advocate referral, while others might simply continue treatment. Many therapists have an upper limit in mind for the length of their treatment. Although these limits may not be clearly stated, the therapeutic subculture into which the patient enters may convey this information. Langs (1974) declared that 5 or 6 years of two to three times per week should be the upper limit, with 2–3 years of psychoanalytically oriented psychotherapy the average (p. 498). Patients may acquire a sense for how long the therapist expects treatment to take and implicitly agree to conform with this time limit.

Patient-Initiated Termination

Patients often leave therapy before therapists are ready to let them go. The average number of visits to a wide variety of clinics over a many-year period was six to eight (Garfield, 1978), reflecting a small number of short-term successes (Malan *et al.* 1975), and a larger number of treatment failures. Once patients commit to therapy, the average number of visits may be close to 20 (Beitman & Maxim, 1984). Major variables in these limits include insurance coverage and willingness to commit personal resources of time, money, and energy.

Goldstein (1973) insisted that premature termination was the therapist's fault:

> When the patient drops out prematurely it is usually possible to determine the therapist's error which led to it. For example, a particular patient quit therapy after three sessions when, upon the therapist's urging, he approached his estranged wife to assert his desire for reconciliation. Her response was a flat refusal. His already weak sense of self-worth was obliterated and he decided that this brand of therapy was not for him. Obviously the therapist

had erred in that the patient was put into a situation in which he was not prepared to handle a possible negative response in an adaptive way. Even when the therapeutic error is not so obvious, dropouts may still be chalked up to the therapist's errors. To blame the patient through rationalizations such as the patient's not being sufficiently motivated or not having enough ego strength to withstand the pressures of therapy is an inexcusable exercise. Therapy is the therapist's responsibility. It is the therapist who at the very least implicitly establishes himself as the expert and any failure is the therapist's failure. (p. 222)

Therapists may not only make technical errors, but may be exploiting their patients in some way. The patient's leaving may be a rational exit for a demeaning situation.

CASE 11.1. A 25-year-old woman described herself as very helpless and bound in her marriage. Her 32-year-old therapist decided to use "psychodrama" and suggested she act like a "bound and helpless" housewife. The therapist instructed the patient to put her hands behind her back, pretend that her mouth was gagged, and struggle to get free. She failed to return after this exercise, perhaps recognizing that she again was being exploited. (adapted from Beitman, 1983b, p. 86)

Premature termination may also, however, reflect the patient's flight from himself; it is the clearest form of resistance to psychological change. While therapists may push too hard sometimes or make other technical errors, the fear of change compels some patients to flee the therapeutic encounter. Seeman (1974) suggested a specific hypothesis. Once clients develop their relationship to their therapists into a pattern that conforms to the style of relationship they had as adolescents about to leave home, they repeat that situation in therapy by premature termination.

CASE 11.2. A 44-year-old woman had left home at age 16 to marry a man of whom her parents strongly disapproved. During their marriage, this man regularly beat her until she finally divorced him and supported herself and her three children. The death of her second husband, after 15 years of marriage, brought her to therapy. Over the course of 3 years of therapy, the patient terminated treatment each time she began an intense sexual relationship. The therapist clearly felt that he was being placed in the role of warning her against self-abusive involvement, much as her parents had warned her against her first marriage. Each relationship ended in disaster and required her to return to therapy. When she finally was able to accept her own parents' concern, she no longer needed to abuse them and herself by selecting abusive men.

Finally, patients initiate premature termination through their own deaths. For any therapist who has received a call from a coroner's office about a now-dead patient, the shock of this kind of premature termination reverberates for many years. Patients may also die of more natural causes. The slow wasting away of a well-known patient/person drastically alters the therapeutic relationship. These premature terminations lend an air of futility to any therapeutic effort.

On the other hand, patients may quit therapy because they know that continuation is unnecessary.

CASE 11.3. A 24-year-old graduate student had overcome his fears of homosexuality and his paranoid thinking about the intentions of others. He felt that he could tackle the fears of his controlling mother and, during therapy, proved it. Although he recognized that more work was needed, he felt he could do it on his own. He reported feeling like an adolescent ready and wanting to leave home. Follow-up indicated that he had joined the Peace Corps and had established a very satisfactory relationship with a woman. The therapist had been very reluctant to let him go.

Therapist-Initiated Termination

Therapists may voluntarily initiate termination when the patient appears to have made sufficient gains but is reluctant to leave, or when therapy is stalemated and there appears no way to overcome the snag. Either situation is potentially laden with therapist distortions. How does one determine when enough is enough? Just as patients may be correct in leaving a badly conducted psychotherapy, so they may be correct in wanting to gain more from an effective one.

Stalemates are more easily detected. No matter what the therapist does, no matter how hard the patient appears to be trying, nothing happens. Rogers (1942) described a specific stalemate:

> The writer recalls one series of contacts with a mother in which the counseling had been badly bungled, as seen in present perspective. Since no progress was being made in the handling of her son, the counselor simply stated that it appeared that the contacts were not fruitful and that perhaps they should be discontinued. The mother seemed to accept this, and the situation apparently was closed, when she remarked, as she got up to go, "do you ever accept adults for treatment?" When the answer was in the affirmative, she sat down again and began to reveal all her marital unhappiness, which was basic to her mishandling of her son, but which she had been

reluctant to reveal as long as her boy constituted the ostensible reason for the clinic contacts. In other words, if the impasse which has been reached is clearly stated and recognized, both client and counselor may be able to accept it without too much emotion and to find the way in which it may be overcome. If not, at least the contacts will be closed without hostility and guilt being uppermost. (pp. 236–237)

The fixing of a termination date sometimes sets in motion efforts to change not evident before. Freud somewhat reluctantly set a termination date in his treatment of a young Russian, spoiled by riches, who had come to Vienna before World War I in a state of helplessness. After some positive steps, therapy came to a halt; the patient appeared quite comfortable in his relationship with Freud and did not want to continue to work. Frustrated, Freud insisted that they terminate after 1 more year. At first the patient did not believe him and then, during the last months, proceeded to participate in the treatment. Freud felt guilty about this "blackmailing" device, but believed, as did the patient's subsequent analyst that this maneuver was the only way to get his patient moving (Freud, 1963, pp. 234–236).

Unfortunately, the setting of a date for ending can evoke "blackmail" from the patients. In the following case, the therapist introduced termination because therapy was "flat" and the patient had made some gains.

CASE 11.4. The patient became increasingly anxious, notably enraged at others, and suicidal. He soon insisted that he was simply not ready to terminate treatment, and that if it were indeed effected, he would retreat to his room, would not function — and would possibly kill himself. The patient did not respond to comments on these behaviors. The therapist, fearing the patient's destructive potential, felt that he was required to continue. (Langs, 1974, p. 507)

Forced Termination

Therapists in training are usually required to terminate some or all therapy relationships when they shift from one service to another. Therapists who are leaving town must terminate with all of their patients. These forced terminations can be painful to both participants. Therapists in training must often choose between patients — which one will I continue to follow and to which ones will I say "I don't have enough time"? Dewald's (1965) study of the reactions of his patients when he moved to St. Louis suggested that arbitrary limit setting has a variety of effects on patients. Of the 12 patients he described, 3 responded negatively, 4 used the experience to promote therapeutic change, and 4 seemed to neither benefit nor suffer from the forced ending. Of those who were able to utilize the forced termination, 1 found the challenge of the set date to be a spur to working, 2 others experienced the emotions of previous losses with which they became better able to deal, and 1 found the opportunity to express many deep and hidden emotions. Of those who responded negatively, all 3 withdrew from therapeutic contact, apparently fearing to invest because of the pain of separation. A tentative conclusion is that the setting of a termination date may not only accelerate therapeutic movement for one-third of patients, but may also be cost-efficient. The important problem is to determine which patients will benefit from this technique.

Therapists force terminations by their own deaths. The sudden, explosive news of a therapist's death may have deep impact upon patients, particularly those who have become deeply attached to him or her and/or have special difficulty with permanent loss. Shwed (1980) suggested that colleagues of the deceased should call his or her patients personally and arrange for immediate meetings. Therapists, like their patients, have difficulty confronting this possibility because the denial of death is an enduring part of Western culture, particularly among its leaders and heroes (Becker, 1973).

The Techniques of Termination

A number of conflicts exist among students of termination about the proper way to do it. Since these conflicts endure, it is likely that each position is correct at some time. Determining which approach with which patients seeing which therapists remains the basic question for psychotherapy researchers.

1. Maintain the same frequency or reduce frequency. Reduced frequency is preferred by many therapists as a way to "wean" their patients by gradually increasing the time between meetings (a kind of systematic desensitization to loss). Others insist that this maneuver allows the patient to avoid the pain of loss and thereby passes up the opportunity to resolve reactions to loss.

2. Set a firm date or remain flexible with willingness to extend. Setting a firm date and keeping to it mirrors the often inevitable limitations and boundaries put onto each of us during life. Allowing flexibility in the termination time, including insisting only that the patient announce his or her desire to leave one session ahead of time (Kopp, 1977) permits the patient greater control over his destiny. What lesson and what experience is the therapist trying to create?

3. *Become more egalitarian or remain reserved.* For those therapists who hold rather firmly to a therapeutic personna, termination offers the choice of maintaining that personna or at this time becoming more "real." Resolution of transference distortions should have made psychodynamic patients more capable of seeing their therapists for who they are, but such resolutions are extremely difficult to achieve. According to Geller and Nash (unpublished), most authors agree that therapists should become more human to their patients, while Langs (1974), representing a classical analytic position, argues that such maneuvers are a hoax.

THE CONTENT OF TERMINATION

As therapy winds down, both participants may note a lack of energy between them. Problems arise but the client handles them without discussion, and are, therefore, simply described as relatively unimportant events. Those therapists seeking to read latent content find the associations flat, metaphors tepid, and what does come up, the patient is able to interpret. Termination may come simply with both people's acknowledgement of success and a quick good-bye. The other alternative, the setting of a date for ending, marks the overt beginning of the termination stage. The content of this stage is perhaps the most predictable of any stage since it mirrors the universal human experience of separation. The intensity of the separation is influenced by the following variables: the patient's previous experiences of loss, meaning and length of the therapeutic relationship, the patient's current experiences of loss and current social network, the method of termination (mutual, patient, or therapist initiated), the stage of therapy in which the patient is told, the amount of time between the announcement of termination and the date of the final meeting, and the apparent ease with which the patient may return (true ending or return if necessary).

Patients react to termination in ways that resemble their reactions to previous separations. Those who have had difficulty saying good-bye to important others, have difficulty saying good-bye to meaningful therapeutic relationships. While length of time in therapy is an important variable in determining patient difficulty in separation, short, or infrequent contacts may also generate highly charged relationships. Frequent contacts over many years do not necessarily mean great problems in separation. Current losses through death, divorce, illness, and geographical dislocation, may sensitize patients to the loss of the therapist. If the patient's social network is minimal, then it is more likely that the therapist has assumed great importance, thereby making the loss yet more difficult. Mutual terminations are probably easiest on both participants while patient-initiated terminations may bother therapists more. Forced therapist terminations probably evoke the greatest amount of patient rage (Langs, 1974). If the patient is told of forced termination at the outset, then termination may not be so difficult as in situations in which the patient is told during an intense middle phase that termination will be forced. If the therapist withholds such information until near the time of a forced good-bye, then patients will feel more betrayed (and rightly so). Often termination in private and institutional practice is not permanent, but, instead, the door is held open for return. Those terminations that are final are likely to cause more pain for both participants.

The many predictable elements of termination are there to see if therapists wish to look for them. They can provide deeper understanding of the patient's fears of attachment to others, provide further evidence of the dysfunctional ways in which clients respond to anxiety-provoking events, and offer useful desensitization to the recurrent human problem of loss.

Some patients respond with flippant, superficial, and reasonable-sounding responses. Do these reactions cover more deeply felt emotions; is this reaction typical of the way in which the patient hides the pain of separation?

CASE 11.5. A 44-year-old veteran was nearing the end of his 6 months of psychotherapy with a first-year trainee at a veteran's hospital. The therapist was deeply sensitive to termination, partially because he was delighted to be leaving his current assignment. He, therefore, carefully searched for signs that the patient was having trouble terminating with him because he felt guilty about having to force the good-bye. After patiently responding in the negative to the therapist's repeated queries about his responses to the impending termination, the patient declared: "I appreciate your concern with my reactions to losing you, but I know I will get another student with me during the next 6 months. You are one of a long line of young therapists whom I try to teach about being homosexual."

This patient was terminating with a therapist, but was not leaving the institution. He had developed an attachment to the VA hospital which superceded his attachment to any one therapist (Reider, 1953).

Sometimes a good-bye is simply a good-bye. Yet, often, much lies below the surface.

CASE 11.6. I met with a 45-year-old woman for 20 sessions to help her resolve her anger at her divorce and her ex-husband's remarriage. During termination, she reported that she had begun an affair with a younger man about my age. Some of his other characteristics matched mine. In the dialogue below, I clumsily attempted during the last few hours to investigate this connection.

PATIENT: Thank you very much. You have been a great help to me and you appear to me to be good at what you do.

THERAPIST: Thank you very much. I'd like to ask you about something perhaps related. I'm surprised you haven't thought of me for a relationship outside the office. I fit the kind of man you describe that you like.

PATIENT: Never crossed my mind. I know often women fall in love with their psychiatrists, but I saw you as a knowledgeable person, a professional who is also a friend. Anyway, I've heard stories of women having sex with their psychiatrists and I think they are awful. They shouldn't do it.

THERAPIST: That psychiatrist who made advances toward seeing you outside the office . . .

PATIENT: He was a jerk. If you would have done that, I wouldn't have come back. I don't have fantasies like that. . . .

My interventions were clumsy because I did not present evidence for the possible connection between her current man friend and me, but instead asked her about it as if she could read her own unconscious strivings. Furthermore, the question may have carried with it an implicit offer on my part to her to consider the possibility. Although we terminated psychotherapy, she kept up some contact with me because she was also taking lithium for manic-depressive illness. When she left town, we had one more meeting during which she berated my treatment of her. When she picked up her treatment in another location, she found numerous reasons to criticize my handling of her case. I believe that some of her feelings were justified because of my inexperience. Some others were related to unresolved termination issues. At the time we officially terminated psychotherapy, I had believed that this was a termination in which there was little below the surface. Follow-up suggested differently.

For most patients, termination represents a real interpersonal loss as well as a stimulus for reexperiencing previous losses. The therapist has become a real part of their lives. What am I going to do on Tuesday at

10:00? One patient's response was to imagine at 10:00 each Tuesday, what she would say to her therapist had she actually seen him (Firestein, 1978). The therapist occupies a unique niche in many patients' lives through the special combination of intimacy without reciprocal emotional responsibility that characterizes the relationship. Therapists share intensely personal experiences, understand elements of the self that no other person may ever comprehend, and help in ways that may never be repeated. Through the therapist's efforts, patients have also gained better self-control, tolerance, and acceptance. These are precious gifts. Therefore, patients react to the loss with the emotions of mourning and their accompanying behaviors, fantasies, thoughts, and dreams.

Not uncommonly, patients in the termination stage experience a recurrence of the symptoms that brought them to therapy. A person presenting with psychosis might reexperience those symptoms, recovered depressed patients may reexperience depressive symptoms, or a patient with panic attacks may reexperience intense anxiety. More often than not, these symptoms are short-lived (Firestein, 1978; Geller & Nash, unpublished; Langs, 1974). While there may be many explanations for this recurrence, perhaps the simplest one is to consider these reactions to be a statement about the patient's fear of being, without the therapist, as he or she had been before therapy began. The rapid remission of these symptoms reflects the patient's ability to grasp the gains more fully into his or her own power without the therapist as intermediary.

Sadness is perhaps the most common response to loss. Often a difficult emotion for therapists to tolerate because their aim is to bring "happiness," sadness is a chief characteristic of the human experience of transition. Anger and hurt may also play realistic roles especially in those instances of forced termination in which the therapist does not want to tell the patient for fear of "hurting." Unfortunately, the shorter the interval between the announcement and the actual termination date, the greater the real betrayal since the therapist has robbed the patient of time in which to accommodate to the loss.

Termination may force new behaviors, some of which may be constructive and some of which may not be. Patients may begin new relationships or may alter old ones.

CASE 11.7. A 44-year-old woman had recurrent depressions, usually triggered by interpersonal losses, especially of men with whom she was intimately involved. When she became depressed she often "faked" it to her friends trying to appear happy as usual. As the forced termination with me approached, she recognized that she would no longer "have Bernie to run to" and made increasingly greater efforts to let down her mask with her parents and friends. She consciously went about replacing my role with these other relationships and stated that had not this termination been forced, she might just let me be the only one to see beneath her depression-hiding facade. In so doing, she realized that the reason she went to bed so quickly with any attractive man who asked her, was not for sex but rather for the implicit acceptance and approval. Since she was now allowing herself to be accepted and approved by her parents and friends, she realized that she no longer needed to desperately cling to any man whom she allowed to take her to bed.

Clients may increase their functioning at work, make employment advances, as well as strengthen their marriages and separate from untenable relationships. They may notice the excessive neediness of other dependent people and realize that young children also need distance (Langs, 1974).

They may also precipitously enter destructive relationships, quit well-paying jobs, and disregard apparently useful changes. Sometimes the constructive value of termination-triggered changes are mixed with destructive ones. Time is then required to pass judgment.

CASE 11.8. A 26-year-old isolated English teacher in her 3rd year of psychoanalysis spent much of each therapy hour speaking in literary tones about herself. The material she evolved in these sessions often served as the basis for short stories. Through a friend, she met an equally isolated medical student. Weekend meetings with her new man friend provided both of these very lonely people newfound comfort. Although they had trouble sexually and emotionally, they decided to get married. The medical student was to graduate and leave for his internship in a distant city, requiring that the analysis be terminated. The patient was delighted to have made this significant emotional advance. Her analyst attended the wedding, also delighted. After 3 months in the distant city, the patient returned home, their marriage in shambles. Divorce proceeded 9 months later. However, through her husband, she met another man with whom she shared many globe-trotting adventures. She entered a second marriage to another man at the death of her father; this marriage also quickly ended in divorce. She subsequently retired to a quiet house in the country to continue her successful efforts at writing and established a weekend relationship similar to that with the medical student. Was her psychoanalysis successful? While therapy may have helped her leave her hometown, she was as yet unable to form a committed heterosexual relationship. She remained relatively isolated. Her biggest change was that she lived in the country and not the city.

Mourning is sometimes part of termination. The mourning process may include attempts to become immortal in the mind of the therapist, to somehow live on in memory. Patients may offer gifts for this purpose or attempt to become therapists themselves, with the idea of someday becoming a colleague. Or they may become experts on the school of therapy espoused by their therapists and, as one patient did, give lectures on Freud as partial payment for the benefits he received from psycho-analysis (Firestein, 1978). Some must mourn the passing of their old selves. As problem-filled as that self might have been, it was still familiar and enduring.

Dreams and fantasies may reflect themes of anger and loss. Patients may recall the birth of siblings, abortions, miscarriages (incomplete ther-apy), and births (termination as rebirth). They may recall deaths of parents or other family members, the helplessness they experienced in previous abandonments. They may also have fantasies about the therapist being destroyed or dead. Some have fantasies of murdering the therapist or people close to him or her (Firestein, 1978; Langs, 1974).

Patients often also say "thank-you" and attempt to convey to ther-apists who have aided them their appreciation for the help. Especially when those relationships have been highly useful, this heartfelt apprecia-tion must be acknowledged for the sincere emotion it is. However, this emotion may also be accompanied by a deep sense of loss over the life that could have been, had therapy been initiated earlier. "Had I only met you earlier in my life, how so much more fulfilling my life would have been up to now" (Davanloo, 1984).

RESISTANCE TO TERMINATION

Any thought, behavior, or emotion may be used by clients to avoid con-frontation with the loss of the therapist. During the termination stage, separation themes should be expected in much of what the patient dis-cusses. The themes may be quite obvious, as, for example, in the case of one person who asked at the outset of a termination-stage interview: "Am I aging?" She was experiencing the passage of time too rapidly. Seconds were dripping by like the sands of time in an hourglass being observed in slow motion. Termination was agonizingly intense and painful.

The heartfelt desire to extend thanks to the therapist may go past words into specific acts. Patients may wish to give their therapists gifts, some of them not inexpensive. To accept such presents is to collude with the patient's desire to hide the negative reactions to termination. To refuse the gifts is to force these reactions into the open. (The refusal need not take the form of an outraged "no!" Instead, the present may be placed aside and as with any behavior worthy of examination, the patient may be asked if he or she would join the therapist in looking at it.) Gifts symbolize the patient's belief that therapy requires more than payment of the bill, but also additional monetary rewards. In most therapeutic relationships, this belief is inaccurate and, therefore, represents a distortion. What is the source of this distortion? There are a number of possibilities. The patient may be wishing to remain immortal to the therapist by having a part of him or her kept on the therapist's shelf. The patient may be hiding anger and resentment for the loss behind the sweet smile of that gift. Or the message might be, "I don't deserve to have changed without having to pay a much larger price." Since the gift is not a necessary part of the therapeutic contract, it may represent an attempt to corrupt the therapist and minimize the change. Therapists may wish to test out these assumptions about gifts. In Case 11.6, in which the patient appeared unresponsive to my questions about termination, she also offered me a gift of expensive cut glass that I accepted. Had I refused, I believe the anger that spilled out much later would have "crystallized" earlier.

In Geller and Nash's (unpublished) study of forced termination, 68% of therapists reported that they observed recurrence of symptoms in one or both patients under scrutiny. Others also report the regular recurrence of presenting symptoms (Firestein, 1978; Langs, 1974). Most often these reactions are short-lived. What do they represent? As resistances, they are calls and pleas to avoid the separation — the patient is challenging the therapeutic success and the therapist is asked to question his or her competence. While such reactions can be frightening to both people, Edelson (1963) suggested that the recurrence of symptoms can remind both participants about how far they have come. Familiar resistances may also recur. A notably quiet patient's silence may be briefly resumed or a vituperative patient's abuse may be reenacted (Firestein, 1978, p. 208). Again, it is the duration of the symptom's reappearance that is most important in determining the level of the therapist's concern.

Patients may present with new problems and convey the feelings that more has yet to be done before termination will be successful. Some will become suicidal, homicidal, or complain of physical symptoms. Each of these reactions can be more frightening. Not uncommonly, some come to their sessions late or fail to come. Others prefer to terminate earlier than the agreed-upon date in order to avoid having to face the terror of interpersonal loss.

Although separation may trigger constructive behaviors, other behaviors (e.g., precipitous marriages, pregnancies, flights into therapy with someone else, sudden terminations of significant relationships) more likely represent defensive reactions to the impending loss of the therapist. During these sometimes tumultuous times, therapists must struggle to keep in mind the termination context as a partial explanation for these behaviors.

TRANSFERENCE REACTIONS TO TERMINATION

The therapist plays two real roles in each client's life. He or she has emerged as a caring person with whom a great deal of pain has been shared and from whom much has been learned. The therapist has assumed this meaning within the context of a professional relationship marked by the paying of fees and the keeping of regular appointments. Successful patients deeply appreciate the skill and resourcefulness of their therapists. Termination marks the end of this professional friendship, this growth-promoting business into which they have entered as unequal partners. The real loss often triggers distortions of the person of the therapist that deserve examination. Those terminations that are not mutually agreed upon may also have real elements that trigger yet greater distortions. The therapist is obligated to attempt to separate the real losses from the distorted ones. Therapists who find their patients howling with painful claims of betrayal, may have had some hand in triggering these reactions. Patients may use any number of "joining" techniques to avoid the loss of the therapist, as suggested by the next case:

CASE 11.9. During the last few sessions of a successful psychotherapy, the 25-year-old woman came to the office with a new hairstyle, different makeup, and new clothes. She looked much prettier than she had during most of therapy, which had focused on her destructive relationship with her man friend who was also a therapist. As a result of therapy, she had broken up with him. The patient had formed a relationship with her man friend that resembled a psychotherapeutic one. She was always at fault and he was always able to point out to her how she was creating the difficulty. He was unwilling to look at his own contributions. The therapist, a 36-year-old man reacted very positively to her new appearance and commented on her attractiveness. She asked softly and indirectly whether there was any chance that they might get together outside the office. He was startled and cut off the discussion, embarrassed because he realized that he had played into her seduction. Unfortunately, they did not examine the manner in which this behavior reflected not only her difficulty in saying good-bye, but also her tendency to want to repeat a rather destructive type of relationship. The reason she had entered the relationship with her man friend was his therapeutic attention; it had continued in part because she had a great sense of guilt that made it easy for her to accept the blame of others for the difficulty in her relationship to them.

Some will ask for medications (Schiff, 1962) in order to prolong the relationship. Some will wish to pay the bill on the installment plan in order to continue the contact after the actual separation. Some will devalue the therapist as a way of minimizing the pain of the loss, while others will aggrandize him or her. The roots of these reactions may be traced to earlier relationships and/or used to highlight current ways of reacting to interpersonal pain. Medications may represent pellets of concern during the time when the therapist is saying good-bye and withdrawing concern. Devaluation of the therapist characterizes those people who cannot admit that someone has been important to them, while the overvaluation reflects a self-image of little significance. The pain of termination evokes characteristic response patterns and may be used to highlight and work through them to practice new ones.

For some, the wish to be in psychotherapy far outweighs the wish to change successfully. They may show small increments of improvement and may terminate in superficially reasonable ways, but they might also go on to other therapists. These people are apparently addicted to psychotherapy, finding it a refuge from the more frightening commitments of real-world relationships. The therapist then represents a bulwark against such commitments. Since other therapists are available, particularly for those who have been through many therapeutic relationships, the transference distortions may be evident, but of little interest to the patient since others will take the place of this one. If the patient is married, perhaps couple's therapy is best considered because it is within that relationship that the problem can be best addressed. The very unreality of therapy may serve to help the patient avoid facing the real fear.

The sudden, unexpected death of a therapist may trigger real and idiosyncratically based reactions. In response to such a loss, one patient reported his disbelief by wanting to just wait in the waiting room until the therapist came out to get him. Several other patients sought consolation through proximity to the tangible possessions of the deceased by asking for a "keepsake." One was particularly disturbed because psychotherapy had focused on the difficulty presented by his hostile and withholding mother. He mumbled to his next therapist "My mother has won" (Shwed, 1980, p. 5).

COUNTERTRANSFERENCE REACTIONS TO TERMINATION

The good-bye of many patients represents a real loss for the therapist as well. In successful therapies, the client's values become more like those of the therapist (Beutler, 1983; Strong, 1978) and, therefore, clients appear to be more attractive. Fantasies of becoming friends or images of marriage (Searles, 1959) may stir within the therapist. These are intimately known people upon whose psyche the therapist has pressed much energy and thought. Few relationships achieve the level of intimacy of a long, successful, therapeutic relationship. The pair have adapted to the interpersonal styles of each other; they have come to appreciate each other's foibles and idiosyncracies. Often such patients express in many different ways a great appreciation for the therapist's efforts and come to idealize his or her person and skill. If such people are also witty and charming and pay their bills on time, hours with them can become a refuge from the storms of anger, tears, and demands characterizing the many other therapeutic hours. Termination represents the loss of a very real ongoing human encounter. Sadness at the loss and frustration with losing people just when they are becoming most attractive seem to be natural responses.

Some patients are in themselves very frustrating. No matter what the therapist attempts to do, success is an elusive ideal. Occasionally, external circumstances force termination of such patients. Loss of the pressure from recurrent confrontation with failure and frustration brings a not-uncommon sigh of relief.

These somewhat expectable reactions can develop into full countertransference reactions as a function of other elements in the therapist's life. Among the variables that can influence each therapist's responses to loss are: previous experiences of loss and the therapist's sensitivity to them, current interpersonal losses, and the specific concerns triggered by the loss of this specific patient.

Guilt

Guilt may be a common motivating factor for those in the helping professions. Often carrying the burden as the "white sheep" rather than the "black sheep" of the family, people helpers may be striving to make up for their failures to make the marriage of their parents happier, or to make their family of origin more cohesive, or to save a parent from alcohol and/or depression. Most terminations are not marked by total and complete "cure" because the process of growth and individuation is ever ongoing. Something can always be improved in one's own psyche or personal life. There is in us a basic greediness that some apply to the acquisition of material goods but is more humanistically applied to the perfection of our psyches and our interpersonal relationships. Therefore, termination marks the incomplete fulfillment of impossible therapeutic ideals. Therapists can easily feel guilty about not living up to these standards.

Forced terminations created by decisions the therapist has made unconnected to therapy can easily augment feelings of guilt. Some patients are deeply hurt by the announcement of the therapist's leaving and in many ways beg that he or she change plans and stay indefinitely. If the therapist is leaving a number of patients at the same time, their collective anguish can make psychotherapy a bath of guilt, hour after hour facing patients squirming in the pain of unpredicted loss. If the therapist is also leaving an institution and the city, then his or her own difficulties with saying good-bye to colleagues and friends increases the pain. Those looks that say, "Why are you leaving me?" come not only from patients, but those others with whom ongoing intimacy was expected to last indefinitely.

Inadequacy

Will the parting patient maintain the gains achieved so far? How do we know which ones will relapse or crumble under the onslaught of new psychic threats? Not uncommonly, therapists wonder about whether their work has been adequate, whether there is any durability to the change.

Anger

Feelings of guilt and inadequacy may manifest themselves in frustration and anger. Therapists generally do not like to admit anger at their patients so the feelings may be expressed in disguised ways.

CASE 11.10. A 31-year-old woman returned to therapy after a 6-year hiatus. When we had last met, she was convinced that joining the Irish Republican Army was to be her salvation and the salvation of freedom-loving people in the world. As with many of her grand ideas, this one had not reached fruition and, instead, she had had to rely on her mother for financial support. During the first sessions of our second round, she was extremely disorganized. I invited her sisters to the office; they helped her to become more able to communicate. Our termination was dictated by welfare considerations; we had both agreed to end therapy when the period of time ran out during which she was to receive state money. During the last few sessions, she became incoherent again. I became frustrated with this turn of events and ended the sessions early. I couldn't stand to see her so unchanged. Only later could I see this reaction as the common recurrence of old interaction patterns. Nevertheless, she had made few significant gains and this recurrence of hard-to-follow fantasy talk served to highlight my own inadequacy in helping her. Perhaps, I mused, I should have pushed neuroleptics harder.

Avoiding the Termination

Therapists also wish to avoid these painful feelings associated with loss and, therefore, engage in behavior to bypass them. There are many ways to do this, the simplest of which is to continue therapy. A symptom recurrence can be viewed as therapeutic failure and therapy can, therefore, be continued. New problems requiring solution can be stirred up. In the following case, I was terminating with a 28-year-old woman who had gained considerably from therapy and taught me a great deal about the process. I was finishing my training and going to another city. She paid me regularly and gratefully, and was very pleasant to know. She introduced the following dream somewhat offhandedly, saying that it was probably unimportant:

CASE 11.11. "I come into your house and there are many people. We go to your office and it is crowded also. You motion for me to follow you into the backyard, but people are talking there, too. You act as if you want us to begin our session, but the noise and confusion bothers me. I find myself becoming angry with you and I get up and leave. I go out the front door and sit on the step. You come to the door. I look up at you. And I woke up."

Rather than discuss the patient's feelings of anger at me about the separation or her sadness about having to lose me, I responded quickly with the suggestion that she could write to me in the new city to which I was going. She was very relieved and said: "Now I will know you are out there someplace." We exchanged some letters and I became tired of reading hers and sending mine. I wanted the relationship to end, but I could not bring myself to do it directly. Instead I sent a letter describing how cool the weather was in my new city and littered the page with other icy references that let her know that I was becoming cold toward her. She never wrote again.

Because of the way I handled this case, our ending was not smooth and clean and direct. The patient would have known I was out there whether I had written to her or not. In this case, the therapist helped the patient to ease his and her difficulty with loss by making a plan that included both of them in the future.

There is no right or wrong about continuing a relationship through letter or telephone. However, in this instance we had reached a position of maximum gain and there was no reason for us to make this plan except to ease our mutual difficulty in separation. I don't believe there was any harm done, however, just energy wasted and lessons left unlearned.

In the following example, I review the multiple reactions I had to the loss of a patient described earlier.

CASE 11.12. We had known each other for a long time. I made the decision to leave and told her that I would be leaving in 6 months. She came to the next session looking as distraught as she had during our first meetings. She was in a great deal of pain, extremely angry at me, suicidal, and helpless. Implicitly, she was asking me to rescue her again. Her despair about my leaving triggered a number of countertransference reactions. I felt guilty about leaving her as well as some of my other patients who had grown very dependent upon me. I remembered how ill-formed my own self-definition was at the time I met her; how I more easily fused with her then, than I would have now. I considered how likely it was that in that self-identity state, I was less aware of my effect on her, so bent was I in becoming useful to this damsel in distress. I felt guilty for my own incompetence. Her suicide talk reminded me of two other patients of mine. One was a very disturbed prostitute who died of an overdose of medications I had prescribed. She too had developed a sexualized dependence on me. In her case, I did not recognize it soon enough. Another patient was the wife of a physician who felt helpless in the pain of divorce. She made a suicide attempt, but realized that she was not trying to kill herself physically, but rather was trying to transform her old self into a new self she dimly perceived but feared becoming.

My patient also reminded me of the difficulties I once had in my marriage when my wife and I were caught in the throes of commitment fears while leaving behind our parental families to make our own. Each of us had reacted with tremendous anger and experiences of vulnerability during the torment of that transition. My patient and her husband appeared to be going through a similar anguish.

Her relationship with me spanned most of my time in this city; her difficulty in letting go of me stimulated to my consciousness the painful psychological experiences of this 10-year period.

Patient Suicide

Of all the types of termination, patient suicide will trigger the most intense and long-lasting responses in therapists. They are painful experiences and strike to the core of therapist self-identity. Goldstein and Buongiorna (1984) reviewed the literature on therapist responses and surveyed a group of psychotherapists, each of whom had experienced a patient suicide. Disbelief, shame, anger, vulnerability, and loss of self-confidence were very common responses. A sense of extreme loneliness enveloped most of the therapists and was accompanied by obsessive questions about what could have been done differently. Whose fault was it? What did I miss? While many experts recommend a psychological autopsy (a review of the case for an examination of cause), only 8 of 20 respondents thought it was a good idea while 12 said it compounded the problem. Seventeen out of 20 said they became more active in exploring suicidal ideation, perhaps because they had previously thought that it could not happen to them. The feelings about the suicide remained with each therapist because each is regularly reminded of the event by current patients talking about similar difficulties. A key element for self-exploration is the grandiose rescue fantasies latent in each therapist who misses the clues that therapy is deteriorating.

TRANSFERENCE–COUNTERTRANSFERENCE
SPIRALS DURING TERMINATION

Since therapist and patient influence each other in small ways that amplify, they sometimes spiral into stalemates. During termination, the pair may evolve a number of predictable patterns.

A clinging therapist ignores the forward steps of a positively changing patient because of a desire to remain involved. The patient is forced to repeatedly acknowledge gratitude and must remain in a dependent stance although progress suggests the contrary. Like a suffocated adolescent or a woman on the verge of liberation, the patient may suddenly break away in an indignant and protesting mood (Levinson, 1977).

Patients may successfully elicit sexual, protective, or frightened responses from their therapists, thus paralyzing them in sexualized, overly nurturing, or defensive stalemates. Complete avoidance of these webs may be impossible. Once entangled, therapists should be able to find their ways out of them.

Termination itself is likely to elicit one of two general responses from either person. Each will either tend to withdraw or to increase intimacy. Perhaps these responses are partially predictable from the style by which each says good-bye at airports. Those who drop off a loved one 30 minutes before the flight and leave or prefer to pay for a taxi to the airport rather than take the person themselves are probably more likely to withdraw. Those who stay until the very moment of disappearance down the ramp to the plane are more likely to draw closer (Geller & Nash, unpublished). There are benefits and problems with each style for therapists.

The withdrawing therapist may precipitate anger in his or her patient that the therapist interprets as sadness for leaving, though the trigger is more likely the therapist's withdrawal. This blaming the patient for a rather normal reaction to the therapist's behavior is an unfortunate hazard of the psychotherapeutic experience. For some patients, the therapist's withdrawal may be quite useful since it reduces the value of the relationship and makes the separation less painful. Therapists who move in the opposite direction, toward greater intimacy, may inhibit the expression of anger and resentment by making the relationship realistically pleasurable. Patients may find themselves burdened with the therapist's own problems in separating and find themselves unable to match the therapist's self-revelations.

MUTUALLY BENEFICIAL TERMINATION SPIRALS

The mutual, heartfelt termination is the ideal of most therapist–patient pairs. Each learns from the other; each grows more respectful of the other's humanity, perseverance, and skills; transference distortions lose their immediacy; the pair find themselves liking each other.

CASE 11.13. A 35-year-old gay man who had four sessions to go before termination dreamed that he had written a play. The central figure was a psychiatrist who had just died. The people at the funeral were all his patients, none of whom had met the others until the funeral. The dreamer described the patients at the funeral as representative of his separate selves who were coming together over the termination process. During the final session, the patient requested a hug. At first the therapist recoiled at the idea of being physically close to him. However, he believed that this request was no longer based upon the patient's sexual fantasies, but instead reflected the liking each felt toward the other.

TERMINATION WITHOUT ENDING

Termination implies the final curtain on an intense relationship, but clients and therapists often find ways to keep contact with each other. These methods range from the very indirect (accepting referral by the terminating therapist to another therapist) to the very direct (getting married). A middle ground, straightforward approach is to agree upon a meeting date in the distant future. Other continuation forms include contact by letter and/or telephone, recurrent fantasies about interaction, and attempts to remain close physically without remaining in therapy. And, of course, therapy itself may never end until death or calamity separates them.

Transfer

Forced terminations and stalemated therapies often imply the need for transfer. Unfortunately, therapists may make reflex recommendations of further treatment without careful evaluation of its true need. Unless the patient is deeply troubled, has gained little from the current psychotherapy, or is on medications that must be monitored on a weekly basis, immediate transfer may be unnecessary. A break from psychotherapy is often quite useful to clients. They can test out new ideas and behaviors on their own without reliance upon therapeutic permission or caution. Therapists and patients may rush into transfer discussion in order to avoid the pain of termination. Nevertheless, transfer does involve termination whether it is discussed or not; unresolved anger and sadness about the loss of the first therapist is likely to carry over into the relationship with the second therapist. Unless adequately addressed, these feelings may inhibit therapeutic progress. Transfer involves a therapeutic triangle in which each member is affected by the other two (Sher, 1970).

THE PATIENT

In addition to the pain of losing an important person, the patient is also exposed by the first therapist's reports to the new therapist. How accurate are those reports, how does the new therapist interpret them? What will the patient choose to modify? What if the new therapist is impossible to like or turns out to be better? As a consequence of these often intensely ambivalent feelings, patients may either idealize or depreciate the departing therapist. Sometimes, however, the new therapist brings fresh perspectives and approaches that serve quite usefully, but would have been difficult for the patient had the departing therapist started their relationship in this way.

CASE 11.14. A 36-year-old woman began psychotherapy and drug therapy with a psychiatrist shortly after being hospitalized for a severe depressive episode. She remained quite depressed, but did not require hospitalization during the 8 years that they saw each other. The therapist's approach was to be passive and empathic. He decided to take a job in another city and transferred the patient to a younger, more aggressive psychiatrist. The patient was tearful during the early sessions with the new therapist, but soon stated her appreciation for his attention to her behavior and thought processes. Over the next 4 years, she made slow and steady changes in her depressogenic thoughts and began to make a few friends, though previously she had had none. She remarked that with her previous therapist, she might not have been able to make even this much change because he was so passive. But his acceptance was very useful to her then. The new therapist's aggressiveness would have been too threatening to her earlier in her treatment course.

THE DEPARTING THERAPIST

Not only does the departing therapist suffer a loss, but he or she also stands exposed to the new therapist. How will my techniques and skills be viewed? What will the patient say about me that I will not be able to defend? These influences may affect the therapist's choice for the referral. He or she may pick a therapist for an especially difficult patient with whom he is competitive, in order to create a struggle and possibly failure. Or he or she may feel indebted to therapists who accept the referral of particularly difficult patients. On the other hand, he or she may wish to give a "present" of a "good" patient to a favorite colleague or one from whom he wants a favor. There may be other motivations. For example, a therapist who was sexually attracted to another therapist referred a client to her who was likely to experience similar sexual fantasies toward her. The referred patient symbolized his own sexual desire for the therapist.

THE NEW THERAPIST

The potential new therapist may have difficulty accepting the referral but feel obligated to do so in order to avoid straining the relationship with the departing therapist. Once having accepted the client, the new therapist must address the patient's possible sorrow and rage at the loss of the departing therapist. If the new therapist has little respect for the old one, then the patient's intense feelings about the loss may be hard to accept. If the new therapist is deeply attached to the departing one, the mourning process may be difficult to encounter.

Continued Contact in Fantasy

Patient and therapist may never see each other, but the relationship may live on in the patient's fantasies. All patients will, ideally, carry forth lessons learned from the therapeutic interaction. Some will personify these lessons in an internal dialogue. I asked a patient whom I saw about once every 18 months after termination of once-weekly psychotherapy to describe his dialogue with an imaginary me:

> "Because of your personality and sense of humor, this imaginary friend became not just a conscious figure, but a much richer entity who could enjoy situations in which I found myself, joke with me about them, and laugh both with me and at me.
>
> An example of this was when I saw the movie "Zelig" and gained much enjoyment from realizing the central character was like me or my tendencies taken to their logical absurdity [Zelig was a chameleon personality adapting to each and every circumstance with a new face]. My enjoyment of the film was heightened both by what it told me about myself and by the thought that if you saw the film you would laugh, realizing it was about me.
>
> Other times I engage in conversations in which I ask, 'What would Beitman say?' In my mind you answer and we carry on interesting and fruitful discussions often peppered with smiles and laughter."

Continued Contact By Letter and Telephone

Although classical analytic technique places high value on keeping the boundaries of the therapeutic relationship intact, in practice many analysts do not say good-bye to their patients and instead communicate by letter and telephone. In a questionnaire study about termination, 26 of 30 respondent psychoanalysts reported that they maintained phone or letter contact with certain patients. These contacts averaged 4 per analyst with a range of 1 to 17 patients (Rosenbaum, 1977). The length of post-termination contact ranged from 1 to 19 years. Of the 15 patients on whom any data was offered, 10 relationships were interrupted because the analyst moved and 5 because the patient moved. In most cases, the patient had refused transfer. The phone calls lasted fewer than 2 minutes and the patients were not charged, except for two instances in which the calls lasted longer and the analysts did charge. These contacts were not regularly scheduled, but initiated at the patient's discretion. Six of the 16 patients had required hospitalization before the interruption, but none were required after termination, which suggests that these limited contacts may have been beneficial (pp. 201–202).

Follow-up and Return Visits

Behavior therapists often prescribe "booster sessions" in order to reinforce the gains of therapy and to maintain them (Fishman & Lubetkin, 1980). Researchers often build in follow-up interviews in order to monitor therapeutic gain although both booster sessions and research follow-up interviews may serve similar functions for the patient.

Despite the best efforts of both patient and therapist, untoward events may precipitate the need for additional therapeutic help. Although each participant may be disappointed at having to see the other, their knowledge of each other can speed resolution of additional difficulties. As long as patient and therapist live near each other, the possibility of return exists. Therapists are like "general practitioners of the mind" to whom certain patients may return again and again. Such therapy may be continuing but interrupted (Bennett, 1983). Figure 9 illustrates the variety of scheduling possibilities. The last line describes the not uncommon practice of ongoing contact at irregular intervals. The "therapist-free intervals" allow clients to consolidate their gains much as does the period of time between transfer from one therapist to the next.

In a follow-up study of 20-session cognitive therapy for depression, 7 of 18 patients received some psychological/psychiatric treatment in the 12 months after termination (Kovacs, Rush, Beck, & Hollon, 1981). In a follow-up study of 8 completed psychoanalyses, 4 sought subsequent psychotherapy (Firestein, 1978). Unless therapists do follow-up studies on their patients, they will not know how many have sought treatment elsewhere.

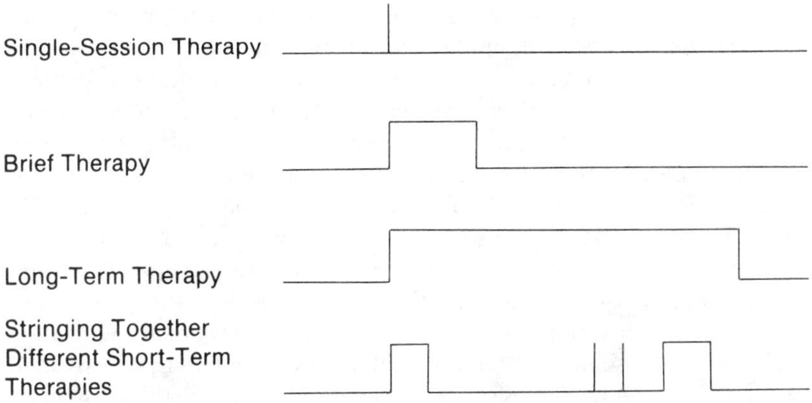

Figure 9. Therapy interval formats (S. Thorpe, personal communication, 1983).

Social Contact After Termination

Two people meet to do business. One is seeking the professional services of the other. They want to see more of each other outside the office. If they were general physician and patient, or lawyer and client, there would be little social repercussion. If they are psychotherapist and patient, then social outrage is more likely, especially if sex becomes part of the relationship. Should physicians or lawyers who develop sexual relationships with their clients also be censured or should psychotherapists be more free to become friends and become sexually involved with their patients?

Most psychotherapists would agree that sex during therapy is to be forbidden at the very least because it ruins the psychotherapeutic relationship. In addition, it also may represent the enactment of a client fantasy that would be better understood than acted out. In many ways, sex between patient and therapist is a form of rape, in which the therapist uses his or her own power to achieve control and obedience. It may also resemble the sexual abuse of children, in that the therapist wins the victim's trust and then exploits it. Through the child's curiosity and need to please, the abuser gains control and obedience. Unlike rape, in which physical threats form the power base, and unlike sexual abuse of children, in which the need to please a trusted other forms the power base, some sexual activity between patient and therapist is engineered knowledgeably and willingly by the patient. Sometimes the therapist is the vulnerable person. Sometimes the therapist is the victim. However, the therapist is always responsible.

CASE 11.15. A prominent psychotherapist was deeply unhappy with his marriage. He was contemplating divorce, but was afraid to act. He was treating a woman 15 years younger than he in intensive psychotherapy three times per week. She was deeply in love with him, coveted his social position, and seemed to recognize his vulnerability. She was also training to be a psychotherapist. As the years of their therapy continued, he began to see her outside the office and they began an affair. The younger of his two adolescent sons became deeply depressed, perhaps sensing that something was amiss with his parents. Each time his mother would complain to his father that she was anxious, he would simply advise her to do relaxation exercises. The son suspected something terrible since his father usually insisted upon talking over problems. The psychotherapist/father referred his son for psychotherapy to his still-secret lover because he was afraid that his colleagues would find out about his affair. Subsequently, the son went to visit his father at his office, only to discover the psychotherapist embracing his father. Shortly thereafter, the father divorced his wife and married his patient. He was censured by many of his colleagues. Four years later, he made a suicide attempt that his new wife discovered but failed to report. A few weeks later he completed his suicide.

This tragedy illustrated for me the need for a strict boundary between professional and personal relationships. I am sure there are instances of happy marriages and good friendships between people who have met as psychotherapist and patient, but I think the probabilities for successes are low. Any therapist who must pick friends and lovers from the ranks of his patients must feel inadequate to the task of meeting others on an equal footing outside the office. This inadequacy suggests the need for personal psychotherapy.

Unending Psychotherapy

Some patients and therapists never stop seeing each other until one of them is dead. Some patients switch therapists but continue as psychotherapy patients for many years of their lives. Like the chronic medical patient who has little biomedical difficulty but is addicted to physicians (Ries, Bokan, Katon, & Kleinman, 1981), some patients are simply addicted to their roles as psychotherapy patients. They have the money, time, and desire to keep the role and find someone to fill it for them. Some are veterans in veterans' hospitals' outpatient departments; some are wealthy, lonely, older people; some are working young professionals afraid to commit; and some are moderately disturbed people who are terribly afraid of changing.

CASE 11.16. A woman was hospitalized for prolonged addiction to drugs and alcohol, phobic withdrawal, and a generally chaotic and disorganized life. Psychoanalysis was tried as a "heroic" measure, but her first analyst soon became convinced that she lacked the ego resources for this procedure, and began using supportive techniques. After his death, a second analyst attempted more intensive work with her, but also shifted to a more supportive procedure. Throughout both treatments, the patient showed significant gains, always limited by an excessively dependent attachment to her therapist. She overcame her drug and alcohol addiction, took a relatively routine secretarial position, and progressively overcame her phobia for driving in unfamiliar places within the city. Though she functioned better than she had for many years prior to treatment, she remained unmarried and led a life of limited gratification. Ten years after treatment had begun, the frequency of appointments had decreased to once per week, but a real termination was nowhere in sight. She appeared to have developed into a therapeutic "lifer." (adapted from L. Horowitz, 1974, pp. 236–237)

12. *After Termination*

Therapists may find it all too easy to stop thinking about patients they no longer see. The rush of new faces and new problems, the desire to attend to the immediate human knots and tangles help to obscure from memory those people no longer asking for help. Researchers and administrators are, however, demanding that attention be paid to the posttermination period to help determine the durability of psychotherapeutic change. This chapter addresses the question of change maintenance and the variables that seem to contribute to it.

MAINTENANCE OF CHANGE

The expectation of long-term improvement in personal adjustment following the completion of psychotherapy remains a tacit and generally untested assumption (Steffen & Karoly, 1980). Except for the obvious evidence to the contrary from many returning patients, psychotherapists appear to believe that once a positive change has been initiated, it will endure. Evidence from psychotherapy research on change maintenance is fragmentary. Researchers have enough difficulty trying to agree upon adequate measures of change from the beginning to the end of therapy. Except for the study of addictive behaviors, measurable, adequate definition of relapse appears elusive and compounds the already difficult problem of adequate posttreatment criteria. For example, a patient's return for therapy may be used as a marker for relapse, but it also may indicate a readiness for further changes. Other follow-up problems include attrition, use of different measures and/or criteria and/or raters at follow-up from those used at treatment termination, and the confounding effects of the events and experiences following termination (Klein & Rabkin, 1984).

The limited evidence from behavioral therapy suggests a consistent trend toward reduction of treatment effect as the length of follow-up increases (Mash & Terdal, 1980). Smith and associates (1980) and Andrews and Harvey (1981) also conclude that the effects of psychotherapy are not permanent and appear to decrease at a regular rate.

Although these conclusions are based upon very limited sample sizes, they are indeed sobering. What are the critical variables influencing the durability of change and how much can therapists do to increase the likelihood of change maintenance? To answer these questions, therapists must conceptualize their clients devoid of therapeutic input by picturing them in their environment, subject to outside influences, buffered only by what they have learned about themselves through previous experience and through therapy.

Among the critical variables in studying the maintenance of change, is the type of problem under examination. The following four different problems illustrate some of these variables: addictive behaviors, agoraphobia, conversion symptoms, and transference distortions.

Addictive Behaviors

The study of the maintenance of behavioral changes has received the most attention in the treatment of addictive behaviors because successful therapy is marked not only by the cessation of the target behavior, but also by continued abstinence or successful moderation over time. "Stopping is easy," say many smokers, "I do it every day." Among the addictive behaviors are all actions culminating in some form of immediate gratification (the pleasure, the "high," tension reduction, surge of self-inflation). The addictions are negatively connoted because the immediate gratification is followed by some negative consequence such as physical discomfort, social disapproval, financial loss, or loss of self-esteem. The more common forms of such behaviors are excessive alcohol consumption, drug abuse, overeating, and smoking. Other behaviors may also be considered part of this definition: wife beating, explosive violence, child abuse, rape, exhibitionism, fetishism, and bulimia. Compulsive promiscuity and repeated extramarital affairs also fit this model because each has high initial gratification (the new physical contact and conquest) followed by potentially negative consequences (failure of long-term commitment) (Marlatt, 1982).

Especially in the treatment of these disorders, therapists must distinguish between efforts to promote cessation of the target behavior from efforts to maintain the change. Cessation may be self-initiated for a variety of reasons (fear of divorce, fear of long-term health consequences, religious conversion, aversion therapy, desire to please a therapist, and so on), but maintenance often requires different strategies. And most important, the variables contributing to relapse must be outlined before adequate models for relapse prevention can be developed.

The definition of relapse itself is a critical element for both helping professionals and clients alike. Does a single drink, or one cigarette, or one binge–vomit episode mean relapse? If the client believes it means relapse, then he or she gives the self license to continue the unwanted behavior. "See, I can't control myself. I must be hopelessly addicted. I may as well do another." This deviation is then amplified into a spiral of full-blown relapse. The abstinence violation effect (AVE) need not have such influence if it is perceived as a predictable event that need not lead to relapse (Marlatt, 1982).

What are the factors leading to that first violation of abstinence? Sometimes the person finds her- or himself in a high-risk situation where she or he is unable to say "no." The recovering alcoholic's wife is out of town; he is visiting a friend of hers because she needed some help with moving; she was lonely and offered him a drink because she wanted some company; they got drunk; she asked him to go to bed. Many times, however, the situation in which the lapse takes place is the final link in a long, casual chain through which the client has, out of his own direct awareness, set up the high-risk situation in which the relapse appears unavoidable. In the preceding example, he may have encouraged his wife to leave town, knowing that her friend would be alone and had plenty of alcohol and was interested in him sexually. The desire to set in motion a series of such events may be initiated by the physiological cravings and urges often associated with drug abuse and sexual behavior of all kinds. As the high-risk situation develops and the client's coping responses are blocked, a decrease in expectations of mastery of the situation is accompanied by increases in the expectation of enjoyment from the forbidden behavior. The abstinence violation effect then leads to full-blown relapse (Marlatt, 1982).

The concept of "attention" placement seems to play a critical part in these developments. For example, focusing attention on one's failure and associated negative affect can increase the likelihood of more failure. "I can't stop anyway and another drink (rape, binge–vomit) may make me feel better for awhile." On the other hand, focusing attention away from the self may decrease self-regulation when social situations are predisposing toward the unwanted behavior. For example, an unexpected lunch meeting may include pressure to have a cocktail. Too much self-confidence about the behavioral control may lead to decrease in attention to self-environmental interaction and also contribute to relapse (Kirschenbaum & Tomarken, 1982).

Agoraphobia

Clinical research trials in the treatment of agoraphobia illustrate the effect of treatment type upon maintenance. In the use of intensive *in vivo* therapist-assisted exposure, continued progress after termination does not occur. On the other hand, trials in which the spouses were directly included produced continuing improvement in follow-up (including spouses also decreased the dropout rate). By including the spouse in a slow, gradual exposure, the dramatic change in the agoraphobic's behavior often achieved by intensive exposure is avoided. This rapid change can easily upset a social equilibrium in which the spouse's behavior is partially determined by the agoraphobic's. If the spouse is included in the change process, he or she can then make the necessary gradual adjustment as the identified patient changes (Barlow & Beck, 1984). In this way, a positive feedback loop is established that can continue into the future without the therapist's intervention.

Conversion Symptoms

Once having targeted a specific behavior, behavioral therapists are often successful in bringing about a desired change. Exposure to feared stimuli, response prevention, stimulus control, and careful manipulation of potent reinforcers are among the many effective principles by which therapists may gain control over another person's actions. Psychoanalysts from Freud to the present have warned about the possibility of symptom substitution. This caveat is based upon the notion that all symptoms are manifestations of underlying intrapsychic conflicts that are not resolved by attention to the surface manifestations. According to this hypothesis, the problem will simply manifest itself in some other way. The same conclusion might also be drawn from a systems perspective. Rather than possessing an intrapsychic function, the symptom might also possess an interpersonal element that gives the patient control over others. The longer the symptom remains part of the patient's life, the more the symptom begins to play an important role in his or her neurotic style and interpersonal relationships.

Naturally, behavioral therapists have argued vehemently against the existence of symptom substitution, while psychoanalysts have confidently warned about the unstable consequences of symptom-focused therapy. The arguments continue because each side has some clinical reality backing its claims. There are times when the treatment of an isolated symptom is effective within a controlled environment, but loses its efficacy when the patient is discharged from therapeutic control. Drug and alcohol addictions are the most obvious examples; hysterical conversion symptoms (the targets of Freud's first therapeutic efforts) also show the instability of symptom change.

CASE 12.1. A 14-year-old girl quarreled with her mother over dating an older cousin. After another argument over household duties, the patient became unable to speak. Their physician recommended that she stay in bed for a few days. The family treated her as a sick person and relieved her of her household duties. The patient returned to school after 5 weeks, although she still did not speak. After being scolded by the teacher, she began to speak normally. After another argument with her mother, her voice was reduced to a whisper. The next day she had sexual intercourse with her cousin. Her mother questioned her sharply about this incident, and she once again became mute. She was then admitted to a psychiatric unit. For 5 days she communicated by writing notes and by nodding her head. Immediately after a program of shaping speech through selective positive reinforcement was explained to her, she began to speak normally. During a 2-day pass, her speech remained normal, but she developed severe headaches. The patient was told that her headaches served the same function as her aphonia. Her headaches disappeared. A 4-month follow-up indicated no return of symptoms or appearance of new ones. (adapted from Blanchard & Hersen, 1976, pp. 121–122)

Apparently this patient was able to utilize the dynamic insight offered her and to find another way to gain control over her environment. Sometimes therapists are unable to find ways to induce increases in self-responsibility although they are able to temporarily alter target behaviors.

CASE 12.2. A 75-year-old woman complained that she was immobilized due to an intense fear of walking, or a fear that she would fall. She remained in bed most of the day unless aided by a relative to walk around. She was admitted to a behavioral treatment unit where she remained in bed for the first few days. The staff realized how much she loved social interaction and, therefore, instructed her that no one would come to visit her in her room. If she wanted social contact, she could come to the dayroom. After a few days, she hobbled out of her room. Later she walked confidently. She was discharged well recovered, much to the delight of her relatives. When she returned home, fewer people came to call, as they had when she was an invalid. Before, her family had gravitated round her like so many moons hovering around the mother planet.

The son, who had never married, had attended to her dutifully. A physiotherapist had visited her three times per week, a cleaning lady had attended to her house, and others had done her shopping and business for her. A few days after being at home, she once again became afraid of falling and returned to bed. Her relatives, though angry, visited her with more regularity and tended to her needs. (Carr & Preston, unpublished)

Transference Distortions

Although patients in psychotherapy obviously do not present themselves for treatment complaining of misperceptions of the person of the therapist, many psychodynamic therapists believe that correction of these distortions leads to enduring change. Inherent in this approach is the belief that fundamental intrapsychic and interpersonal difficulties emerge within these distortions and that their correction leads to fundamental change. While little systematic evidence to support this hypothesis has emerged from classical psychoanalysis, in which transference interpretation is the "ultimate and decisive instrument" (Greenson, 1967, p. 39), Malan (1976a) has offered some evidence from short-term dynamic approaches. He and his colleagues studied 60 short-term therapies with follow-ups extending more than 10 years in some cases. Successful psychodynamic change was correlated with early and thorough interpretation about transference, particularly links between feelings about the therapist and feelings about parents. Unfortunately, serious methodological problems limit the credibility of these findings (Frances & Perry, 1983). Yet transference interpretation appeals to many clinicians as the royal road to durable psychotherapeutic change.

The Menninger Foundation Psychotherapy Research Project raised doubts among psychoanalysts about the effectiveness of classical transference interpretations in bringing about lasting change. These researchers studied 42 patients whose primary treatment was either classical psychoanalysis with some parameters or supportive psychotherapy. They attempted to test many psychoanalytic assumptions, including the necessity for conflict resolution through insight as the primary mode of durable change. They were able to confirm that in four of six successful psychoanalytic cases, gains were maintained and consolidated. In the other two with only partial conflict resolution, some symptoms returned.

Much to the surprise of the predictors, a number of patients in supportive therapy not only improved but maintained their gains. (During their form of supportive therapy, the patient was encouraged to develop more effective means of coping with internal and external pressures through a wide variety of mechanisms all depending upon a strong trusting relationship with the therapist. In a general way, it resembled cognitive–behavioral approaches.) Nine of 10 patients who showed significant improvement with supportive treatment maintained their gains during the 2-year follow-up.

Furthermore, two patients in supportive treatment who showed no gains at termination showed significant improvement at follow-up. One of these cases is summarized here because it illustrates how far afield from psychoanalytic treatment a patient–therapist pair may range and still achieve durable change. It is all the more significant because it took place within a study designed to test (and confirm) basic psychoanalytic hypotheses.

CASE 12.3. The patient started in classical psychoanalysis, but after 6 months switched to supportive treatment lasting 4½ years. Her phobia for closed places and for driving each had diminished significantly, she no longer hyperventilated, and her somatic symptoms essentially ceased. [Had she been experiencing panic attacks?] Rages at her husband had also diminished significantly. This psychotherapy had been explicitly conducted along lines of a "mutual friendship" model. Not only did the therapist convey a warm, genuine, concernerd attitude, but he attempted to engender a free, two-way expression of feeling. The therapist was open, honest, and direct in stating his own emotional responses and in answering all questions, frankly, even about his personal life. After termination, the patient made further gains in symptom reduction and in relieving problems in interpersonal relationships. Two factors may have contributed to the post-termination gains. The patient and her family returned to their home city and once again lived close to her mother and other family members. The therapist and patient also continued contact through regular correspondence — three to four times per year from each of them. On one occasion when the therapist had not heard from her for an extended period of time, he placed a long-distance call to find out how she was doing. (adapted from L. Horowitz, 1974, pp. 241–243)

The Menninger study has been challenged on a number of methodological grounds. The outcome measures were global, lacking specificity. The differences between the two treatment groups were not clearly marked, but rather were played out on a continuum. There were no control groups. Nevertheless, it has served to clarify basic psychoanalytic assumptions and, thereby, open psychoanalytic practice to a greater number of potentially effective change and maintenance mechanisms.

MAINTENANCE VARIABLES

Each symptom is embedded in a biological–intrapsychic–interpersonal–social–political–developmental context. Each of these categories of influence has influential subdivisions. They have been organized under the construct of general systems theory (Miller, 1975) and brought into medicine as the biopsychosocial model (Engel, 1977). This attempt to conceptualize the human condition as a multilayered context of contexts, as interdependent systems functioning within each other, provides a foothold toward understanding the problem of change maintenance. A second useful construct is deviation amplifying feedback (DAF), the snowball effect. Taken together, they offer a broad outline of change maintenance as an interactive set of forces operating between systems, over time. There are many powerful forces operating to disrupt any equilibrium as well as many powerful forces operating to maintain it. Any patient who seeks treatment has exhausted his or her resources in disrupting an unwanted equilibrium. He or she would like to alter the current set of forces in a desirable direction and to maintain the change. Following is an overview of the critical variables leading to change and its maintenance based on the notions of DAF and general systems theory.

Biological Variables

The limits of psychotherapeutic knowledge are obvious when the patient dies and ceases to function as a biological entity. Alzheimer's disease, that tragic transformation of a personality into a walking non-person, illustrates the necessity of proper brain function for psychological change. Manic–depressive illness and schizophrenia generally require treatment by medications first, although psychotherapy can be a useful adjunct.

Once a medication is introduced into a human system, it can operate as a crucial deviation from current equilibrium, leading to a new and more desirable homeostasis. For one manic–depressive patient who was depressed far more frequently than manic, lithium treatment caused a major realignment in her family structure. Her husband and children required many months before they could adjust to her loss of depression. The cessation of medications can also have strongly deleterious effects by shifting patients back into old equilibria.

Medications are simple, concrete interventions, the presence or absence of which is easily determined. Other interventions and events are less concrete, but serve similar functions — to shift over time from one homeostatic level to another and often to maintain it.

Time and Development

The passage of time brings aging and change. The only true constant is change. When 20-year-old heroin–cocaine addicts become 40, they run out of the old energy and hustle and often must shift to the more conventional alcohol. Athletes once full of youthful energy must shift to less vigorous activities over the same time frame. Beauty often fades; attractiveness must be measured in other terms. Some never make this time-forced transition and continue in the old ways, suffering more pain because their behaviors do not bring the same consequences. The aging beauty and aging athlete are not successful anymore. Loss can bring maturity or devastation. Relationships end; people die. New vistas appear; will they be grasped? These events, too, are outside the control of psychotherapists. Normal individual development requires adaptation to change and, if possible, embracing it, learning from it, growing with it.

Conscious Attitude

A most critical variable under individual control is one's own conscious attitude toward the self-in-life. Among the most important elements of one's own personal philosophy is a sense of self-mastery (Frank, 1974) or self-efficacy (Bandura, 1977). In a study of 45 patients who had but one psychiatric contact in their entire lives, 11 were genuinely improved over a 2- to 8-year follow-up, in part because of that one contact. All 11 shared the belief that they could manage their lives without psychotherapy (Malan *et al.*, 1975).

Purpose in life may also aid in the maintenance of change. Belief in the possibility that one matters, that one's efforts have a positive effect on others, and that some section of the world might somehow be better off because "I am," give the future meaning. The specifics will vary with the stages of the life cycle: 45-year-old males may become more sympathetic, giving, productive, and dependable than they were at age 30, a change that suggests a shift from self-centered pursuit to the active nurturing of others. Middle-aged women who for the most part were asked to devote their lives to marriage and motherhood may be turning away from altruism and focusing more intensively upon their own needs (Yalom, 1980). Each individual must balance the shifts in developmental values with the roles and needs of the social fabric within which he or she is enmeshed in order to maintain a positive life meaning. The inability to maintain this flexibility leads to decompensation at retirement or at the last child's departure.

Unconscious Attitudes

Buried under an easy awareness of our own selves are myriads of thought circuits and reflex arcs predetermined by genetic and environmental interactions. Sections of these circuits operate critical stimulus–response patterns and are, therefore, the objectives of much psychotherapeutic effort. Attitudes toward authority, toward intimacy, and toward self-preservation are located deeply within. If these basic images, schemata, constructs can be altered, then perhaps long-lasting change will follow. By failing to respond with old patterns, patients with basic alterations in constructs about self, intimacy, and authority may prevent a negative DAF from dumping them into a negative equilibrium. A woman, for example, who finally learns that she has married men who abuse her because of some desire to find their goodness and develop it, may look more carefully at her next selection.

Psychotherapeutic Learning

If one discovers personal responsibility by noticing how one contributes to a recurrent problem, this discovery represents psychotherapeutic learning. If one is able to anticipate entrance into a recurrent problem before the situation has developed, this anticipation is psychotherapeutic learning. If one is also able to say "No! I will not behave that old way in this situation," then this ability is a form of psychotherapeutic learning. If one is able to generate a more adaptive response at this decision point, then the selection of the new alternative represents the product psychotherapeutic learning. If one is able to apply some principle to the situation in order to learn yet more adaptive perspectives and behaviors, one has learned how to learn psychotherapeutically. Each psychotherapy school and each therapist has developed some of these: feeling awareness and expression, problem-solving procedures, synchronicity, repetition compulsion; the knowledge that consequences determine behavior, that "perseverance furthers," that "it all depends on how you look at it," that "love is all there is"; and that it is vital to "be here, now." Many of these ideas are not original to psychotherapy nor do people discover them only during psychotherapy, rather, they represent distillations of some of the wisdom of the world applicable to daily life. Are there a limited number of basic principles that may be taught in an effort to make psychotherapists obsolete?

Life-style

The choices each person makes about how to conduct daily schedules create a repeated pattern forming a life-style. Where drug addiction or boredom are the only choices, energetic people will opt for the adventure of dealing and shooting. Where one's life is filled with demands of work and family with little sense of self-indulgence, affairs and alcoholism are likely to thrive. If the friends one chooses to see are all drug abusers or alcoholics, social pressure is likely to increase relapse.

Particularly in the treatment of addictive behaviors, life-style changes appear to be essential to change maintenance. Schedules may need changing, social contacts altered, obligations reduced, and "positive addictions" like meditation, jogging, and other body-oriented pursuits begun (Marlatt, 1982). Such changes may need to be fashioned as "obsessive–compulsive self-regulation." Each client may be required to encourage repetitively into consciousness, thoughts and images that counter tendencies toward unwanted thoughts and behaviors. Furthermore, clients may be required to engage in multiple "rituals" (e.g., exercise, diaries, reminders) (Kirschenbaum & Tomarken, 1982). Although less obvious, many other problems like depression, personality disorders, and agoraphobia probably require some form of careful preventative self-regulation in order to maintain gains of therapy.

Psychotherapeutic Spouses and Friends

Among the more effective change-maintenance forces are close personal relationships that have psychotherapeutic elements. If a positive psychotherapeutic change is warmly received by a spouse the change will more likely endure. If the spouse also changes positively, they will enter into a DAF leading them to a happier equilibrium, perhaps where positive change is part of their ongoing interaction.

Interpersonal and Geographical Changes

Spouses may not adjust to individual changes in their partners. Divorce is a not-uncommon consequence of individual psychotherapy because the spouse not in therapy is generally committed to the status quo, often for neurotic reasons. Perhaps therapists should help their clients be more aware of the social consequences of their altered behaviors (DeVoge, 1980). For some, drastic social-context shifts are absolutely essential. The paranoid, depressed, isolated individual may require a group home simply to eat as well as to discover the value of human contact. The drug-abusing prostitute will be required to leave the drug and abuse-filled life if she is to gain any positive sense of self. In a study of opioid drug addicts in San Antonio, this hypothesis was firmly supported. During relocation to other towns and cities, the subjects were voluntarily abstinent 54% of the time and only 12% of the time while living in San Antonio. Relocation was correlated with 1-year abstinence three times more often than were treatment and correctional interactions (17% vs. 6%). When abstinent subjects returned to San Antonio, a great majority resumed opioid use within 1 month (Maddux & Desmond, 1982).

Social, Cultural, and Economic Shifts

War disrupts all of the previously mentioned variables and can, thereby, lead to devastating psychological changes. Cultural revolutions may neutralize basic values and institutions, rendering some people hopeless and lost. Economic disasters, recessions, and other out-of-control reductions in perceived economic requirements lead to the loss of psychological gains. Social stability aids in the maintenance of psychotherapeutic changes. Peace in a context of individual freedom and social responsibility is an effective agent in the maintenance of change.

13. *Reflections*

As this project comes to an end, I look back over the book and forward to the future of psychotherapy.

CONCEPTUAL WEAKNESSES

I wish that this book could have been more than it is. It may prove to be a foundation for organizing our concepts of psychotherapy, and it may help to provide a rallying point for those psychotherapists interested in finding connections between themselves and other practitioners. It lacks, however, some vital links for a solid conceptualization of the psychotherapeutic process. My failure to prescribe "what to do when" is not a true failure because a major underlying premise behind the book is the belief that the personality of the therapist and the personality of the client usually provide too much variability to actually predict the best single technique. However, there are many other problems:

1. What is to be done about theories of psychopathology? Deviation amplifying feedback is a very useful construct as is $S \rightarrow O \rightarrow R$, but these process configurations are content neutral. What is human psychopathology? What is human wellness? Defenses, coping styles, character patterns, operants, metacommunications, and security operations cover much of the same territory. They are predominantly descriptions of thought–behavior complexes accompanied by conflicting notions of causes. None is sufficient, but each contributes some idea about what is "good" and what is "bad." I place these words in quotes to emphasize that psychotherapists have tended to avoid making value judgments. For this reason, theories of psychological dysfunction have been manacled. They cannot be constructed without direct attention to questions of value. The term "dysfunction," for example, implies that something is wrong and is therefore not right. The often-used term "inappropriate" is a veiled criticism of certain behaviors — a judgment, a value. Religions are replete with dicta of

correct and acceptable behavior, but in the attempts of psychotherapists to avoid being associated with religious doctrine, they have avoided direct statements of their beliefs about what is right and good, except, of course, the relief of symptoms.

2. Closely tied to the failure to articulate a useful theory of psychopathology is the failure to define the ingredients of optimal human functioning. While few will deny, for example, that most agoraphobics are better off being able to leave home, the question of when the ailment is best left unchanged is left unaddressed. How does a psychotherapist define the limits of self-responsibility? Should a criminal be taught self-forgiveness for crimes of murder or rape? How do therapists decide the optimal functioning for a specific patient? What standards are to be used, and how are they to be adjusted to the individual? What is the place of theology in the practice of therapy? What about the problems of war, of economic imperatives, of capitalism, of male dominance, of gay rights? What are therapists to do with shifting moral and political climates that change values? What are psychotherapists truly trying to teach?

3. Between theories of psychopathology and valued outcomes lie the techniques and process of change. I have broken the change process into three substages and gathered together a number of often-used techniques for promoting movement through these stages. The product of these efforts offers a potential foundation for future conceptualization, but needs clarification and extension. This book is published at a time of transition for psychotherapy not unlike the transition of the psychotherapy client caught between giving up old patterns and beginning new ones. We are leaving behind the competing schools and traveling on to a clearer, more scientifically grounded, concept. We are crossing the narrow footbridge between the two states. Some will retreat back to the old ways. Others will charge ahead to grasp pieces of new possibilities. Others will remain paralyzed on the narrow footbridge swinging in the heavy winds pouring through the abyss. They will wait for the signal to move on. As we study the transition from the old to the new in psychotherapy concepts, perhaps we will understand more fully the process of individual change.

The weaknesses of this book reflect the weaknesses of our concepts of psychotherapy. We do not sufficiently grasp the human mind, either in wellness or in disorder. We do not comprehend the process of change, although we use theoretical phrases and technical terms to cover over our ignorance. Yes, exposure seems to work for phobias, but of what else can we be even half as certain? We do not accept our personal judgments about the rights and wrongs of human behavior. In our attempts to be value free, we have become value blind.

MY OWN STYLE OF THERAPY

While I have attempted to be "generic" about psychotherapy, to define it in objective terms removed from personal bias, I am certain that I have not succeeded in this goal. I too hold some notions more dearly than others, feel more comfortable with certain concepts and techniques than others. At the outset, I did not know what kind of psychotherapist I was. While writing this book, the answers became clearer.

Before I became a psychotherapist, I was an athlete. As an athlete, deeds spoke much louder to me than words; I could never score a touchdown by saying I wanted one (although wishing and imagining seemed to be very helpful in accomplishing that goal). I transferred this thinking to the game of life: action, behavior change, doing something was the ultimate prize. I was raised by parents who rarely asked me about myself, so I did not learn to speak about myself until years after separating from them. To satisfy my intense need for self-expression during high school, I followed Anne Frank's (1952) observation: "Paper is patient." I wrote my thoughts, sometimes staining the pages with tears born from unrequited teenage love. Through these experiences, I came to appreciate the value of diaries in carrying out the objectives of psychotherapy. I went to medical school, where I was exposed to psychoanalytic thinking. My reaction was powerfully ambivalent. I developed a tremendous fascination with the cult figure of Freud, found some of his discoveries compelling, but came to despise the hypocrisy of his followers. As an aspiring psychiatrist, I came to know a few analysts very well and, since they seemed to have obvious character flaws, could not help but question the effectiveness of their techniques. There had to be more. I loved George Kelly's (1955) ideas of personal constructs and have ever since learned to study the maps of reality each person/patient carries into my office. In addition, war, theology, existential philosophy, and my religion have compelled me to question the meaning of existence and the manner in which each person is capable of determining his or her own world view.

I have come to see myself as an existential–cognitive–behavioral–psychodynamic–systems therapist trying to fit the understanding and techniques I possess to the world view and needs of the person in front of me. I loved the introductory courses in college because they were overviews of new areas of knowledge. They suffered from a necessary superficiality. My touching upon the various schools of psychotherapy may also reflect a certain superficiality, but I have yet to be convinced that most schools have not made too much of some very good but limited ideas.

THE FUTURE OF PSYCHOTHERAPY

A colleague of mine attended a 1985 family therapy conference and during it was struck by two presentations:

1. A well-respected family therapist proclaimed that she knew how to treat schizophrenia. She had treated 19 families in her own very specific way. All those attending should follow her lead because most of the 19 had been cured.

2. An anthropologist who had some psychotherapy research experience but no clinical experience insisted that psychiatrists were interested only in drugs, diagnosis, and money. When the money ran out, they sent the patient to "us" (apparently referring to the social workers who composed most of the audience). The listeners applauded.

Some psychotherapists will continue to proclaim the right and true path for treatment. Others will follow. Such therapists perform a useful function for the rest of us because through their intense self-belief they become willing to expose themselves to the scrutiny of others. They challenge cherished beliefs; they force listeners to think again about what they are doing. But the era of charismatic leaders for large groups of therapists appears to be coming to an end. There are too many right and true ways for any of them to be universally applicable. Family therapy is the latest, and perhaps the last, cure-all. The next decades are likely to show incremental contributions to a clear conceptualization of the psychotherapeutic enterprise. The territory has been outlined during the last 100 years. Now the spaces must be filled in.

The psychotherapy professions war with each other. These wars need not continue. Some of the conflicts are as sticky as those between the Palestinians and the Israelis. Should not professions whose avowed aim includes the reduction of interpersonal conflict and the achievement of better coping be able to apply their techniques to interprofessional rivalries? Certainly no single profession is better trained in psychotherapy than the others. Psychiatrists in training are receiving less psychotherapy training but are immersed in much psychotherapy practice. Psychologists receive much seminar material but relatively little client contact. Social work training in psychotherapy is quite variable and more site dependent than in psychiatry and psychology. Ministers tend to receive no formal training as part of their education. The training for a master's degree in psychiatric nursing is likely to include some psychotherapy experience. The counseling profession may receive the most consistent master's level training (Beitman, 1983c). And there are many people with extremely varied backgrounds who simply declare themselves to be psychotherapists.

The biggest problem among the multiple professions practicing psycho-therapy is that professional affiliation is likely to be quite useless in pre-dicting psychotherapeutic effectiveness.

The problem of interprofessional rivalry may be related to the wars between charismatic leaders of different psychotherapy schools. Without a clear, formal definition of psychotherapeutic practice and some means to measure effectiveness, one's claim to be a psychotherapist cannot be refuted. This book is intended to help to develop a clear concept of psychotherapy that may lead to a reduction in these intergroup wars.

References

Adler, G. The borderline narcissistic personality disorder continuum. *American Journal of Psychiatry*, 1981, *138*, 46–50.

Agel, J. (Ed.). *The radical therapist*. New York: Ballantine, 1971.

Agras, W. S. *Behavior modification*. Boston: Little, Brown, 1972.

Ajaya, S. *Psychotherapy east and west, a unifying paradigm*. Honesdale, Pa: Himalayan Publishers, 1984.

Alexander, F. The dynamics of psychotherapy in the light of learning theory. In J. Marmor & S. M. Woods (Eds.), *The interface between the psychodynamic and behavioral therapies*. New York: Plenum, 1980.

Alexander, F., & French, T. M. *Psychoanalytic therapy*. New York: Ronald, 1946.

Altschul, V. The so-called boring patient. *American Journal of Psychotherapy*, 1977, *31*, 533–545.

Amada, G. The interlude between short- and long-term psychotherapy. *American Journal of Psychotherapy*, 1983, *37*, 357–364.

American Psychiatric Association Commission on Psychotherapies. *Psychotherapy research: Methodological and efficacy issues*. Washington D.C.: American Psychiatric Association, 1982.

Andrews, G., & Harvey, R. Does psychotherapy benefit neurotic patients? *Archives of General Psychiatry*, 1981, *38*, 1203–1208.

Applebaum, S. A. The idealization of insight. *International Journal of Psychoanalytic Psychotherapy*, 1975, *4*, 272–302.

Bachrach, H. M. Empathy. *Archives of General Psychiatry*, 1976, *33*, 35–38.

Bandler, R., & Grinder, J. *Frogs into princes*. Moab, Utah: Real People, 1979.

Bandura, A. *Principles of behavior modification*. New York: Holt, Rinehart & Winston, 1969.

Bandura, A. Social learning perspective on behavior change. In A. Burton (Ed.), *What makes behavior change possible?* New York: Brunner/Mazel, 1976.

Bandura, A. Self-efficacy: Toward a unifying theory of behavioral change. *Psychological Review*, 1977, *54*, 191–215.

Bank, S. P., & Kahn, M. D. *The sibling bond*. New York: Basic Books, 1982.

Barlow, D. H., & Beck, J. G. The psychosocial treatment of anxiety disorders: Current status, future directions. In J. B. W. Williams & R. L. Spitzer (Eds.), *Psychotherapy research: Where are we and where should we go*. New York: Guilford, 1984.

Bart, P. B. Ideologies and utopias of psychotherapy. In P. M. Roman & H. M. Trice (Eds.), *The sociology of psychotherapy*. New York: Jason Aronson, 1974.

Basch, M. F. Dynamic psychotherapy and its frustrations. In P. L. Wachtel (Ed.), *Resistance*. New York: Plenum, 1982.

Beahrs, J. O. *Unity and multiplicity: Multilevel consciousness of self in hypnosis, psychiatric disorder and mental health.* New York: Brunner/Mazel, 1982.

Beck, A. T. *Cognitive therapy and the emotional disorders.* New York: International Universities Press, 1976.

Beck, A. T., & Emery, G. *Anxiety disorders and phobias: A cognitive perspective.* New York: Basic Books, 1985.

Beck, A. T., Rush, A. J., Shaw, B. F., & Emery, G. *Cognitive therapy of depression.* New York: Guilford, 1979.

Becker, E. *The denial of death.* New York: Free Press, 1973.

Beebe, J. E., & Rosenbaum, C. P. The use of dreams in psychotherapy. In C. P. Rosenbaum & J. E. Beebe (Eds.), *Psychiatric treatment: Crisis/clinic/consultation.* New York: McGraw-Hill, 1975.

Beitman, B. D. Engagement techniques for individual psychotherapy. *Social Casework,* 1979, *60,* 306–309.

Beitman, B. D. Pharmacotherapy as an intervention during the stages of psychotherapy. *American Journal of Psychotherapy,* 1981, *35,* 206–214.

Beitman, B. D. Comparing psychotherapies by the stages of the process. *Journal of Operational Psychiatry,* 1983(a), *14,* 20–28.

Beitman, B. D. Categories of countertransference. *Journal of Operational Psychiatry,* 1983(b), *14,* 82–90.

Beitman, B. D. The demographics of American psychotherapists: A pilot study. *American Journal of Psychotherapy,* 1983(c), *37,* 37–49.

Beitman, B. D. Introducing medications during psychotherapy. In B. D. Beitman & G. L. Klerman (Eds.), *Combining psychotherapy and drug therapy in clinical practice.* New York: Spectrum, 1984.

Beitman, B. D. Two episodes of depression treated by very brief psychotherapy: An example of systematic technical eclecticism. In J. Norcross (Ed.), *The casebook of eclectic psychotherapy.* New York: Brunner/Mazel, 1986.

Beitman, B. D., Chiles, J. S., & Carlin, A. The pharmacotherapy-psychotherapy triangle. *Journal of Clinical Psychiatry,* 1984, *45,* 458–459.

Beitman, B. D., & Maxim, P. E. A survey of psychiatric practice: Implications for residency training. *Journal of Psychiatric Education,* 1984, *8,* 149–153.

Bennett, M. J. Focal psychotherapy — terminable and interminable. *American Journal of Psychotherapy,* 1983, *37,* 365–375.

Bergin, A. E., & Strupp, H. H. *Changing frontiers in the science of psychotherapy.* Chicago: Aldine, 1972.

Berne, E. *Transactional analysis in psychotherapy.* New York: Grove, 1961.

Berne, E. *Games people play.* New York: Grove, 1967.

Beutler, L. E. *Eclectic psychotherapy.* New York: Pergamon, 1983.

Bieber, I. *Cognitive psychoanalysis.* New York: Jason Aronson, 1980.

Birk, L., & Brinkley-Birk, A. W. Psychoanalysis and behavior therapy. *American Journal of Psychiatry,* 1974, *131,* 499–510.

Blackburn, I. M., Bishop, S., Glen, A. I. M., Whalley, L. S., & Christie, J. E. The efficacy of cognitive therapy in depression. *British Journal of Psychiatry,* 1981, *139,* 181–189.

Blanchard, E. B., & Hersen, M. Behavioral treatment of hysterical neurosis: Symptom substitute and symptom return reconsidered. *Psychiatry,* 1976, *39,* 118–129.

Bloch, S. Assessment of patients for psychotherapy. *British Journal of Psychiatry,* 1979, *135,* 193–208.

Bolen, J. S. *The Tao of psychology: Synchronicity and the self.* San Francisco: Harper & Row, 1979.

Bonime, W. *The clinical use of dreams.* New York: Basic Books, 1962.

Boszormenyi-Nagy, I. Behavior change through family change. In A. Burton (Ed.), *What makes behavior change possible?* New York: Brunner/Mazel, 1976.

Brady, J. P. Social skills training for psychiatric patients. I. Concepts, methods and clinical results. *American Journal of Psychiatry,* 1984, *141,* 333–340.

Brinkley, J. R., Beitman, B. D., & Friedel, R. O. Low-dose neuroleptic regimes in the treatment of borderline patients. *Archives of General Psychiatry,* 1979, *36,* 319–323.

Brown, M. The new body therapies. In H. H. Strupp & A. E. Bergin (Eds.). *Psychotherapy and behavior change.* Chicago: Aldine, 1974.

Bruch, H. *Learning psychotherapy.* Boston: Harvard University Press, 1974.

Buckley, P., Karasu, T. B., Charles, E., & Stein, S. Theory and practice in psychotherapy. *Journal of Nervous and Mental Disease,* 1979, *167,* 218–223.

Burton, A. (Ed.). *What makes behavior change possible?* New York: Brunner/Mazel, 1976.

Campbell, D. T. On the conflicts between biological and social evolution and between psychology and moral tradition. *American Psychologist,* 1975, *30,* 1103–1126.

Carr, J. E., & Preston, C. E. Behavior modification and the aged: A case study in failure. (Unpublished manuscript. University of Washington.)

Cashdan, S. *Interactional psychotherapy.* New York: Grune & Stratton, 1973.

Chessick, R. *Intensive psychotherapy of the borderline patient.* New York: Jason Aronson, 1977.

Chessick, R. D. Psychoanalytic listening. *Contemporary Psychoanalysis,* 1982, *18,* 613–634. (a)

Chessick, R. D. Current issues in intensive psychotherapy. *American Journal of Psychotherapy,* 1982, *36,* 438–449. (b)

Cohen, J. [Review of *Benefits of psychotherapy*]. *Psychiatry,* 1981, *44,* 177–181.

Colarusso, C. A., & Nemiroff, R. A. *Adult development.* New York: Plenum, 1981.

Cornsweet, C. Nonspecific factors and theoretical choice. *Psychotherapy: Theory Research and Practice,* 1983, *20,* 307–313.

Coyne, J. C., & Lazarus, R. S. Cognitive style, stress perception and coping. In I. L. Kutash *& L. B. Schlesinger (Eds.), Handbook of stress and anxiety.* San Francisco: Jossey-Bass, 1980.

Davanloo, H. (Ed.) *Basic principles and techniques in short-term dynamic psychotherapy.* New York: Spectrum, 1978.

Davanloo, H. *Short-term dynamic psychotherapy.* Audiovisual presentation at the meeting of the Washington State Psychiatric Association, Seattle, September, 1984.

Derogatis, L. R. *SCL-90: Administration, scoring and procedures manual for the revised version.* Baltimore: Clinical Psychometric Research, 1977.

DeRubeis, R. J., Hollon, S. D., Evans, M. D., & Bernis, K. M. Can psychotherapies for depression be discriminated? A systematic investigation of cognitive therapy and interpersonal therapy. *Journal of Consulting and Clinical Psychology,* 1982, *50,* 744–756.

DeVoge, J. T. Reciprocal role training. In P. Karoly & J. J. Steffen (Eds.), *Improving the long-term effects of psychotherapy.* New York: Gardner, 1980.

Dewald, P. A. Reactions to forced termination of therapy. *Psychiatric Quarterly,* 1965, *39,* 102–126.

Dewald, P. A. Toward a general concept of the therapeutic process. *International Journal of Psychoanalytic Psychotherapy,* 1976, *5,* 283–299.

Dickes, R. Technical considerations of the therapeutic and working alliances. *International Journal of Psychoanalytic Psychotherapy,* 1975, *4,* 1–24.

Docherty, J. P. [Introduction to section V.: The therapeutic alliance and treatment outcome]. In R. E. Hales & A. J. Frances (Eds.), *American Psychiatric Association Annual Review (Vol. 4)*. Washington: American Psychiatric Press, 1985.

Driscoll, R. H. *Pragmatic psychotherapy*. New York: Van Nostrand Reinhold, 1984.

Eckert, E. D., & Halmi, K. A. Anorexia nervosa: Psychological therapies and pharmacotherapy. In B. D. Beitman & G. L. Klerman (Eds.), *Combining psychotherapy and drug therapy in clinical practice*. New York: Spectrum, 1984.

Edelson, M. *The termination of intensive psychotherapy*. Springfield, Ill.: Charles C. Thomas, 1963.

Eisler, R. M. The behavioral assessment of social skills. In M. Hersen & A. S. Bellack (Eds.), *Behavioral assessment*. New York: Pergamon, 1976.

Ellis, A. *Reason and emotion in psychotherapy*. New York: Lyle Stuart, 1962.

Ellis, A. *Humanistic psychotherapy*. New York: McGraw-Hill, 1973. (a)

Ellis, A. Rational-emotive therapy. In R. Corsini (Ed.), *Current psychotherapies*. Itasca, Ill.: F. E. Peacock, 1973. (b)/(Third edition, 1984).

Engel, G. L. The need for a new medical model: A challenge for biomedicine. *Science*, 1977, *196*, 129.

Erickson, M. H., Rossi, E. L., & Rossi, S. I. *Hypnotic realities*. New York: Wiley, 1976.

Erikson, E. H. *Childhood and society* (2nd Ed.). New York: W. W. Norton, 1963.

Fagan, J., & Shepherd, E. L. (Eds.). *Gestalt therapy now*. New York: Harper & Row, 1970.

Favazza, A. R., & Oman, M. Overview: Foundations of cultural psychiatry. *American Journal of Psychiatry*, 1978, *35*, 293–303.

Fenichel, O. *The psychoanalytic theory of neurosis*. New York: W. W. Norton, 1945.

Fensterheim, H., & Glazer, H. I. (Eds.). *Behavioral psychotherapy: Basic principles and case studies in an integrative clinical model*. New York: Brunner/Mazel, 1983.

Fine, R. Psychoanalysis. In R. Corsini (Ed.), *Current Psychotherapies*. Itasca, Ill.: F. E. Peacock, 1973.

Firestein, S. K. *Termination in psychoanalysis*. New York: International Universities Press, 1978.

Fishman, S. T., & Lubetkin, B. S. Maintenance and generalization of individual behavior therapy programs: Clinical observations. In P. Karoly & J. J. Steffen (Eds.), *Improving the long-term effects of psychotherapy*. New York: Gardner, 1980.

Frances, A., & Perry, S. Transference interpretations in focal therapy. *American Journal of Psychiatry*, 1983, *140*, 405–409.

Frank, A. *Diary of a young girl*. New York: Doubleday, 1952.

Frank, J. *Persuasion and healing*. Baltimore: John Hopkins Press, 1961.

Frank, J. D. Psychotherapy: The restoration of morale. *American Journal of Psychiatry*, 1974, 131–134.

Frank, J. D. Restoration of morale and behavior change. In A. Burton (Ed.), *What makes behavior change possible*. New York: Brunner/Mazel, 1976.

Frank, J. D., Hoehn-Saric, R., Imber, S. D., Liberman, B. L., & Stone, A. R. *Effective ingredients of successful psychotherapy*. New York: Brunner/Mazel, 1978.

Frankl, V. E. *The doctor, and the soul*. New York: Knopf, 1955.

Frankl, V. E. *Man's search for meaning*. New York: Washington Square, 1959.

Frankl, V. E. Paradoxical intention: A logotherapeutic technique. *American Journal of Psychotherapy*, 1960, *14*, 520–531.

Freud, A. [Annual Freud lecture at the New York Psychoanalytic Institute]. Reprinted in *Newsweek*, April 4, 1968.

Freud, A. *The ego and the mechanisms of defense*. New York: International Universities Press, 1971.

Freud, S. The future prospects for the psychoanalytic movement. *Standard edition*, 1910, *11*, 141–151.

Freud, S. Civilization and its discontents. *Standard edition*, 1933, *21*, 59–145.

Freud, S. *The interpretation of dreams.* New York: Random House, 1938. (original work published 1900)

Freud, S. *Collected papers* (Vol. 2). London: Hogarth, 1950.

Freud, S. *Therapy and technique* (Philip Rieff, Ed.). New York: Collier, 1963.

Fromm-Reichman, F. *Principles of intensive psychotherapy.* Chicago: University of Chicago Press, 1961.

Garfield, S. L. Research on client variables in psychotherapy. In S. L. Garfield & A. E. Bergin (Eds.), *Handbook of psychotherapy and behavioral change.* New York: Wiley, 1978.

Garfield, S. L. *Psychotherapy: An eclectic approach.* New York: Wiley, 1980.

Garfield, S. L., & Kurtz, R. A. A survey of clinical psychologists: Characteristics, activities and orientations. *The Clinical Psychologist*, 1974, *28*, 7–10.

Gedo, J., & Goldberg, A. *Models of the mind.* Chicago: University of Chicago Press, 1973.

Geller, J. D., & Nash, V. Termination from psychotherapy as viewed by psychiatric residents. (Unpublished manuscript. New Haven.)

Givelber, F., & Simon, B. A death in the life of a therapist and its impact on the therapy. *Psychiatry*, 1981, *44*, 141–149.

Goldberg, A. Narcissism and the readiness for psychotherapy termination. *Archives of General Psychiatry*, 1975, *32*, 695–699.

Goldfried, M. R., & Davison, G. C. *Clinical behavior therapy.* New York: Holt, Rinehart & Winston, 1976.

Goldfried, M. R. Resistance and clinical behavior therapy. In P. L. Wachtel (Ed.), *Resistance.* New York: Plenum, 1982.

Goldfried, M. R., & Padawar, W. Current status and future directions in psychotherapy. In M. R. Goldfried (Ed.), *Converging themes in psychotherapy.* New York: Springer, 1982.

Goldstein, A. Behavior therapy. In R. Corsini (Ed.), *Current psychotherapies.* Itasca, Ill.: F. E. Peacock, 1973.

Goldstein, L. S., & Buongiorna, P. A. Psychotherapists as suicide survivors. *American Journal of Psychotherapy*, 1984, *38*, 392–398.

Goldstein, M. J. Schizophrenia: The interaction of family and neuroleptic therapy. In B. D. Beitman & G. L. Klerman (Eds.), *Combining psychotherapy and drug therapy in clinical practice.* New York: Spectrum, 1984.

Gomes-Schwartz, B., Hadley, S. W., & Strupp, H. H. Individual psychotherapy and behavior therapy. *Annual Review of Psychology*, 1978, *29*, 437–471.

Grant, B., Katon, W., & Beitman, B. D. Panic disorder. *Journal of Family Practice*, 1983, *17*, 907–914.

Greenberg, L. S. A task analysis of intrapersonal conflict resolution. In L. N. Rice & L. S. Greenberg (Eds.), *Patterns of change.* New York: Guilford, 1984.

Greenberg, R. P., & Pies, R. Is paradoxical intention risk-free?: A review and case report. *Journal of Clinical Psychiatry*, 1983, *44*, 66–69.

Greenson, R. R. *The technique and practice of psychoanalysis* (Vol. I). New York: International Universities Press, 1967.

Griffith, M. S. The influences of race on the psychotherapeutic relationship. *Psychiatry*, 1977, *40*, 27–39.

Grof, S. *Realms of the human unconscious.* New York: Viking, 1975.

Grotstein, J. S. *Disorders of self-regulation.* (Unpublished manuscript. Los Angeles, 1983.)

Gunderson, J., & Singer, N. Defining borderline patients. *American Journal of Psychiatry*, 1975, *132*, 1–10.

Gurman, A. S. The patient's perception of the therapeutic relationship. In A. S. Gurman & A. M. Razin (Eds.), *Effective psychotherapy: A handbook of research*. New York: Pergamon, 1977.

Hales, R. E., & Frances, A. J. (Eds.). *Annual review (Vol. 4)*. Washington, D.C.: American Psychiatric Press, 1985.

Haley, J. *Strategies of psychotherapy*. New York: Grune & Stratton, 1963.

Haley, J. *Uncommon therapy*. New York: Norton, 1973.

Hall, R. C. W., Gardner, E. R., Popkin, M. K., LeCann, A. F., & Stickney, S. K. Unrecognized physical illness prompting psychiatric admission: A prospective study. *American Journal of Psychiatry*, 1981, *138*, 629–635.

Harper, R., Bauer, R., & Kannankist, J. Learning theory and Gestalt therapy. *American Journal of Psychotherapy*, 1976, *30*, 55–72.

Harris, T. A. *I'm O.K. – You're O.K.* New York: Avon, 1967.

Hart, J. *Modern eclectic therapy*. New York: Plenum, 1983.

Hartley, D. E. Research on the therapeutic alliance in psychotherapy. In R. E. Hales & A. J. Frances (Eds.), *American Psychiatric Association annual review* (Vol. 4). Washington, D.C.: American Psychiatric Press, 1985.

Hatterer, M. S. The problems of women married to homosexual men. *American Journal of Psychiatry*, 1974, *131*, 275–278.

Havens, L. Existential use of the self. *American Journal of Psychiatry*, 1974, *131*, 1–10.

Hersen, M., & Bellack, A. S. (Eds.). *Behavioral assessment*. New York: Pergamon, 1976.

Hersen, M., Bellak, A. S., Himmelhoch, J. M., & Thase, M. E. Effects of social skill training, amitriptyline and psychotherapy in unipolar depressed women. *Behavior Therapy*, 1984, *15*, 21–40.

Hill, C. Panel on integrative psychotherapy research: Conceptual and methodological issues. Meeting of the Society for the Exploration of Psychotherapy Integration. Annapolis, June, 1985.

Hine, F. R., Werman, D. S., & Simpson, D. M. Effectiveness of psychotherapy: Problems on research of complex phenomena. *American Journal of Psychiatry*, 1982, *139*, 204–208.

Hollon, S. Cognitive therapy seminar. University of Washington, 1982.

Hollon, S. Cognitive therapy. Grand rounds, University of Washington, September 1983.

Horwitz, L. *Clinical prediction in psychotherapy*. New York: Jason Aronson, 1974.

Horowitz, M. Microanalysis of working through in psychotherapy. *American Journal of Psychiatry*, 1974, *131*, 1208–1210.

Horowitz, M. J., Marmar, C., Weiss, D. S., Dewitt, K. N., & Rosenbaum, R. Brief psychotherapy of bereavement reactions. *Archives of General Psychiatry*, 1984, *41*, 438–448.

Jamison, K. R., & Goodwin, F. K. Psychotherapeutic treatment of manic–depressive patients on lithium. In M. H. Greenhill & A. Gralnick (Eds.), *Psychopharmacology and psychotherapy*. New York: Free Press, 1983.

Jung, C. G. *The practice of psychotherapy*. New York: Pantheon, 1954.

Jung, C. G. *Man and his symbols*. Garden City, N.Y.: Doubleday, 1964.

Jung, C. G. *Analytical psychology*. New York: Vintage Books, 1968.

Jung, C. G. *Synchronicity*. Princeton: Bollingen, 1973.

Kaiser, H. Emergency. *Psychiatry*, 1962, *20*, 97–118.

Karoly, P. Person variables in therapeutic change and development. In P. Karoly & J. J. Steffen (Eds.), *Improving the long-term effects of psychotherapy*. New York: Gardner, 1980.

Karoly, P., & Steffen, J. J. *Improving the long-term effects of psychotherapy*. New York: Gardner, 1980.

Kelly, G. A. *A theory of personality*. New York: Norton, 1955.

Kernberg, O. *Borderline conditions and pathological narcissism*. New York: Jason Aronson, 1975.

Kirschenbaum, D. S., & Tomarken, A. J. Self-regulatory failure. In P. C. Kendall (Ed.), *Advances in cognitive behavioral research and therapy* (Vol. 1). New York: Academic, 1982.

Klein, D. F., Gittelman, R., Quitkin, F., & Ritkin, A. (Eds.). *Diagnosis and drug treatment of psychiatric disorders: Adults and children* (2nd ed.). Baltimore: Williams & Wilkins, 1980.

Klein, D. F., & Rabkin, J. G. Specificity and strategy in psychotherapy research and practice. In J. B. W. Williams & R. L. Spitzer (Eds.), *Psychotherapy research: Where are we and where should we go?* New York: Guilford, 1984.

Klein, M. *The psychoanalysis of children*. London: Hogarth, 1932.

Kleinman, A., Eisenberg, L., & Good, B. Culture, illness and care. *Annals of Internal Medicine*, 1978, *88*, 251–254.

Klerman, G. L., Weissman, M. M., Rounsaville, B. J., & Chevron, E. S. *Interpersonal psychotherapy of depression*. New York: Basic Books, 1984.

Koestler, A. *The roots of coincidence*. New York: Random House, 1972.

Kohut, H. The psychoanalytic treatment of narcissistic personality disorders. *Psychoanalytic Study of the Child*, 1968, *23*, 86–113.

Kopp, S. *Back to one*. Palo Alto: Science & Behavior Books, 1977.

Kovacs, M., & Beck, A. T. Maladaptive cognitive structures in depression. *American Journal of Psychiatry*, 1978, *135*, 525–533.

Kovacs, M., Rush, A. J., Beck, A. T., & Hollon, S. D. Depressed outpatients treated with cognitive therapy or pharmacotherapy. *Archives of General Psychiatry*, 1981, *38*, 33–39.

Kuhn, T. S. *The structure of scientific revolutions*. Chicago: University of Chicago Press, 1962.

Langs, R. *The technique of psychoanalytic psychotherapy* (Vol. 1 and 2). New York: Jason Aronson, 1973, 1974.

Langs, R. *The therapeutic interaction* (2 vols.). New York: Jason Aronson, 1976.

Lazare, A., Eisenthal, S., & Wasserman, L. The customer approach to patienthood. *Archives of General Psychiatry*, 1975, *32*, 553–558.

Lazarus, A. *Behavior therapy and beyond*. New York: McGraw-Hill, 1971.

Lazarus, A. *Multi-modal behavior therapy*. New York: Springer, 1976.

Lazarus, A., & Fay, A. Resistance or rationalization? A cognitive-behavioral perspective. In P. L. Wachtel (Ed.), *Resistance*. New York: Plenum, 1982.

Lazarus, R. S. The stress and coping paradigm. In C. Eisdorfer, D. Cohen, A. K. Kleinman, & P. E. Maxim (Eds.), *Models for clinical psychopathology*. New York: Spectrum, 1981.

Leuner, H. Basic principles and therapeutic efficacy of guided affective imagery (GAI). In J. L. Singer & K. S. Pope (Eds.), *The power of human imagination*. New York: Plenum, 1978.

Levinson, H. L. Termination of psychotherapy: Some salient issues. *Social Casework*, 1977, *58*, 480–489.

Lewis, J. M. *To be a therapist*. New York: Brunner/Mazel, 1978.

Lilly, J. C. *Programming and metaprogramming in the human biocomputer*. New York: Julian, 1972.

Lipton, J. E. *The cave man and the bomb: Human nature, evolution and nuclear war.* New York: McGraw-Hill, 1985.

Loewald, H. H. Psychoanalytic theory and psychoanalytic process. *Psychoanalytic Study of the Child,* 1970, *25,* 45–68.

Luborsky, L. Helping alliances in psychotherapy. In J. L. Klaghorn (Ed.), *Successful psychotherapy.* New York: Brunner/Mazel, 1976.

Luborsky, L., & Auerbach, A. H. The therapeutic relationship in psychodynamic psychotherapy: The research evidence and its meaning for practice. In. R. E. Hales & A. J. Frances (Eds.), *American Psychiatric Association annual review* (Vol. 4). Washington, D.C.: American Psychiatric Press, 1985.

Luborsky, L., Singer, B., & Luborsky, L. Comparative studies of psychotherapy. *Archives of General Psychiatry,* 1975, *32,* 995–1012.

Luborsky, L., Woody, G. E., McLellan, A. J., & O'Brien, C. P. Can independent judges recognize different psychotherapies? An experience with manual-guided therapies. *Journal of Consulting and Clinical Psychology,* 1982, *50,* 49–62.

Maddux, J. F., & Desmond, D. P. Residence relocation inhibits opioid dependence. *Archives of General Psychiatry,* 1982, *39,* 1313–1317.

Mahoney, M. J., & Arnkoff, D. Cognitive and self-control therapies. In S. L. Garfield & A. E. Bergin (Eds.), *Handbook of Psychotherapy and Behavioral Change.* New York: Wiley, 1978.

Malan, D. H. *A study of brief psychotherapy.* New York: Plenum, 1963.

Malan, D. H. *Toward the validation of dynamic therapy: A replication.* New York: Plenum, 1976. (a)

Malan, D. H. *The frontier of brief psychotherapy.* New York: Plenum, 1976 (b)

Malan, D. H. *Individual psychotherapy and the science of psychodynamics.* London: Butterworths, 1979.

Malan, D. H., Heath, E. S., Bacal, H. A., & Balfour, F. H. G. Psychodynamic changes in untreated neurotic patients. *Archives of General Psychiatry,* 1975, *32,* 110–126.

Mann, J. *Time-limited psychotherapy.* Cambridge: Harvard University Press, 1973.

Marks, I. M. The current status of behavioral psychotherapy. *American Journal of Psychiatry,* 1976, *133,* 253–261.

Marks, I. M. Behavioral psychotherapy of adult neurosis. In S. L. Garfield & A. E. Bergin (Eds.), *Handbook of psychotherapy and behavioral change.* New York: Wiley, 1978.

Marks, I. M., & Mathews, A. M. Brief standard self-rating for phobic patients. *Behavioral Research and Therapy,* 1979, *17,* 263–267.

Marlatt, G. A. Relapse prevention: A self-control program for the treatment of addictive behaviors. In R. B. Stuart (Ed.), *Adherence, compliance, and generalization in behavioral medicine.* New York: Brunner/Mazel, 1982.

Marmar, C. R., Wilner, N., & Horowitz, M. J. Recurrent client states in psychotherapy. In L. N. Rice & L. S. Greenberg (Eds.), *Patterns of change.* New York: Guilford, 1984.

Marmor, J. Common operational factors in diverse approaches. In A. Burton (Ed.), *What makes behavior change possible?* New York: Brunner/Mazel, 1976.

Marmor, J., & Woods, S. M. (Eds.) *The interface between the psychodynamic and behavioral therapies.* New York: Plenum, 1980.

Marziali, E., Marmar, C., & Krupnick, J. Therapeutic alliance scales: Development and relationship to therapeutic outcome. *American Journal of Psychiatry,* 1981, *138,* 361–364.

Mash, E. S., & Terdal, L. J. Follow-up assessments in behavioral therapy. In P. Karoly & J. Steffen (Eds.), *Improving the long-term effects of psychotherapy.* New York: Gardner, 1980.

Mavissakalian, M. R. Agoraphobia: Behavioral therapy and pharmacotherapy. In B. D. Beitman & G. L. Klerman (Eds.), *Combining psychotherapy and drug therapy in clinical practice*. New York: Spectrum, 1984.

May, R. Values, myths and symbols. *American Journal of Psychiatry*, 1975, *132*, 703–706.

McConnaughy, E. A., Prochaska, J. O., & Velicer, W. F. Stages of change in psychotherapy: Measurement and sample profiles. *Psychotherapy: Theory Research and Practice*, 1983, *20*, 368–375.

McGlashan, T. H., & Miller, G. H. The goals of psychoanalysis and psychoanalytic psychotherapy. *Archives of General Psychiatry*, 1982, *39*, 377–388.

Meador, B. D., & Rogers, C. R. Client-centered therapy. In R. Corsini (Ed.), *Current psychotherapies*. Itasca, Ill.: F. E. Peacock, 1973.

Meichenbaum, D. *Cognitive-behavior modification*. New York: Plenum, 1977.

Meichenbaum, D., & Gilmore, J. B. Resistance from a cognitive–behavioral perspective. In P. L. Wachtel (Ed.), *Resistance*. New York: Plenum, 1982.

Meissner, W. W., Mack, J. E., & Semrad, E. V. Classical psychoanalysis. In A. E. Freedman, H. I. Kaplan, & B. J. Sadock (Eds.), *Comprehensive textbook of psychiatry/II* (Vol. 1). Baltimore: Williams & Wilkins, 1975.

Melges, F. T. Future-oriented psychotherapy. *American Journal of Psychotherapy*, 1972, *26*, 22–33.

Melges, F. T. *Time and the personal future*. New York: Wiley, 1982.

Mendel, W. M. Interpretation and working through. *American Journal of Psychotherapy*, 1975, *29*, 409–414.

Menninger, K. *Theory of psychoanalytic technique*. New York: Basic Books, 1958.

Miller, J. G. General systems theory. In A. M. Freedman, H. I. Kaplan, & B. J. Sadock (Eds.), *Comprehensive textbook of psychiatry/II*. Baltimore: Williams & Wilkins, 1975.

Morgenstern, A. Reliving the last goodbye: The psychotherapy of an almost silent patient. *Psychiatry*, 1980, *43*, 251–258.

Mumford, E., Schlesinger, H. J., Glass, G. V., Patrick, C., & Cuerdon, T. A new look at evidence about reduced cost of medical utilization following mental health treatment. *American Journal of Psychiatry*, 1984, *141*, 1145–1158.

Murphy, G. E., Simons, A. D., Wetzel, R. D., & Lustman, P. J. Cognitive therapy and pharmacotherapy. *Archives of General Psychiatry*, 1984, *41*, 33–41.

Murray, J. E., & Jacobson, L. I. Cognition and learning in traditional and behavioral psychotherapy. In S. L. Garfield & A. E. Bengin (Eds.), *Handbook of psychotherapy and behavioral change*. New York: Wiley, 1978.

Norcross, J., & Prochaska, J. A national survey of clinical psychologists: Affiliations and orientations. *The Clinical Psychologist*, 1982, *39*, 1–6.

Orlinsky, D. E., & Howard, K. I. The relation of process to outcome in psychotherapy. In S. L. Garfield & A. E. Bengin (Eds.), *Handbook of psychotherapy and behavioral change*. New York: Wiley, 1978.

Parloff, M. B., Waskow, I. E., & Wolf, B. E. Research on therapist variables in relation to process and outcome. In S. L. Garfield & A. E. Bergin (Eds.), *Handbook of psychotherapy and behavior change*. New York: Wiley, 1978.

Peake, T. H., & Egli, D. The language of feelings. *Journal of Contemporary Psychotherapy*, 1982, *13*, 162–174.

Pentony, P. *Models of influence in psychotherapy*. New York: Free Press, 1981.

Perls, F. S. *Gestalt therapy verbatim*. Lafayette, Calif.: Real People, 1969.

Perls, F. *The Gestalt approach and eye witness to therapy*. Ben Lomond, Calif.: Science & Behavior Books, 1973.

Polster, E., & Polster, M. *Gestalt therapy integrated*. New York: Brunner/Mazel, 1973.

Potter, N. D., & Evans, F. B. Experience of certainty and despair in the beginning psychotherapist. *Voices*, 1983, *19*, 42–50.

Prochaska, J. O., & DiClemente, C. C. Transtheoretical therapy: Toward a more integrative model of change. *Psychotherapy: Theory, Research and Practice*, 1982, *19*, 276–288.

Prochaska, J. O., & DiClemente, C. C. *The transtheoretical approach.* Homewood, Ill.: Dorsey, 1984.

Racker, H. *Transference and countertransference.* New York: International Universities Press, 1968.

Raimy, V. *Misunderstandings of the self.* San Francisco: Jossey-Bass, 1975.

Rank, O. *The trauma of birth.* New York: Harper & Row, 1973. (First published, 1929)

Regier, D. A., Goldberg, I. D., & Taube, C. A. The de facto U.S. mental health services system. *Archives of General Psychiatry*, 1975, *35*, 685–689.

Reich, A. On counter transference. *International Journal of Psychoanalysis*, 1951, *32*, 25–31.

Reich, W. *Character analysis.* New York: Simon & Schuster, 1945.

Reich, W. *Selected writings.* New York: Farrar, Straus & Cudahy, 1961.

Reider, N. A type of transference to institutions. *Bulletin of the Menninger Clinic*, 1953, *17*, 58.

Richert, A. Differential prescription for psychotherapy on the basis of client role preferences. *Psychotherapy: Theory, Research and Practice*, 1983, *20*, 321–329.

Ries, R. K., Bokan, J. A. Katon, W. J., & Kleinman, A. The medical care abuser: Differential diagnosis and management. *Journal of Family Practice*, 1981, *13*, 257.

Rockwell, W. J. K., & Pinkerton, R. S. Single session psychotherapy. *American Journal of Psychotherapy*, 1982, *36*, 32–40.

Rogers, C. R. *Counseling and psychotherapy.* Boston: Houghton Mifflin, 1942.

Rogers, C. *Client-centered psychotherapy.* Boston: Houghton Mifflin, 1951.

Rogers, C. R. *On becoming a person.* Boston: Houghton Mifflin, 1961.

Rokeach, M. *Beliefs, attitudes and values.* San Francisco: Jossey-Bass, 1972.

Rosenbaum, M. Premature interruption of psychotherapy: Continuation of contact by telephone and correspondence. *American Journal of Psychiatry*, 1977, *134*, 200–202.

Rosenbaum, R. L., & Horowitz, M. J. Motivation for psychotherapy: A factorial and conceptual analysis. *Psychotherapy: Theory, Research and Practice*, 1983, *20*, 346–354.

Rush, A. J., Beck, A. T., Kovacs, M., & Hollon, S. Comparative efficacy of cognitive therapy and pharmacotherapy in the treatment of depressed outpatients. *Cognitive Therapy Research*, 1977, *1*, 17–37.

Sander, F. M. Other determinants of therapeutic modality choice. [Letter to the editor]. *American Journal of Psychiatry*, 1984, *141*, 1493–1494.

Sandler, J., Dare, C., & Holder, A. Basic psychoanalytic concepts: 3. Transference. *British Journal of Psychiatry*, 1970, *116*, 667–672. (a)

Sandler, J., Dare, C., & Holder, A. Basic psychoanalytic concepts: 8. Special forms of transference. *British Journal of Psychiatry*, 1970, *117*, 561–567. (b)

Sandler, J., Dare, C., & Holder, A. Basic psychoanalytic concepts: 9. Working through. *British Journal of Psychiatry*, 1970, *117*, 617–621. (c)

Sandler, J., Dare, C., & Holder, A. Basic psychoanalytic concepts: 10. Interpretations and other interventions. *British Journal of Psychiatry*, 1971, *118*, 53–59.

Sandler, J., Holder, A., & Dare, C. Basic psychoanalytic concepts: 2. The treatment alliance. *British Journal of Psychiatry*, 1970, *116*, 555–558. (a).

Sandler, J., Holder, A., & Dare, C. Basic psychoanalytic concepts: 4. Counter transference. *British Journal of Psychiatry*, 1970, *117*, 83–88. (b)

Sandler, J., Holder, A., & Dare, C. Basic psychoanalytic concepts: 5. Resistance. *British Journal of Psychiatry*, 1970, *117*, 215–221. (c)

Satir, V. *Conjoint family therapy.* Palo Alto, Calif.: *Science & Behavior Books*, 1967.

Schiff, S. K. Termination of therapy. *Archives of General Psychiatry*, 1962, *6*, 77–98.

Schlessinger, N., & Robbins, F. P. *A developmental view of the psychoanalytic process.* New York: International Universities Press, 1983.

Schneidman, E. S. *Deaths of man.* New York: Quadrangle, 1973.

Schorr, J. E. Clinical use of categories of therapeutic imagery. In J. L. Singer & K. S. Pope (Eds.), *The power of human imagination.* New York: Plenum, 1978.

Searles, H. F. Oedipal love in the countertransference. *International Journal of Psychoanalysis*, 1959, *40*, 180–190.

Searles, H. F. The patient as therapist to his analyst. In P. L. Giovacchini (Ed.), *Tactics and techniques in psychoanalytic therapy: Vol. 2. Countertransference.* New York: Jason Aronson, 1975.

Seeman, M. Patients who abandon psychotherapy. *Archives of General Psychiatry*, 1974, *32*, 486–491.

Shapiro, A. K., Struening, E., Shapiro, E., & Barton, H. Prognostic correlates of psychotherapy in psychiatric outpatients. *American Journal of Psychiatry*, 1976, *133*, 802–808.

Shear, K. Psychotherapeutic approaches to panic attacks [Panel on agoraphobia]. First Annual Meeting of the Society for the Exploration of Psychotherapy Integration, Annapolis, June, 1985.

Shelton, J. L., & Levy, R. L. Behavioral assignments and treatment compliance. Champaign, Ill.: Research, 1981.

Sher, M. The process of changing therapists. *American Journal of Psychotherapy*, 1970, *25*, 278–286.

Shwed, H. S. When a psychiatrist suddenly dies . . . making provisions for patients [Roche Reprint]. *Frontiers of Psychiatry*, 1980, *10*, 4–5.

Sifneos, P. E. Short-term anxiety provoking psychotherapy. *Seminars in Psychiatry*, 1969, *1*, 389–399.

Sifneos, P. *Short-term psychotherapy and emotional crises.* Cambridge: Harvard University Press, 1972.

Sifneos, P. Conference on short-term dynamic psychotherapy, Montreal, 1976.

Simons, A. D., Garfield, S. L., & Murphy, G. E. The process of change in cognitive therapy and pharmacotherapy for depression. *Archives of General Psychiatry*, 1984, *41*, 45–51.

Singer, B. A., & Luborsky, L. Counter transference: The status of clinical versus quantitative research. In A. S. Gurman & A. M. Razin (Eds.), *Effective psychotherapy.* New York: Pergamon, 1977.

Singer, J. L., & Pope, K. S. The use of imagery and fantasy techniques in psychotherapy. In J. L. Singer & K. S. Pope (Eds.), *The power of human imagination.* New York: Plenum, 1978.

Sloane, R. B., Cristol, A. H., Pepernik, M. C., & Whipple, K. Role preparation and expectation of improvement in psychotherapy. *Journal of Nervous and Mental Disease*, 1970, *150*, 18–26.

Sloane, R. B., Staples, F. R., Cristol, A. H., Yorkston, N. J., & Whipple, K. *Psychotherapy versus behavior therapy.* Cambridge: Harvard University Press, 1975.

Smith, M. L., Glass, G. V., & Miller, T. *The benefits of psychotherapy.* Baltimore: Johns Hopkins University Press, 1980.

Stampfl, G. Implosive therapy: Staring down your nightmares. *Psychology Today*, 1975, *8*(9), 66–73.

Steffen, J. J., & Karoly, P. Toward a psychology of therapeutic persistence. In P. Karoly & J. J. Steffen (Eds.), *Improving the long-term effects of psychotherapy*. New York: Gardner, 1980.

Stewart, R. L. Psychoanalysis and psychoanalytic therapy. In A. M. Freedman, H. I. Kaplan, & B. J. Sadock (Eds.), *Comprehensive textbook of psychiatry*. Baltimore: Williams and Wilkins, 1975.

Stone, A. S. Suicide precipitated by psychotherapy. *American Journal of Psychotherapy*, 1971, *25*, 18–26.

Strauss, J. S., & Hisham, H. Clinical questions and "real" research. *American Journal of Psychiatry*, 1981, *12*, 1592–1597.

Strong, S. R. Social psychological approach to psychotherapy research. In S. L. Garfield & A. E. Bergin (Eds.), *Handbook of psychotherapy and behavior change*. New York: Wiley, 1978.

Strupp, H. H. Toward a reformulation of the psychotherapeutic influence. *International Journal of Psychiatry*, 1973, *11*, 263–365.

Strupp, H. H. Psychoanalysis, "focal psychotherapy," and the nature of the therapeutic influence. *Archives of General Psychiatry*, 1975, *32*, 127–135.

Strupp, H. H. The nature of the therapeutic influence and its basic ingredients. In A. Burton (Ed.), *What makes behavior change possible?* New York: Brunner/Mazel, 1976.

Strupp, H. H., & Hadley, S. W. A tripartite model of mental health and therapeutic outcomes. *American Psychologist*, March 1977, 187–196.

Sullivan, H. S. *The psychotherapeutic interview*. New York: Norton, 1954.

Tauber, E. Exploring the therapeutic use of counter transference data. *Psychiatry*, 1954, *17*, 331–336.

Therapist–patient sex: Survey findings speak. *Psychiatric News*, October 1, 1976, 28–29.

Truax, C. B. Reinforcement and nonreinforcement in Rogerian psychotherapy. *Journal of Abnormal Psychology*, 1966, *71*, 1–7.

Ulman, R. B., & Stolorow, R. D. The transference–countertransference neurosis in psychoanalysis. *Bulletin of the Menninger Clinic*, 1985, *49*, 37–51.

Wachtel, P. L. *Psychoanalysis and behavior therapy*. New York: Basic Books, 1977.

Wachtel, P. L. (Ed.) *Resistance*. New York: Plenum, 1982.

Wachtel, P. L. Comments made at First Annual Meeting of the Society for Psychotherapy Integration, Annapolis, 1985.

Waldinger, R. J., & Gunderson, J. G. Completed psychotherapies with borderline patients. *American Journal of Psychotherapy*, 1984, *38*, 190–202.

Wallach, M. A., & Wallach, L. *Psychology's sanction for selfishness: The error of egoism in theory and therapy*. San Francisco: W. H. Freeman, 1983.

Wapnick, K. (Letter to the editor). *American Academy of Psychotherapists Newsletter*, February 1984, p. 1.

Ward, N. Psychological aspects of medication management. In B. D. Beitman & G. L. Klerman (Eds.), *Combining psychotherapy and drug therapy in clinical practice*. New York: Spectrum, 1984.

Watters, W. W., Bellissimo, A., & Rubenstein, J. S. Teaching individual psychotherapy: Learning objectives in communication. *Canadian Journal of Psychiatry*, 1982, 27, 263–269.

Watzlawick, P., Beavin, J. H., & Jackson, D. D. *Pragmatics of human communication*. New York: Norton, 1967.

Watzlawick, P., Weakland, J., & Fisch, R. *Change*, New York: W. W. Norton, 1974.

Weigert, E. Counter transference and self-analysis of the psychoanalyst. *International Journal of Psychoanalysis*, 1954, *35*, 242–246.

Weigert, E. Existential psychoanalysis. In A. M. Freedman & H. I. Kaplan (Eds.), *Comprehensive textbook of psychiatry*. Baltimore: Williams & Wilkins, 1967.

Weiner, I. B. *Principles of psychotherapy*. New York: Wiley, 1975.

Weiner, M. F. *Therapist disclosure*. Baltimore: University Park, 1983.

Weissman, M. M. The psychological treatment of depression: An update of clinical trials. In J. B. W. Williams & R. L. Spitzer (Eds.), *Psychotherapy research: Where are we and where should we be going*. New York: Guilford, 1984.

Weissman, M. M., & Bothwell, S. Assessment of social adjustment by patient self-report. *Archives of General Psychiatry*, 1976, *33*, 1111–1115.

Winnicott, D. *The motivational process and the facilitating environment*. New York: International Universities Press, 1965.

Wolberg, L. R. *The technique of psychotherapy* (Vol. 2). New York: Grune & Stratton, 1967.

Wolpe, J. *The practice of behavior therapy* (2nd ed.). New York: Pergamon, 1973.

Wolpe, J. Conditioning is the basis of all psychotherapeutic change. In A. Burton (Ed.), *What makes behavior change possible?* New York: Brunner/Mazel, 1976.

Yalom, I. *The theory and practice of group psychotherapy*. New York: Basic Books, 1970.

Yalom, I. *Existential psychotherapy*. New York: Basic Books, 1980.

Yalom, I. D. *Inpatient group psychotherapy*. New York: Basic Books, 1983.

Yates, A. J. *Theory and practice in behavior therapy*. New York: Wiley, 1975.

Zung, W. K. Assessment of anxiety disorder: Qualitative and quantitative approaches. In W. E. Fann *et al.* (Eds.), *Phenomenology and treatment of anxiety disorders*. New York: Spectrum, 1979.

Weigert, E. Existential psychoanalysis. In A. M. Freedman & H. I. Kaplan (Eds.), *Comprehensive textbook of psychiatry*. Baltimore: Williams & Wilkins, 1967.

Weiner, I. B. *Principles of psychotherapy*. New York: Wiley, 1975.

Weiner, M. F. *Therapist disclosure*. Baltimore: University Park, 1983.

Weissman, M. M. The psychological treatment of depression: An update of clinical trials. In J. B. W. Williams & R. L. Spitzer (Eds.), *Psychotherapy research: Where are we and where should we be going*. New York: Guilford, 1984.

Weissman, M. M., & Bothwell, S. Assessment of social adjustment by patient self-report. *Archives of General Psychiatry*, 1976, *33*, 1111–1115.

Winnicott, D. *The motivational process and the facilitating environment*. New York: International Universities Press, 1965.

Wolberg, L. R. *The technique of psychotherapy* (Vol. 2). New York: Grune & Stratton, 1967.

Wolpe, J. *The practice of behavior therapy* (2nd ed.). New York: Pergamon, 1973.

Wolpe, J. Conditioning is the basis of all psychotherapeutic change. In A. Burton (Ed.), *What makes behavior change possible?* New York: Brunner/Mazel, 1976.

Yalom, I. *The theory and practice of group psychotherapy*. New York: Basic Books, 1970.

Yalom, I. *Existential psychotherapy*. New York: Basic Books, 1980.

Yalom, I. D. *Inpatient group psychotherapy*. New York: Basic Books, 1983.

Yates, A. J. *Theory and practice in behavior therapy*. New York: Wiley, 1975.

Zung, W. K. Assessment of anxiety disorder: Qualitative and quantitative approaches. In W. E. Fann *et al.* (Eds.), *Phenomenology and treatment of anxiety disorders*. New York: Spectrum, 1979.

Index

Numbers in italics indicate material in figures and tables.